INTRODUCTION
TO NUTRITION
AND METABOLISM

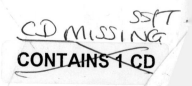

INTRODUCTION

TO NUTRITION

AND METABOLISM

THIRD EDITION

DAVID A BENDER

SENIOR LECTURER IN BIOCHEMISTRY
UNIVERSITY COLLEGE LONDON

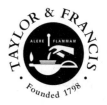

First published 2002 by Taylor & Francis
11 New Fetter Lane, London EC4P 4EE

Simultaneously published in the USA and Canada
by Taylor & Francis Inc
29 West 35th Street, New York, NY 10001

Taylor & Francis is an imprint of the Taylor & Francis Group

© 2002 David A Bender

Typeset in Copperplate Gothic and Garamond by
Prepress Projects Ltd, Perth, Scotland
Printed and bound in Great Britain by
TJ International Ltd, Padstow, Cornwall

British Library Cataloguing in Publication Data
A catalogue record for this book is available from the British Library

Library of Congress Cataloging in Publication Data

Bender, David A.
    Introduction to nutrition and metabolism/David A. Bender.–3rd ed.
      p. cm.
    Includes bibliographical references and index.
    1. Nutrition. 2. Metabolism. I. Title.
    QP141 .B38 2002
    612.3′9–dc21   2001052290

    ISBN 0–415–25798–0 (hbk)
    ISBN 0–415–25799–9 (pbk)

Contents

Preface

The food we eat has a major effect on our physical health and psychological wellbeing. An understanding of the way in which nutrients are metabolized, and hence of the principles of biochemistry, is essential for an understanding of the scientific basis of what we would call a prudent or healthy diet.

My aim in the following pages is to explain both the conclusions of the many expert committees that have deliberated on the problems of nutritional requirements, diet and health over the years and also the scientific basis on which these experts have reached their conclusions. Much what is now presented as 'facts' will be proven to be incorrect in years to come. This book is intended to provide a foundation of scientific knowledge and understanding from which to interpret and evaluate future advances in nutrition and health sciences.

Nutrition is one of the basic sciences that underlie a proper understanding of health and human sciences and the ways in which human beings and their environment interact. In its turn, the science of nutrition is based on both biochemistry and physiology, on the one hand, and the social and behavioural sciences on the other. This book contains such biochemistry as is essential to an understanding of the science of nutrition.

In a book of this kind, which is an *introduction* to nutrition and metabolism, it is not appropriate to cite the original scientific literature which provides the (sometimes conflicting) evidence for the statements made; in the clinical problems and some of the tables of data I have acknowledged my sources of data as a simple courtesy to my follow scientists, and also to guide readers to the original sources of information. Otherwise, the suggestions for further reading and Internet sites listed under additional resources are intended to provide an entry to the scientific literature.

Two of my colleagues have provided especially helpful comments: Dr Derek Evered, Emeritus Reader in Biochemistry at Chelsea College, University of London, and Professor Keith Frayn (University of Oxford). I would like to thank them for their kind and constructive criticisms of the second edition of this book. I am grateful to those of my students whose perceptive questions have helped me to formulate and clarify my thoughts, and especially those who responded to my enquiry as to what they would like to see (for the benefit of future generations of students) in this new edition.

This book is dedicated to those who will use it as a part of their studies, in the hope that they will be able, in their turn, to advance the frontiers of knowledge, and help their clients, patients and students to understand the basis of the advice they offer.

David A Bender
December 2001

Additional resources

At the end of each chapter there is a list of the additional resources that are available on the CD that accompanies this book. All of these can be run directly from the CD, or may be copied onto a hard disk or network, for internal use only, in educational institutions – instructions for installation are included in the ReadMe file on the CD. To access the resources listed here you will require an IBM-compatible PC running Windows 95, 98 or higher.

The resources on the CD consist of the following.

PowerPoint presentations to accompany each chapter

If you have Microsoft PowerPoint 2000 installed on your computer then you can view these presentations immediately. If not, the PowerPoint viewer is also on the CD and can be installed by running Ppview32.exe from the folder 'extra files'.

Teachers are welcome to use these PowerPoint presentations, or parts of them, in their lectures, provided that due acknowledgement is made; they are copyright David A Bender 2002 (and some of the figures are copyright Taylor & Francis 2002), and may not be published for profit in any form.

Self-assessment quizzes

For most chapters there is a computer-based self-assessment quiz on the CD. This consists of a series of statements to be marked true or false; you assess your confidence in your answer, and gain marks for being correct, or lose marks for being incorrect, scaled according to your confidence in your answer.

These quizzes are accessed from the program Testme.exe on the CD.

Simulations of laboratory experiments

There are a number of simulations of laboratory experiments on the CD; they are accessed by name – e.g. the Enzyme Assay program (Chapter 2) is accessed from the Enzyme Assay icon.

Problems at the end of chapters

At the end of most chapters there are problems to be considered. These are of various kinds:

- open-ended problems to be thought about;
- defined calculation problems to which there is a correct answer (but the answer is not provided here);
- problems of data interpretation, in which you are guided through sets of data and prompted to draw conclusions (again, deliberately, no answers to these problems are provided);
- clinical problems in which you are given information about a patient and expected to deduce the underlying biochemical basis of the problem, and explain how the defect causes the metabolic disturbances.

Other resources

NUTRITION BOOKS

Bender AE and Bender DA, *Food Tables and Labelling*, Oxford University Press, Oxford, 1998.

Bender DA and Bender AE, *Benders' Dictionary of Nutrition and Food Technology*, Woodhead Publishing, Cambridge, 1999.

Bender DA and Bender AE, *Nutrition: a Reference Handbook*, Oxford University Press, Oxford, 1997.

Garrow JS, James WPT and Ralph A, *Human Nutrition and Dietetics*, 10th edn, Churchill Livingstone, Edinburgh, 2000.

Holland B, Welch AA, Unwin D, Buss DH, Paul AA and Southgate DAT (eds), *McCance & Widdowson's The Composition of Foods*, 5th edn, RSC/HMSO, London, 1991.

BIOCHEMISTRY BOOKS

Campbell PN and Smith AD. *Biochemistry Illustrated*, 4th edn, Churchill Livingstone, Edinburgh, 2000.

Champe PC and Harvey RA. *Lippincott's Illustrated Reviews, Biochemistry*, 2nd edn, Lippincott-Raven, Philadelphia, 1994.

Elliott WH and Elliott DC. *Biochemistry and Molecular Biology*. Oxford University Press, Oxford, 1997.

Frayn KN. *Metabolic Regulation: A Human Perspective*. Portland Press, London, 1996.

Gillham B, Papachristodoulou DK and Thomas JH. *Wills' Biochemical Basis of Medicine*. 3rd edn, Butterworth-Heinemann, Oxford, 1997.

Marks DB, Marks AD and Smith CM. *Basic Medical Biochemistry: A Clinical Approach*. Williams & Wilkins, Baltimore, 1996.

Stryer L. *Biochemistry*, 4th edn, Freeman, New York,1995.

Voet D and Voet JG. *Biochemistry*, 2nd edn, John Wiley, New York, 1995.

Zubay GL, Parson WW and Vance DE. *Principles of Biochemistry*, William C Brown, Dubuque, IA, 1995.

REVIEW JOURNALS

Nutrition Research Reviews, published biannually by CABI Publishing, Wallington, Oxford, for the Nutrition Society.

Nutrition Reviews, published monthly by the International Life Sciences Institute, Washington, DC.

Annual Reviews of Biochemistry and *Annual Reviews of Nutrition*, published annually by Annuals Reviews Inc.

If you have problems with some of the chemistry in this book, try the following:

Wood EJ and Myers A, *Essential Chemistry for Biochemistry*, 2nd edn, The Biochemical Society/Portland Press, London, 1991.

INTERNET LINKS

Professional organizations and learned societies

American Council on Science and Health: http://www.acsh.org/

American Society for Nutritional Sciences: http://www.nutrition.org

Association for the Study of Obesity: http://www.aso.org.uk

Biochemical Society: http://www.biochemsoc.org.uk/default.htm

British Association for the Advancement of Science: http://www.britassoc.org.uk/info/scan5.html

British Dietetic Association: http://www.bda.uk.com

British Nutrition Foundation: http://ww.nutrition.org.uk

COPUS (Committee on Public Understanding of Science): http://www.royalsoc.ac.uk/st_cop01.htm

International Society for the Study of Obesity: http://www.iaso.org/home.html

International Union of Nutritional Sciences home page: http://www.monash.edu.au/IUNS/

Learning and Teaching Support Network, bioscience: http://ltsn.ac.uk/NV/bioframes.htm

National Sports Medicine Institute: http://nsmi.org.uk/

North American Association for the Study of Obesity: http://www.naaso.org

Nutrition Society: http://www.nutsoc.org

Information about nutrition and food

Arbor Nutrition Guide: http://arborcom.com/

Eat Well, Live Well Research and Information Centre, Monash University: http://www.healthyeating.org

Food and Nutrition Information Center, US Department of Agriculture: http://www.nal.usda.gov/fnic/

International Food Information Service: http://www.ifis.org/

Martindale's Virtual Nutrition Center: http://www.sci.lib.uci.edu/HSG/Nutrition.html

Nutrition web sites reviewed from Tufts University: http://navigator.tufts.edu

General research tools and information

Cornell Cooperative Extension – a useful source of information on nutrition and agriculture: http://www.cce.cornell.edu/

Enzyme database: http://www.expasy.ch/enzyme/

Glossary of biochemistry and molecular biology online: http://db.portlandpress.com/db.htm

ILSI (International Life Sciences Institute) – publishers of *Nutrition Reviews*: http://www.ilsi.org

MedBioWorld – links to nutrition-related journals available on-line: http://www.sciencekomm.at/journals/food.html

Medline: http://www.nlm.nih.gov/PubMed/

MedWeb Biomedical Internet Resources from Emory University: http://www.cc.emory.edu/WHSCL/medweb.html

OMNI (Organising Medical Networked Information): http://www.omni.ac.uk

On-Line Mendelian Inheritance in Man (OMIM): http://www3.ncbi.nih.gov.Omim/

Government and international sites

Department of Environment, Food and Rural Affairs, UK: http://www.maff.gov.uk/defra/default.htm

Department of Health, UK: http://www.open.gov.uk/doh/dhhome.htm

FAO Food and Agriculture Organization of the UN: http://www.fao.org

FDA Consumer – the consumer bulletin of the US Food and Drug Administration: http://www.fda.gov/fdac/796_toc.html

Food and Nutrition Information Center: http://www.nal.usda.gov/fnic/

Food Standards Agency (UK): http://www.foodstandards.gov.uk

Health Canada Nutrition: http://www.hc-sc.gc.ca/hppb/nutrition

IUNS (International Union of Nutritional Sciences): http://www.monash.edu.au/

NHS Direct Online – UK government site providing advice and information about illnesses: http://www.nhsdirect.nhs.uk

United Nations and other international organizations:http://www.undcp.org/unlinks.html

US Food and Drug Administration: http://www.fda.gov.default.htm
WHO World Health Organization: http://www.who.int/home-page/

Just for fun

David Bender's home page: http://www.biochem.ucl.ac.uk/~dab/dab.html

CHAPTER **1**

Why eat?

An adult eats about a tonne of food a year. This book attempts to answer the question 'why?' – by exploring the need for food and the uses to which that food is put in the body. Some discussion of chemistry and biochemistry is obviously essential in order to investigate the fate of food in the body, and why there is a continuous need for food throughout life. Therefore, in the following chapters various aspects of biochemistry and metabolism will be discussed. This should provide not only the basis of our present understanding, knowledge and concepts in nutrition, but also, more importantly, a basis from which to interpret future research findings and evaluate new ideas and hypotheses as they are formulated.

We eat because we are hungry. Why have we evolved complex physiological and psychological mechanisms to control not only hunger, but also our appetite for different types of food? Why do meals form such an important part of our life?

Objectives

After reading this chapter you should be able to:

- describe the need for metabolic fuels and, in outline, the relationship between food intake, energy expenditure and body weight;
- describe in outline the importance of an appropriate intake of dietary fat;
- describe the mechanisms involved in short-term and long-term control of food intake;
- describe in outline the mechanisms involved in the sense of taste;
- explain the various factors that influence people's choices of foods.

1.1 *The need for energy*

There is an obvious need for energy to perform physical work. Work has to be done to lift a load against the force of gravity, and there must be a source of energy to perform that work. As discussed in section 5.1, the energy used in various activities can readily be measured, as can the metabolic energy yield of the foods that are the fuel for that work (see Table 1.1). This means that it is possible to calculate a balance between the intake of energy, as metabolic fuels, and the body's energy expenditure. Obviously, energy intake has to be appropriate for the level of energy expenditure; as discussed in Chapters 6, and 8 neither excess intake nor a deficiency is desirable.

Figure 1.1 shows the relationship between food intake, physical work and changes in body reserves of metabolic fuels, as shown by changes in body weight. This study was carried out in Germany at the end of the Second World War, when there was a great deal of rubble from bomb damaged buildings to be cleared, and a large number of people to be fed and found employment. Increasing food intake resulted in an increase in work output – initially with an increase in body weight, indicating that the food supply was greater than required to meet the (increased) work output. When a financial reward was offered as well, the work output increased to such an extent that people now drew on their (sparse) reserves of metabolic fuel, and there was a loss of body weight.

Quite apart from obvious work output, the body has a considerable requirement for energy, even at rest. Only about one-third of the average person's energy expenditure is for voluntary work (section 5.1.3). Two-thirds is required for maintenance of the body's functions, homeostasis of the internal environment and metabolic integrity.

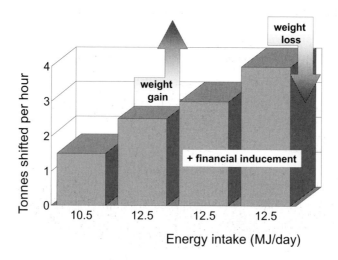

FIGURE 1.1 *The relationship between food intake, work output and body weight (Wuppertal data). From data reported by Widdowson EM, MRC Special Report series no. 275, HMSO, 1951.*

As shown in Figure 1.2, about 20% of total energy expenditure is required to maintain the electrical activity of the brain and nervous system. This energy requirement, the basal metabolic rate (BMR; section 5.1.3.1) can be measured by the output of heat, or the consumption of oxygen, when the subject is completely at rest.

Part of this basal energy requirement is obvious – the heart beats to circulate the blood; respiration continues; and there is considerable electrical activity in nerves and muscles, whether they are 'working' or not. These processes require a metabolic energy source. Less obviously, there is also a requirement for energy for the wide variety of biochemical reactions occurring all the time in the body: laying down reserves of fat and carbohydrate (section 5.6); turnover of tissue proteins (section 9.2.3.3); transport of substrates into, and products out of, cells (section 3.2.2); and the production and secretion of hormones and neurotransmitters.

1.1.1 UNITS OF ENERGY

Energy expenditure is measured by the output of heat from the body (section 5.1). The unit of heat used in the early studies was the calorie – the amount of heat required to raise the temperature of 1 gram of water by 1 degree Celsius. The calorie is still used to some extent in nutrition; in biological systems the kilocalorie, kcal (sometimes written as Calorie with a capital C) is used. One kilocalorie is 1000 calories (10^3 cal), and hence the amount of heat required to raise the temperature of 1 kg of water through 1 degree Celsius.

Correctly, the joule is used as the unit of energy. The joule is an SI unit, named after James Prescott Joule (1818–89), who first showed the equivalence of heat, mechanical work and other forms of energy. In biological systems, the kilojoule (kJ $= 10^3$ J $=$ 1000 J) and megajoule (1 MJ $= 10^6$ J $= 1,000,000$ J) are used.

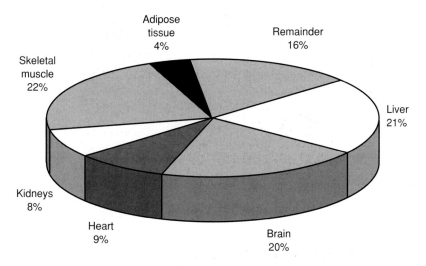

FIGURE 1.2 *Percentage of total energy expenditure by different organs of the body.*

To convert between calories and joules:

1 kcal = 4.186 kJ (normally rounded off to 4.2 kJ)

1 kJ = 0.239 kcal (normally rounded off to 0.24 kcal)

As discussed in section 5.1.3, average energy expenditure of adults is between 7.5 and 10 MJ/day for women and between 8 and 12 MJ/day for men.

1.2 *Metabolic fuels*

The dietary sources of metabolic energy (the metabolic fuels) are carbohydrates, fats, protein and alcohol. The metabolism of these fuels results in the production of carbon dioxide and water (and also urea in the case of proteins; section 9.3.1.4). They can be converted to the same end-products chemically, by burning in air. Although the process of metabolism in the body is more complex, it is a fundamental law of chemistry that, if the starting material and end-products are the same, the energy yield is the same, regardless of the route taken. Therefore, the energy yield of foodstuffs can be determined by measuring the heat produced when they are burnt in air, making allowance for the extent to which they are digested and absorbed from foods. The energy yields of the metabolic fuels in the body, allowing for digestion and absorption, are shown in Table 1.1.

1.2.1 THE NEED FOR CARBOHYDRATE AND FAT

Although there is a requirement for energy sources in the diet, it does not matter unduly how that requirement is met. There is no requirement for a dietary source of carbohydrate – as discussed in section 5.7, the body can make as much carbohydrate as is required from proteins. Similarly, there is no requirement for a dietary source of fat, apart from the essential fatty acids (section 4.3.1.1), and there is certainly no requirement for a dietary source of alcohol. However, as discussed in section 7.3.2, diets that provide more than about 35–40% of energy from fat are associated with increased risk of heart disease and some cancers, and there is some evidence that diets that provide more than about 20% of energy from protein are also associated with health problems. Therefore, as discussed in section 7.3, the general consensus is that diets should provide about 55% of energy from carbohydrates, 30% from fat and 15% from protein.

Although there is no requirement for fat in the diet, fats are nutritionally important and, as discussed in section 1.3.3.1, there is a specific mechanism for detecting the taste of fats in foods.

TABLE 1.1 *The energy yield of metabolic fuels*

	kcal/g	kJ/g
Carbohydrate	4	17
Protein	4	16
Fat	9	37
Alcohol	7	29

1 kcal = 4.186 kJ or 1 kJ = 0.239 kcal

- It is difficult to eat enough of a very low-fat diet to meet energy requirements. As shown in Table 1.1, the energy yield per gram of fat is more than twice that of carbohydrate or protein. The problem in many less developed countries, where undernutrition is a problem (see Chapter 8), is that diets provide only 10–15% of energy from fat, and it is difficult to consume a sufficient bulk of food to meet energy requirements. By contrast, the problem in Western countries is an undesirably high intake of fat, contributing to the development of obesity (see Chapter 6) and the diseases of affluence (see section 7.3.1).
- Four of the vitamins, A, D, E and K (see Chapter 11), are fat soluble, and are found in fatty and oily foods. More importantly, because they are absorbed dissolved in fat, their absorption requires an adequate intake of fat. On a very low-fat diet the absorption of these vitamins may be inadequate to meet requirements.
- There is a requirement for small amounts of two fatty acids which are required for specific functions; these are the so-called essential fatty acids (section 4.3.1.1). They cannot be formed in the body, but must be provided in the diet.
- In many foods, a great deal of the flavour (and hence the pleasure of eating) is carried in the fat.
- Fats lubricate food, and make it easier to chew and swallow.

1.2.2 THE NEED FOR PROTEIN

Unlike fats and carbohydrates, there is a requirement for protein in the diet. In a growing child this need is obvious. As the child grows, and the size of its body increases, so there is an increase in the total amount of protein in the body.

Adults also require protein in the diet. There is a continuous small loss of protein from the body, for example in hair, shed skin cells, enzymes and other proteins secreted into the gut and not completely digested. More importantly, there is turnover of tissue proteins, which are continually being broken down and replaced. Although there is no change in the total amount of protein in the body, an adult with an inadequate intake of protein will be unable to replace this loss, and will lose tissue protein. Protein turnover and requirements are discussed in Chapter 9.

1.2.3 THE NEED FOR MICRONUTRIENTS — MINERALS AND VITAMINS

In addition to metabolic fuels and protein, the body has a requirement for a variety of mineral salts, in small amounts. Obviously, if a metal or ion has a function in the body, it must be provided by the diet, as the different elements cannot be interconverted. Again, the need is obvious for a growing child; as the body grows in size, so the total amounts of minerals in the body will increase. In adults, there is a turnover of minerals in the body, and losses must be replaced from the diet.

There is a requirement for a different group of nutrients, also in very small amounts – the vitamins. These are organic compounds that have a variety of functions in metabolic processes. They cannot be synthesized in the body, and so must be provided by the diet. There is turnover of the vitamins, so there must be replacement of the losses. Vitamins and minerals are discussed in Chapter 11.

1.3 Hunger and appetite

Human beings have evolved an elaborate system of physiological and psychological mechanisms to ensure that the body's needs for metabolic fuels and nutrients are met.

1.3.1 HUNGER AND SATIETY — SHORT-TERM CONTROL OF FEEDING

As shown in Figure 1.3, there are hunger and satiety centres in the brain, which stimulate us to begin eating (the hunger centres in the lateral hypothalamus) and to to stop eating when hunger has been satisfied (the satiety centres in the ventromedial hypothalamus). A great deal is known about the role of these brain centres in controlling food intake, and there are a number of drugs which modify responses to hunger and satiety. Such drugs can be used to reduce appetite in the treatment of obesity (section 6.3.3) or to stimulate it in people with loss of appetite or anorexia.

What is not known is what signals hunger or satiety to these hypothalamic centres. It may be the relative concentrations of glucose, triacylglycerols, non-esterified fatty acids and ketone bodies available as metabolic fuels in the fed and fasting states (section 5.3). Equally, the relative concentrations of the hormones insulin and glucagon (section 5.3 and section 10.5) and some of the peptide hormones secreted by the gastrointestinal tract during digestion of food may be important. There is also evidence that the amount of the amino acid tryptophan available for uptake into the brain may be important; tryptophan availability to the brain is controlled by both the concentration of tryptophan relative to other large neutral amino acids (section 4.4.1) and the extent

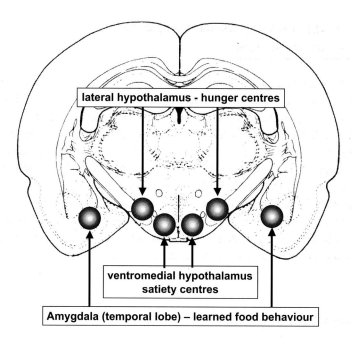

FIGURE 1.3 *Hypothalamic appetite control centres.*

to which it is bound to serum albumin – non-esterified fatty acids displace tryptophan from albumin binding, making it more readily available for brain uptake.

There is experimental evidence that the liver may play a key role in controlling appetite. In the fasting state there is a considerable increase in citric acid cycle activity in the liver (section 5.4.4) as the liver metabolizes fatty acids and other fuels to provide the adenosine triphosphate (ATP) required for synthesis of glucose from amino acids and other non-carbohydrate precursors (the process of gluconeogenesis; section 5.7) in order to maintain the plasma concentration of glucose. This hepatic 'energy flow' hypothesis still begs the question of what provides the signal from the liver to the central nervous system; although there are sensory neuronal pathways from the liver, lesioning them does not affect feeding behaviour in experimental animals.

The hypothalamic hunger and satiety centres control food intake remarkably precisely. Without conscious effort, most people can regulate their food intake to match energy expenditure very closely – they neither waste away from lack of metabolic fuel for physical activity nor lay down excessively large reserves of fat. Even people who have excessive reserves of body fat and can be considered to be so overweight or obese as to be putting their health at risk (section 6.2.2) balance their energy intake and expenditure relatively well considering that the average intake is a tonne of food a year, whereas the record obese people weigh about 250 kg (compared with average weights between 60 and 100 kg), and it takes many years to achieve such a weight. A gain or loss of 5 kg body weight over 6 months would require only a 1% difference between food intake and energy expenditure per day (section 5.2).

1.3.2 Long-term control of food intake and energy expenditure

In addition to the immediate control of feeding by hunger and satiety, there is also long-term control of food intake and energy expenditure, in response to the state of body fat reserves. In 1994 it was shown that the normal product of the gene that is defective in the homozygous recessive mutant (*ob/ob*) obese mouse is a small peptide that is secreted by adipose tissue. Administration of the synthetic peptide to genetically obese mice caused them to lose weight, and administration of excessive amounts of the peptide to normal mice also caused weight loss. It was called leptin, from the Greek λεπτοσ – lean or thin.

Further studies showed that the administration of leptin to the genetically obese diabetic (*fa/fa*) rat had no effect on body weight, and indeed these rats secreted a normal or greater than normal amount of leptin. The defect in these animals is a mutation in the membrane receptor for leptin.

Initially, the leptin receptor was found in the hypothalamus, and because the circulating concentration of leptin is determined largely by the mass of adipose tissue in the body, it was assumed that the function of leptin is to signal the size of fat reserves in the body to the hypothalamus, in order to control appetite. Interestingly, subcutaneous adipose tissue secretes more leptin than does abdominal adipose tissue, which may be an important factor in the difference in health risks associated with central (abdominal) obesity and hip–thigh obesity, which is due to subcutaneous fat (section 6.3.2).

Control of food intake is certainly one of the functions of leptin – reduced food intake can be observed in response to direct injection of the peptide into the central nervous system, and in response to leptin there is increased secretion of a number of peptide neurotransmitters that are known to be involved in regulation of feeding behaviour. However, the weight loss seen in response to leptin is greater than can be accounted for by the reduced food intake alone. Furthermore, in response to leptin there is a specific loss of adipose tissue, whereas, as discussed in section 8.2, in response to reduced food intake there is a loss of both adipose tissue and lean tissue.

Leptin receptors are also found in a variety of tissues other than the hypothalamus, including muscle and adipose tissue itself. Leptin has a number of actions in addition to its action in the hypothalamus, which result in increased energy expenditure and loss of adipose tissue:

- It causes increased expression of uncoupling protein (section 3.3.1.4) in adipose tissue and muscle. This results in relatively uncontrolled oxidation of metabolic fuel, unrelated to requirements for physical and chemical work, and increased heat output from the body (thermogenesis).
- It increases the activity of lipase in adipose tissue (section 10.5.1), resulting in the breakdown of triacylglycerol reserves and release of non-esterified fatty acids for oxidation.

- It decreases the expression of acetyl CoA carboxylase in adipose tissue (section 5.6.1). This results in both decreased synthesis of fatty acids and increased oxidation of fatty acids as a consequence of decreased formation of malonyl CoA (section 5.6.1 and section 10.5.2).
- There is some evidence that leptin also promotes apoptosis (programmed cell death) specifically in adipose tissue, thus reducing the number of adipocytes available for storage of fat in the body.

The result of these actions of leptin on adipose tissue and muscle is that there is a considerable increase in metabolic rate, and an increase in energy expenditure, as well as a reduction in food intake.

Although most leptin is secreted by adipose tissue, it is also secreted by muscle and the gastric mucosa. The role of leptin secretion by muscle is unclear, but in response to a meal there is a small increase in circulating leptin, presumably from the gastric mucosa. This suggests that, in addition to its role in long-term control of food intake and energy expenditure, leptin may be important in responses to food intake. Insulin (which is secreted mainly in response to food intake; section 5.3.1) stimulates the synthesis and secretion of leptin in adipose tissue.

There is also a circadian variation in leptin secretion, with an increase during the night. This is in response to the glucocorticoid hormones, which are secreted in increased amount during the night. It is likely that the loss of appetite and weight loss associated with chronic stress, when there is increased secretion of glucocorticoid hormones, is mediated by the effect of these hormones on leptin synthesis and secretion.

When leptin was first discovered, there was great hope that, as in the obese mouse, human obesity (see Chapter 6) might be due to a failure of leptin synthesis or secretion, and that administration of synthetic leptin might be a useful treatment for severe obesity. However, most obese people secrete more leptin than lean people (because they have more adipose tissue), and it is likely that the problem is due not to lack of leptin, but rather to a loss of sensitivity of the leptin receptors. Only in a very small number of people has obesity been found to be genetically determined by a mutation in the leptin gene.

1.3.3 APPETITE

In addition to hunger and satiety, which are basic physiological responses, food intake is controlled by appetite, which is related not only to physiological need, but also to the pleasure of eating – flavour and texture, and a host of social and psychological factors.

1.3.3.1 Taste and flavour

Taste buds on the tongue can distinguish five basic tastes – salt, savouriness, sweet, bitter and sour – as well as having a less well-understood ability to taste fat. The ability to taste salt, sweetness, savouriness and fat permits detection of nutrients; the ability to taste sourness and bitterness permits avoidance of toxins in foods.

Salt (correctly the mineral sodium) is essential to life, and wild animals will travel great distances to a salt lick. Like other animals, human beings have evolved a pleasurable response to salty flavours – this ensures that physiological needs are met. There is evidence that sensitivity to salt changes in response to the state of sodium balance in the body, with an increased number of active salt receptors (see below) on the tongue at times of sodium depletion. However, there is no shortage of salt in developed countries and, as discussed in section 7.3.4, average intakes of salt are considerably greater than requirements, and may pose a hazard to health.

The sensation of savouriness is distinct from that of saltiness, and is sometimes called *umami* (the Japanese for savoury). It is largely due to the presence of free amino acids in foods, and hence permits detection of protein-rich foods. Stimulation of the umami receptors of the tongue is the basis of flavour enhancers such as monosodium glutamate, which is an important constituent of traditional oriental condiments, and is widely used in manufactured foods.

The other instinctively pleasurable taste is sweetness, which permits detection of carbohydrates, and hence energy sources. While it is only sugars (section 4.2.1) that have a sweet taste, human beings (and a few other animals) secrete the enzyme amylase in saliva (section 4.2.21); amylase catalyses the hydrolysis of starch, which is the major dietary carbohydrate, to sweet-tasting sugars while the food is being chewed.

The tongue is sensitive to the taste not of triacylglycerols, but rather of free fatty acids, and especially polyunsaturated fatty acids (section 4.3.1.1). This suggests that the lipase secreted by the tongue has a role in permitting the detection of fatty foods as an energy source, in addition to its role in fat digestion (section 4.3.2).

Sourness and bitterness are instinctively unpleasant sensations; many of the toxins that occur in foods have a bitter or sour flavour. Learned behaviour will overcome the instinctive aversion, but this is a process of learning or acquiring tastes, not an innate or instinctive response.

The receptors for salt, sourness and savouriness (umami) all act as ion channels, transporting sodium ions, protons or glutamate ions respectively into the cells of the taste buds.

The receptors for sweetness and bitterness act via cell-surface receptors linked to intracellular formation second messengers. There is evidence that both cyclic adenosine monophosphate (cAMP) (section 1.3.2) and inositol trisphosphate (section 10.3.3) mechanisms are involved, and more than one signal transduction pathway may be involved in the responses to sweetness or sourness of different compounds. Some compounds may activate more than one type of receptor.

In addition to the sensations of taste provided by the taste-buds on the tongue, a great many flavours can be distinguished by the sense of smell. Again some flavours and aromas (fruity flavours, fresh coffee and, at least to a non-vegetarian, the smell of roasting meat) are pleasurable, tempting people to eat and stimulating appetite. Other flavours and aromas are repulsive, warning us not to eat the food. Again this can be seen as a warning of possible danger – the smell of decaying meat or fish tells us that it is not safe to eat.

Like the acquisition of a taste for bitter or sour foods, a taste for foods with what would seem at first to be an unpleasant aroma or flavour can also be acquired. Here things become more complex – a pleasant smell to one person may be repulsive to another. Some people enjoy the smell of cooked cabbage and sprouts, whereas others can hardly bear to be in the same room. The durian fruit is a highly prized delicacy in South-East Asia, yet to the uninitiated it smells of sewage or faeces – hardly an appetizing aroma.

1.3.4 WHY DO PEOPLE EAT WHAT THEY DO?

People have different responses to the same taste or flavour. This may be explained in terms of childhood memories, pleasurable or otherwise. An aversion to the smell of a food may protect someone who has a specific allergy or intolerance (although sometimes people have a craving for the foods of which they are intolerant). Most often, we simply cannot explain why some people dislike foods that others eat with great relish.

A number of factors may influence why people choose to eat particular foods.

1.3.4.1 The availability and cost of food

In developed countries the simple availability of food is not a constraint on choice. There is a wide variety of foods available, and when fruits and vegetables are out of season at home they are imported; frozen, canned and dried foods are widespread. By contrast, in developing countries, the availability of food is a major constraint on what people choose. Little food is imported, and what is available will depend on the local soil and climate. In normal times the choice of foods may be very limited, while in times of drought there may be little or no food available at all, and what little is available will be very much more expensive than most people can afford.

Even in developed countries, the cost of food may be important and, for the most disadvantaged members of the community, poverty may impose severe constraints on the choice of foods. In developing countries, cost is the major problem.

1.3.4.2 Religion, habit and tradition

Religious and ethical considerations are important in determining the choice of foods. Observant Jews and Muslims will eat meat only from animals that have cloven hooves and chew the cud. The words *kosher* in Jewish law and *hallal* in Islamic law both mean clean; the meat of other animals, which are scavenging animals, birds of prey and detritus-feeding fish, is regarded as unclean (*traife* or *haram*). We now know that many of these forbidden animals carry parasites that can infect human beings, so these ancient prohibitions are based on food hygiene.

Hindus will not eat beef. The reason for this is that the cow is far too valuable, as a source of milk and dung (as manure and fuel) and as a beast of burden, for it to be killed just as a source of meat.

Many people refrain from eating meat as a result of humanitarian concern for the animals involved, or because of real or perceived health benefits. Vegetarians can be divided into a variety of groups, according to the strictness of their diet:

- Some avoid red meat but eat poultry and fish.
- Some specifically avoid beef because of the potential risk of contracting variant Creutzfeldt–Jakob disease (vCJD) from eating meat infected with bovine spongiform encephalitis (BSE).
- Some (pescetarians) eat fish, but not meat or poultry.
- Ovo-lacto-vegetarians eat eggs and milk but not meat.
- Lacto-vegetarians eat milk but not eggs.
- Vegans eat only plant foods, and no foods of animal origin.

Perhaps the strictest of all vegetarians are the Jains (originally from Gujarat in India), whose religion not only prohibits the consumption of meat, but extends the sanctity of life to insects and grubs as well – an observant Jain will not eat any vegetable that has grown underground, lest an insect was killed in harvesting it.

Foods that are commonly eaten in one area may be little eaten elsewhere, even though they are available, simply because people have not been accustomed to eating them. To a very great extent, eating habits as adults continue the habits learned as children.

Haggis and oatcakes rarely travel south from Scotland, except as speciality items; black pudding is a staple of northern British breakfasts but is rarely seen in the south-east of England. Until the 1960s yoghurt was almost unknown in Britain, eaten only by a few health food 'cranks' and immigrants from Eastern Europe. Many British children believe that fish comes only as rectangular fish fingers, whereas children in inland Spain may eat fish and other seafood three or four times a week. The French mock the British habit of eating lamb with mint sauce – and the average British reaction to such French delicacies as frogs' legs and snails in garlic sauce is one of horror. The British eat their cabbage well boiled; the Germans and Dutch ferment it to produce sauerkraut.

This regional and cultural diversity of foods provides one of the pleasures of travel. As people travel more frequently, and become (perhaps grudgingly) more adventurous in their choice of foods, so they create a demand for different foods at home, and there is an increasing variety of foods available in shops and restaurants.

A further factor which has increased the range of foods available has been immigration of people from a variety of different backgrounds, all of whom have, as they have become established, introduced their traditional foods to their new homes. It is hard to believe that in the 1960s there were only a handful of tandoori restaurants in the whole of Britain and that pizza was something seen only in southern Italy and a few specialist restaurants, or that Balti cooking was unknown until the 1990s.

Some people are naturally adventurous and will try a new food just because they have never eaten it before. Others are more conservative and will try a new food only when they see someone else eating it safely and with enjoyment. Others are yet more conservative in their food choices; the most conservative eaters 'know' that they do not like a new food because they have never eaten it before.

1.3.4.3 Luxury status of scarce and expensive foods

Foods that are scarce or expensive have a certain appeal of fashion or style; they are (rightly) regarded as luxuries for special occasions rather than everyday meals. Conversely, foods that are widespread and cheap have less appeal.

In the nineteenth century, salmon and oysters were so cheap that the Articles of apprentices in London specified that they should not be given salmon more than three times a week, while oysters were eaten by the poor. Through much of the twentieth century, salmon was scarce and a prized luxury food; however, fish farming has increased the supply of salmon to such an extent that it is again a (relatively) inexpensive food. Chicken, turkey, guinea fowl and trout, which were expensive luxury foods in the 1950s, are now widely available as a result of changes in farming practice, and they form the basis of inexpensive meals.

By contrast, fish such as cod and herring, once the basis of cheap meals, are now becoming scarce and expensive as a result of depletion of fish stocks by overexploitation.

1.3.2.4 The social functions of food

Human beings are essentially social animals, and meals are important social functions. People eating in a group are likely to eat better, or at least to have a wider variety of foods and a more lavish and luxurious meal, than people eating alone. Entertaining guests may be an excuse to eat foods that we know to be nutritionally undesirable, and perhaps to eat to excess. The greater the variety of dishes offered, the more people are likely to eat. As we reach satiety with one food, so another, different, flavour is offered to stimulate appetite. A number of studies have shown that, faced with only one food, people tend to reach satiety sooner than when a variety of different foods is on offer. This is the difference between hunger and appetite – even when we are satiated, we can still 'find room' to try something different.

Conversely, and more importantly, many lonely single people (and especially the bereaved elderly) have little incentive to prepare meals and no stimulus to appetite. Although poverty may be a factor, apathy (and frequently, especially in the case of widowed men, ignorance) severely limits the range of foods eaten, possibly leading to undernutrition. When these problems are added to the problems of infirmity, ill-fitting dentures (which make eating painful) and arthritis (which makes handling many foods difficult) and the difficulty of carrying food home from the shops, it is not surprising that we include the elderly among those vulnerable groups of the population who are at risk of undernutrition.

In hospitals and other institutions there is a further problem. People who are unwell may have low physical activity, but they have higher than normal requirements for energy, and nutrients, as a part of the process of replacing tissue in convalescence (section 9.1.2.2), or as a result of fever or the metabolic effects of cancer (section 8.4). At the same time, illness impairs appetite, and a side-effect of many drugs is to distort the sense of taste, depress appetite or cause nausea. It is difficult to provide a range of exciting and attractive foods under institutional conditions, yet this is what is needed to tempt the patient's appetite.

Additional resources

PowerPoint presentation 1 on the CD.

CHAPTER **2**

Enzymes and metabolic pathways

All metabolic processes depend on reaction between molecules, with breaking of some covalent bonds and the formation of others, yielding compounds that are different from the starting materials. In order to understand nutrition and metabolism it is therefore essential to understand how chemical reactions occur, how they are catalysed by enzymes and how enzyme activity can be regulated and controlled.

Objectives

After reading this chapter you should be able to:

* explain how covalent bonds are broken and formed, what is meant by thermoneutral, endothermic and exothermic reactions and how reactions come to equilibrium;
* explain how a catalyst increases the rate at which a reaction comes to equilibrium and how enzymes act as catalysts;
* explain how an enzyme exhibits specificity for both the substrates bound and the reaction catalysed;
* define a unit of enzyme activity;
* explain how pH, temperature and concentration of enzyme affect the rate of reaction;

- describe and explain the dependence of the rate of reaction on concentration of substrate, define the kinetic parameters K_m and V_{max} and explain how they are determined experimentally;
- explain how enzymes may show cooperative binding of substrate and how this affects the substrate dependence of activity;
- describe the difference between irreversible and reversible inhibitors of enzymes, their clinical relevance and how they may be distinguished experimentally;
- describe the difference between competitive and non-competitive reversible inhibitors of enzymes, their clinical relevance and how they may be distinguished experimentally;
- explain what is meant by the terms coenzyme and prosthetic group, apoenzyme and holoenzyme and describe the roles of coenzymes in oxidation and reduction reactions;
- describe the classification of enzymes on the basis of the reaction catalysed;
- describe and explain what is meant by a metabolic pathway and by linear, branched, spiral (looped) and cyclic pathways.

2.1 *Chemical reactions: breaking and making covalent bonds*

Breaking covalent bonds requires an initial input of energy in some form – normally as heat, but in some cases also light or other radiation. This is the activation energy of the reaction. The process of breaking a bond requires activation of the electrons forming the bond – a temporary shift of electrons from orbitals in which they have a stable configuration to other orbitals, further from the nucleus. Electrons that have been excited in this way have an unstable configuration, and the covalent bonds they had contributed to are broken. Electrons cannot remain in this excited state for more than a fraction of a second. Sometimes they simply return to their original unexcited state, emitting the same energy as was taken up to excite them, but usually as a series of small steps, rather than as a single step. Overall there is no change when this occurs.

More commonly, the excited electrons may adopt a different stable configuration, by interacting with electrons associated with different atoms and molecules. The result is the formation of new covalent bonds, and hence the formation of new compounds. In this case, there are three possibilities (as shown in Figure 2.1):

- There may be an output of energy equal to the activation energy of the reaction, so that the energy level of the products is the same as that of the starting materials. Such a reaction is energetically neutral (thermoneutral).
- There may be an output of energy greater than the activation energy of the reaction, so that the energy level of the products is lower than that of the starting materials. This is an exothermic reaction – it proceeds with the output of heat. An exothermic reaction will proceed spontaneously once the initial activation energy has been provided.

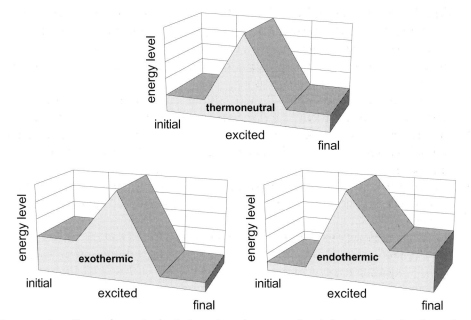

FIGURE 2.1 *Energy changes in chemical reactions: thermoneutral, endothermic and exothermic reactions.*

- There may be an output of energy less than the activation energy, so that the energy level of the products is higher than that of the starting materials. The solution will take up heat from its surroundings and will have to be heated for the reaction to proceed. This is an endothermic reaction.

In general, reactions in which relatively large complex molecules are broken down to smaller molecules are exothermic, whereas reactions that involve the synthesis of larger molecules from smaller ones are endothermic.

2.1.1 EQUILIBRIUM

Some reactions, such as the burning of a hydrocarbon in air to form carbon dioxide and water, are highly exothermic, and the products of the reaction are widely dispersed. Such reactions proceed essentially in one direction only. However, most reactions do not proceed in only one direction. If two compounds, A and B, can react together to form X and Y, then X and Y can react to form A and B. The reactions can be written as:

(1) $A + B \rightarrow X + Y$

(2) $X + Y \rightarrow A + B$

Starting with only A and B in the solution, at first only reaction (1) will occur, forming X and Y. However, as X and Y accumulate, so they will undergo reaction (2), forming A and B. Similarly, starting with X and Y, at first only reaction (2) will occur, forming A and B. As A and B accumulate, so they will undergo reaction (1), forming X and Y.

In both cases, the final result will be a solution containing A, B, X, and Y. The relative amounts of [A+B] and [X+Y] will be the same regardless of whether the starting compounds (substrates) were A and B or X and Y. At this stage the rate of reaction (1) forming X and Y, and reaction (2) forming A and B, will be equal. This is equilibrium, and the reaction can be written as:

$$A + B \rightleftharpoons X + Y$$

If there is a large difference in energy level between [A+B] and [X+Y] – i.e. if the reaction is exothermic in one direction (and therefore endothermic in the other direction) – then the position of the equilibrium will reflect this. If reaction (1) above is exothermic, then at equilibrium there will be very little A and B remaining – most will have been converted to X and Y. Conversely, if reaction (1) is endothermic, then relatively little of the substrates will be converted to X and Y at equilibrium.

At equilibrium the ratio of [A+B]/[X+Y] is a constant for any given reaction, depending on the temperature. This means that a constant addition of substrates will disturb the equilibrium and increase the amount of product formed. Constant removal of products will similarly disturb the equilibrium and increase the rate at which substrate is removed.

2.1.2 CATALYSTS

A catalyst is a compound that increases the rate at which a reaction comes to equilibrium without itself being consumed in the reaction, so that a small amount of catalyst can affect the reaction of many thousands of molecules of substrate. Although a catalyst increases the rate at which a reaction comes to equilibrium, it does not affect the position of the equilibrium. Catalysts affect the rate at which equilibrium is achieved in three main ways:

- By providing a surface on which the molecules that are to undergo reaction can come together in higher concentration than would be possible in free solution, thus increasing the probability of them colliding and reacting. Binding also aligns the substrates in the correct orientation to undergo reaction.
- By providing a microenvironment for the reactants that is different from the solution as a whole.
- By participating in the reaction by withdrawing electrons from, or donating electrons to, covalent bonds. This enhances the breaking of bonds that is the prerequisite for chemical reaction and lowers the activation energy of the reaction.

2.2 *Enzymes*

Enzymes are proteins that catalyse metabolic reactions. There are also a number of enzymes that are not proteins but are catalytic molecules of RNA (section 9.2.2) – these are sometimes referred to as ribozymes.

As discussed in section 4.4.2, proteins are linear polymers of amino acids. Any protein adopts a characteristic pattern of folding, determined largely by the order of the different amino acids in its sequence. This folding of the protein chain results in reactive groups from a variety of amino acids, which might be widely separated in the primary sequence, coming together at the surface and creating a site that has a defined shape and array of chemically reactive groups. This is the active site of the enzyme. It is the site that both binds the compounds which are to undergo reaction (the substrates) and catalyses the reaction.

Many enzymes also have a non-protein component of the catalytic site; this may be a metal ion, an organic compound that contains a metal ion (e.g. haem; section 3.3.1.2), or an organic compound, which may be derived from a vitamin (see Chapter 11) or readily synthesized in the body. This non-protein part of the active site may be covalently bound, in which case it is generally referred to as a prosthetic group, or may be tightly, but not covalently, bound, in which case it is usually referred to as a coenzyme (section 2.4).

Amino acid side-chains at the active site provide chemically reactive groups which can facilitate the making or breaking of specific chemical bonds in the substrate by donating or withdrawing electrons. In this way, the enzyme can lower the activation energy of a chemical reaction (Figure 2.2) and so increase the speed at which the reaction attains equilibrium under much milder conditions than are required for a simple chemical catalyst. In order to hydrolyse a protein into its constituent amino acids in the laboratory, it is necessary to use concentrated acid as a catalyst and to heat the sample at 105 °C overnight to provide the activation energy of the hydrolysis. As discussed in section 4.4.3, this is the process of digestion of proteins, which occurs in the human gut under relatively mild acid or alkaline conditions, at 37 °C, and is complete within a few hours of eating a meal.

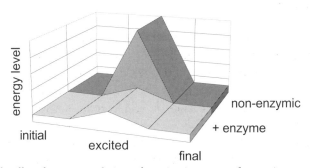

FIGURE 2.2 *The effect of enzyme catalysis on the activation energy of a reaction.*

2.2.1 SPECIFICITY OF ENZYMES

The binding of substrates to enzymes involves interactions between the substrates and reactive groups of the amino acid side-chains that make up the active site of the enzyme. This means that enzymes show a considerable specificity for the substrates they bind. Normally, several different interactions must occur before the substrate can bind in the correct orientation to undergo reaction, and binding of the substrate often causes a change in the shape of the active site, bringing reactive groups closer to the substrate.

Figure 2.3 shows the active sites of three enzymes that catalyse the same reaction – hydrolysis of a peptide bond in a protein (section 4.4.3). The three enzymes show different specificity for the bond that they hydrolyse:

- Trypsin catalyses cleavage of the esters of basic amino acids.
- Chymotrypsin catalyses hydrolysis of the esters of aromatic amino acids.
- Elastase catalyses hydrolysis of the esters of small neutral amino acids.

This difference in specificity for the bond hydrolysed is explained by differences in the substrate binding sites of the three enzymes. In all three enzymes, the substrate binds in a groove at the surface, in such as way as to bring the bond to be cleaved over the serine residue that initiates the catalysis. The amino acid providing the carboxyl side of the peptide bond to be cleaved sits in a pocket below this groove, and it is the nature of the amino acids that line this pocket that determines the specificity of the enzymes:

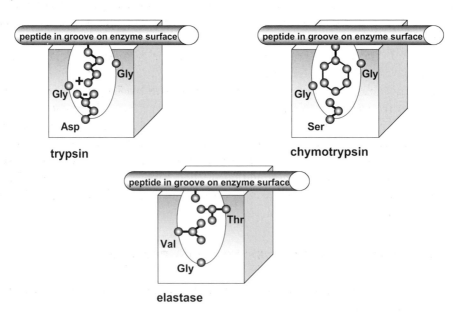

FIGURE 2.3 *Enzyme specificity – the substrate binding sites of trypsin, chymotrypsin and elastase.*

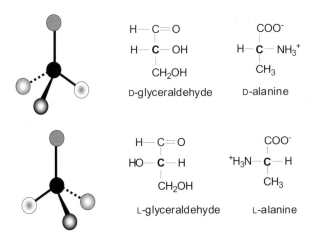

H—C=O
H—C—OH
CH₂OH

D-glyceraldehyde

COO⁻
H—C—NH₃⁺
CH₃

D-alanine

H—C=O
HO—C—H
CH₂OH

L-glyceraldehyde

COO⁻
⁺H₃N—C—H
CH₃

L-alanine

FIGURE 2.4 *DL-isomerism.*

- In trypsin there is an acidic group (from aspartate) at the base of the pocket – this will attract a basic amino acid side-chain.
- In chymotrypsin the pocket is lined by small neutral amino acids, so that a relatively large aromatic group can fit in.
- In elastase there are two bulky amino acid side-chains in the pocket, so that only a small neutral side-chain can fit it.

The specificity of enzymes is such that they distinguish between the D- and L-isomers (Figure 2.4), and between the *cis-* and *trans-*isomers (Figure 2.5 and section 4.3.1.1), of the substrate. This is because the isomers have different shapes. In non-enzymic chemical reactions they may behave identically, and it may be difficult to distinguish between them. The shape and conformation of the substrate are critically important for binding to an enzyme.

The participation of reactive groups at the active site provides specificity not only for the substrates that will bind, but also for the reaction that will be catalysed. For example, in a non-enzymic model system, an amino acid may undergo α-decarboxylation to yield an amine, transfer of the α-amino group and replacement with an oxo-group (section 9.3.1.2), isomerization between the D- and L-isomers, or a variety of reactions involving elimination or replacement of the side-chain. In an enzyme-catalysed reaction only one of the possible reactions will be catalysed by any given enzyme.

2.2.2 STAGES IN AN ENZYME-CATALYSED REACTION

An enzyme-catalysed reaction can be considered to occur in three distinct steps, all of which are reversible:

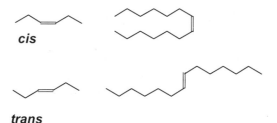

cis

trans

FIGURE 2.5   Cis/trans *isomerism.*

- Binding of the substrate (S) to the enzyme, to form the enzyme–substrate complex:

  Enz + S ⇌ Enz – S

- Reaction of the enzyme-substrate complex to form the enzyme–product complex:

  Enz – S ⇌ Enz – P

- Breakdown of the enzyme–product complex, with release of the product (P):

  Enz – P ⇌ Enz + P

Hence, overall, the process can be written as:

  Enz + S ⇌ Enz – S ⇌ Enz–P ⇌ Enz + P

where Enz is the enzyme, S the substrate and P the product. The reaction occurs in three stages, all of which are reversible.

2.2.3 UNITS OF ENZYME ACTIVITY

When an enzyme has been purified, it is possible to express the amount of enzyme in tissues or plasma as the number of moles of enzyme protein present. However, what is more important is not how much of the enzyme protein is present in the cell, but how much catalytic activity there is – how much substrate can be converted to product in a given time. Therefore, amounts of enzymes are usually expressed in units of activity.

The SI unit of catalysis is the katal = 1 mole of substrate converted per second. However, enzyme activity is usually expressed as the number of micromoles (μmol) of substrate converted (or of product formed) per minute. This is the standard unit of enzyme activity, determined under specified optimum conditions for that enzyme, at 30 °C. This temperature is a compromise between mammalian biochemists, who would work at body temperature (37 °C for human beings) and microbiological biochemists, who would normally work at 20 °C.

2.3 *Factors affecting enzyme activity*

Any given enzyme has an innate activity – for many enzymes the catalytic rate constant is of the order of 4–5000 mol of substrate converted per mole of enzyme per second or higher. However, a number of factors affect the activity of enzymes.

2.3.1 EFFECT OF PH

Both the binding of the substrate to the enzyme and catalysis of the reaction depend on interactions between the substrates and reactive groups in the amino acid side-chains which make up the active site. They have to be in the appropriate ionization state for binding and reaction to occur – this depends on the pH of the medium. Any enzyme will have maximum activity at a specific pH – the optimum pH for that enzyme. As the pH rises or falls away from the optimum, so the activity of the enzyme will decrease. Most enzymes have little or no activity 2–3 pH units away from their pH optimum. Figure 2.6 shows the activity of two enzymes that are found in plasma and which catalyse the same reaction, hydrolysis of a phosphate ester; enzyme A is acid phosphatase (released from the prostate gland, with a pH optimum around 3.5) and enzyme B is alkaline phosphatase (released from bone, with a pH optimum around 9.0). Neither has any significant activity at pH 7.35–7.45, which is the normal range of plasma pH. However, alkaline phosphatase is significantly active in the alkaline microenvironment at cell surfaces, and is important, for example, in the hydrolysis of pyridoxal phosphate (the main form of vitamin B_6 in plasma; section 11.9) to free pyridoxal for uptake into tissues.

2.3.2 EFFECT OF TEMPERATURE

Chemical reactions proceed faster at higher temperatures, for two reasons:

- Molecules move faster at higher temperatures, and hence have a greater chance of colliding to undergo reaction.
- At a higher temperature it is also easier for electrons to gain activation energy, and hence become excited into unstable orbitals to undergo reaction.

With enzyme-catalysed reactions, although the rate at which the reaction comes to equilibrium increases with temperature, there is a second effect of temperature – denaturation of the enzyme protein, leading to irreversible loss of activity (section 4.4.2. As the temperature increases, so the movement of parts of the protein molecules relative to each other increases, leading eventually to disruption of the hydrogen bonds that maintain the folded structure of the protein. When this happens, the protein chain unfolds and the active site is lost. As the temperature increases further, so the denatured protein becomes insoluble, and precipitates out of solution.

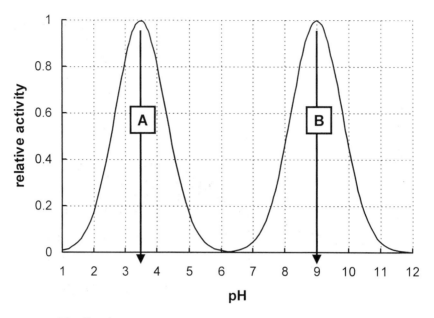

FIGURE 2.6 *The effect of pH on enzyme activity. Enzyme A has a pH optimum of 3.5, enzyme B a pH optimum of 9.0.*

As shown in Figure 2.7, temperature thus has two opposing effects on enzyme activity. At relatively low temperatures (up to about 50–55 °C), increasing temperature results in an increase in the rate of reaction. However, as the temperature increases further, so denaturation of the enzyme protein becomes increasingly important, resulting in a rapid fall in activity at higher temperatures. The rate of increase in the rate of reaction with increasing temperature depends on the activation energy of the reaction being catalysed; the rate of decrease in activity at higher temperatures is a characteristic of the enzyme itself.

The apparent temperature optimum of an enzyme-catalysed reaction depends on the time for which the enzyme is incubated. As shown in Figure 2.7, during a short incubation (e.g. 1 min) there is negligible denaturation, and so the apparent optimum temperature is relatively high, whereas during a longer incubation denaturation is important, and so the apparent optimum temperature is lower.

The effect of temperature is not normally important physiologically, as body temperature is normally maintained close to 37 °C. However, some of the effects of fever (when body temperature may rise to 40 °C) may be due to changes in the rates of enzyme-catalysed reactions. Because different enzymes respond differently to changes in temperature, there can be a considerable loss of the normal integration between different enzymic reactions and metabolic pathways.

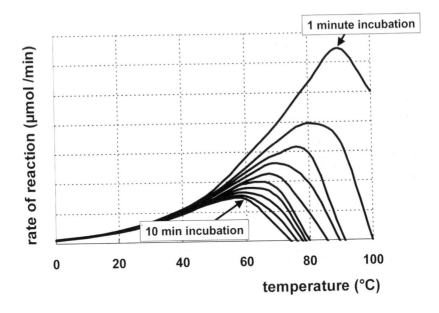

FIGURE 2.7 *The temperature dependence of enzyme activity. In a short (1 min) incubation the enzyme may have an optimum temperature as high as 90 °C, but in longer incubations this falls, so that in a 10-min incubation the optimum temperature is about 55 °C.*

2.3.3 EFFECT OF SUBSTRATE CONCENTRATION

In a simple chemical reaction involving a single substrate, the rate at which product is formed increases linearly as the concentration of the substrate increases. When more substrate is available, more will undergo reaction.

With enzyme-catalysed reactions, the change in the rate of formation of product with increasing concentration of substrate is not linear, but hyperbolic, as shown in Figure 2.8. At relatively low concentrations of substrate (region A in Figure 2.8), the catalytic site of the enzyme may be empty at times, until more substrate binds to undergo reaction. Under these conditions, the rate of formation of product is limited by the time taken for another molecule of substrate to bind to the enzyme. A relatively small change in the concentration of substrate has a large effect on the rate at which product is formed in this region of the curve.

At high concentrations of substrate (region B in Figure 2.8), as product leaves the catalytic site, another molecule of substrate binds more or less immediately, and the enzyme is saturated with substrate. The limiting factor in the formation of product is now the rate at which the enzyme can catalyse the reaction, and not the availability of substrate. The enzyme is acting at or near its maximum rate (or maximum velocity, usually abbreviated to V_{max}). Even a relatively large change in the concentration of substrate has little effect on the rate of formation of product in this region of the curve.

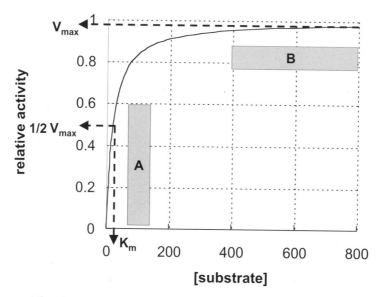

FIGURE 2.8 *The substrate dependence of an enzyme-catalysed reaction. In region A the enzyme is very unsaturated with substrate, and the rate of reaction increases sharply with increasing concentration of substrate. In region B the enzyme is almost saturated with substrate, and there is little change in the rate of reaction with increasing substrate.*

From a graph of the rate of formation of product versus the concentration of substrate (Figure 2.8), it is easy to estimate the maximum rate of reaction that an enzyme can achieve (V_{max}) when it is saturated with substrate. However, it is not possible to determine from this graph the concentration of substrate required to achieve saturation, because the enzyme gradually approaches V_{max} as the concentration of substrate increases.

It is easy to estimate the concentration of substrate at which the enzyme has achieved half its maximum rate of reaction. The concentration of substrate to achieve half V_{max} is called the Michaelis constant of the enzyme (abbreviated to K_m), to commemorate Michaelis, who, together with Menten, first formulated a mathematical model of the dependence of the rate of enzymic reactions on the concentration of substrate.

The K_m of an enzyme is not affected by the amount of the enzyme protein that is present. It is an (inverse) index of the affinity of the enzyme for its substrate. An enzyme which has a high K_m has a relatively low affinity for its substrate compared with an enzyme which has a lower K_m. The higher the value of K_m, the greater is the concentration of substrate required to achieve half-saturation of the enzyme.

In general, enzymes that have a low K_m compared with the normal concentration of substrate in the cell are likely to be acting at or near their maximum rate, and hence to have a more or less constant rate of reaction despite (modest) changes in the concentration of substrate. By contrast, an enzyme which has a high K_m compared with the normal concentration of substrate in the cell will show a large change in the rate of reaction with relatively small changes in the concentration of substrate.

If two enzymes in a cell can both act on the same substrate, catalysing different reactions, the enzyme with the lower K_m will be able to bind more substrate, and therefore its reaction will be favoured at relatively low concentrations of substrate. Thus, knowing the values of K_m and V_{max} for two enzymes, for example at a branch point in a metabolic pathway (see Figure 2.18), it is possible to predict whether one branch or the other will predominate in the presence of different amounts of the substrate.

2.3.3.1 Experimental determination of K_m and V_{max}

Plotting the graph of rate of reaction against substrate concentration, as in Figure 2.8, permits only an approximate determination of the values of K_m and V_{max}, and a number of methods have been developed to convert this hyperbolic relationship into a linear relationship, to permit more precise fitting of a line to the experimental points, and hence more precise estimation of K_m and V_{max}.

The most widely used such linearization of the data is the Lineweaver–Burk double-reciprocal plot of 1/rate of reaction versus 1/[substrate], as shown in Figure 2.9. This has an intercept on the y (1/v) axis $= 1/V_{max}$ when 1/$s = 0$ (i.e. at an infinite concentration of substrate), and an intercept on the x (1/s) axis $= -1/K_m$.

Experimentally, the values of K_m and V_{max} are determined by incubating the enzyme (at optimum pH) with a range of concentrations of substrate, plotting the graph shown in Figure 2.9 and extrapolating back from the experimental points to determine the intercepts.

The Michaelis–Menten equation that describes the dependence of rate of reaction on concentration of substrate is:

$$v = (V_{max} \times [S])/([S] + K_m)$$

One of the underlying assumptions of the Michaelis–Menten model is that there is no change in the concentration of substrate – this means that what should be measured is the initial rate of reaction. This is usually estimated by determining the amount of product formed at a series of short time intervals after the initiation of the reaction, then plotting a rate curve (product formed versus time incubated) and estimating the tangent to this curve as the initial rate of reaction.

2.3.3.2 Enzymes with two substrates

Most enzyme-catalysed reactions involve two substrates; it is only enzymes catalysing lysis of a molecule or an isomerization reaction (section 2.5) that have only a single substrate.

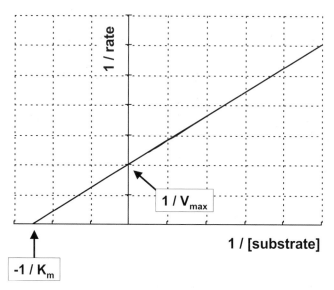

For a reaction involving two substrates (and two products):

$$A + B \rightleftharpoons C + D$$

the enzyme may act by either:

- an ordered mechanism, in which each substrate binds in turn:

    $$A + Enz \rightleftharpoons A\text{–}Enz$$

    $$A\text{–}Enz + B \rightleftharpoons A\text{–}Enz\text{–}B \rightleftharpoons C\text{–}Enz\text{–}D \rightleftharpoons C\text{–}Enz + D$$

    $$C\text{–}Enz \rightleftharpoons Enz + C$$

- a ping-pong mechanism in which one substrate undergoes reaction, modifying the enzyme and releasing product, then the second substrate binds, reacts with the modified enzyme and restores it to the original state:

    $$A + Enz \rightleftharpoons A\text{–}Enz \rightleftharpoons C\text{–}Enz^* \rightleftharpoons C + Enz^*$$

    $$B + Enz^* \rightleftharpoons B\text{–}Enz^* \rightleftharpoons D\text{–}Enz \rightleftharpoons D + Enz$$

These two different mechanisms can be distinguished by plotting $1/v$ vs. 1[substrate A] at several different concentrations of substrate B; as shown in Figure 2.10, the lines converge if the mechanism is ordered but are parallel for a ping-pong reaction.

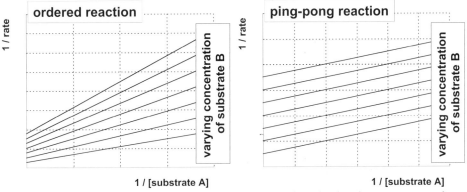

FIGURE 2.10 *The Lineweaver–Burk double-reciprocal plots for ordered and ping-pong two-substrate reactions.*

2.3.3.3 Cooperative (allosteric) enzymes

Not all enzymes show the simple hyperbolic dependence of rate of reaction on substrate concentration shown in Figure 2.8. Some enzymes consist of several separate protein chains, each with an active site. In many such enzymes, the binding of substrate to one active site causes changes in the conformation not only of that active site, but of the whole multi-subunit array. This change in conformation affects the other active sites, altering the ease with which substrate can bind to the other active sites. This is cooperativity – the different subunits of the complete enzyme cooperate with each other. Because there is a change in the conformation (or shape) of the enzyme molecule, the phenomenon is also called allostericity (from the Greek for 'different shape'), and such enzymes are called allosteric enzymes.

Figure 2.11 shows the change in rate of reaction with increasing concentration of substrate for an enzyme that displays substrate cooperativity. At low concentrations of substrate, the enzyme has little activity. When one of the binding sites becomes occupied, this causes a conformational change in the enzyme and so increases the ease with which the other sites can bind substrate. Therefore, there is a steep increase in the rate of reaction with increasing concentration of substrate. Of course, once all the sites become saturated, the rate of reaction cannot increase any further with increasing concentration of substrate; the enzyme achieves its maximum rate of reaction.

Enzymes that display substrate cooperativity are often important in controlling the overall rate of metabolic pathways (section 10.2.1). Their rate of reaction is extremely sensitive to the concentration of substrate. Furthermore, this sensitivity can readily be modified by a variety of compounds that bind to specific regulator sites on the enzyme and affect its conformation, so affecting the conformation of all of the active sites of the multi-subunit complex, and either activating the enzyme at low concentrations of substrate by decreasing cooperativity or inhibiting it by increasing cooperativity.

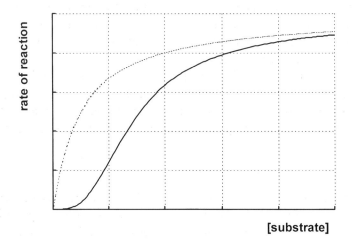

FIGURE 2.11 *The substrate dependence of an enzyme showing subunit cooperativity – a sigmoid curve. For comparison the hyperbolic substrate dependence of an enzyme not showing substrate cooperativity is shown as a dotted line.*

2.3.4 INHIBITION OF ENZYME ACTIVITY

Inhibition of the activity of key enzymes in metabolic pathways by end-products or other metabolic intermediates is an important part of metabolic integration and control (section 10.2). In addition, many of the drugs used to treat diseases are inhibitors of enzymes. Some act by inhibiting the patient's enzyme, so altering metabolic regulation; others act by preferentially inhibiting key enzymes in the bacteria or other organisms that are causing disease.

2.3.4.1 Irreversible inhibitors

Compounds that inhibit enzymes may either act reversibly, so that the inhibition gradually wears off as the inhibitor is metabolized, or irreversibly, causing chemical modification of the enzyme protein, so that the effect of the inhibitor is prolonged, and only diminishes gradually as the enzyme protein is catabolized and replaced (section 9.1.1).

It is important when designing drugs to know whether they act as reversible or irreversible inhibitors. An irreversible inhibitor may only need to be administered every few days; however, it is more difficult to adjust the dose of an irreversible inhibitor to match the patient's needs, because of the long duration of action. By contrast, it is easy to adjust the dose of a reversible inhibitor to produce the desired effect, but such a compound may have to be taken several times a day, depending on the rate at which it is metabolized and excreted from the body.

Irreversible inhibitors are chemical analogues of the substrate, and bind to the enzyme in the same way as does the substrate, then undergo part of the reaction sequence of the normal reaction. However, at some stage they form a covalent bond to a reactive group in the active site, resulting in inactivation of the enzyme. Such inhibitors are sometimes called mechanism-dependent inhibitors, or suicide inhibitors, because they cause the enzyme to commit suicide.

Experimentally, it is simple to distinguish between irreversible and reversible inhibitors; a reversible inhibitor can be removed from the enzyme (for example by dialysis), and this will restore activity. By contrast, an irreversible inhibitor, being covalently bound, cannot be removed by dialysis, and so activity cannot be restored.

2.3.4.2 Competitive reversible inhibitors

A competitive inhibitor is a compound that binds to the active site of the enzyme in competition with the substrate. Commonly, but not always, such compounds are chemical analogues of the substrate. Although a competitive inhibitor binds to the active site, it does not undergo reaction, or, if it does, not to yield the product that would have been obtained by reaction of the normal substrate.

A competitive inhibitor reduces the rate of reaction because at any time some molecules of the enzyme have bound the inhibitor, and therefore are not free to bind the substrate. However, the binding of the inhibitor to the enzyme is reversible, and therefore there is competition between the substrate and the inhibitor for the enzyme. This means that the sequence of the reaction in the presence of a competitive inhibitor can be shown as:

$$\text{Enz} + \text{S} + \text{I} \rightleftharpoons \text{Enz–I}$$

$$\text{Enz} + \text{S} + \text{I} \rightleftharpoons \text{Enz–S} \rightleftharpoons \text{Enz–P} \rightleftharpoons \text{Enz} + \text{P}$$

Figure 2.12 shows the s/v and double-reciprocal plots for an enzyme incubated with various concentrations of a competitive inhibitor. If the concentration of substrate is increased, it will compete more effectively with the inhibitor for the active site of the enzyme. This means that at high concentrations of substrate the enzyme will achieve the same maximum rate of reaction (V_{max}) in the presence or absence of inhibitor. It is simply that in the presence of inhibitor the enzyme requires a higher concentration of substrate to achieve saturation – in other words, the K_m of the enzyme is higher in the presence of a competitive inhibitor.

The effect of a drug that is a competitive inhibitor is that the rate at which product is formed is unchanged, but there is an increase in the concentration of the substrate of the inhibited enzyme in the cell. As the inhibitor acts, so it will cause an increase in the concentration of substrate in the cell, and eventually this will rise high enough for the enzyme to reach a more or less normal rate of reaction. This means that a competitive inhibitor is appropriate for use as a drug where the aim is to increase the available pool of substrate (perhaps so as to allow an alternative reaction to proceed), but inappropriate if the aim is to reduce the amount of product formed.

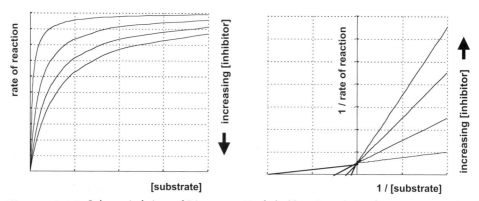

FIGURE 2.12 *Substrate/velocity and Lineweaver–Burk double-reciprocal plots for an enzyme incubated with varying concentrations of a competitive inhibitor.*

2.3.4.3 Non-competitive reversible inhibitors

Compounds that are non-competitive inhibitors bind to the enzyme–substrate complex, rather than to the enzyme itself. The enzyme–substrate–inhibitor complex reacts only slowly to form enzyme–product–inhibitor, so the effect of a non-competitive inhibitor is to slow down the rate at which the enzyme catalyses the formation of product. The reaction sequence can be written as:

$$\text{Enz} + \text{S} + \text{I} \rightleftharpoons \text{Enz–S} + \text{I} \rightleftharpoons \text{Enz–S–I} \rightleftharpoons \text{Enz–P–I} \rightleftharpoons \text{Enz} + \text{P} + \text{I}$$

Because there is no competition between the inhibitor and the substrate for binding to the enzyme, increasing the concentration of substrate has no effect on the activity of the enzyme in the presence of a non-competitive inhibitor. The K_m of the enzyme is unaffected by a non-competitive inhibitor, but the V_{max} is reduced. Figure 2.13 shows the s/v and double-reciprocal plots for an enzyme incubated with several concentrations of a non-competitive inhibitor.

A non-competitive inhibitor would be the choice for use as a drug when the aim is either to increase the concentration of substrate in the cell or to reduce the rate at which the product is formed, as, unlike a competitive inhibitor, the accumulation of substrate has no effect on the extent of inhibition.

2.4 COENZYMES AND PROSTHETIC GROUPS

Although most enzymes are proteins, many contain small non-protein molecules as an integral part of their structure. These may be organic compounds or metal ions. In either case, they are essential to the function of the enzyme, and the enzyme has no activity in the absence of the metal ion or coenzyme.

When an organic compound or metal ion is covalently bound to the active site of the enzyme it is usually referred to as a prosthetic group; compounds that are tightly

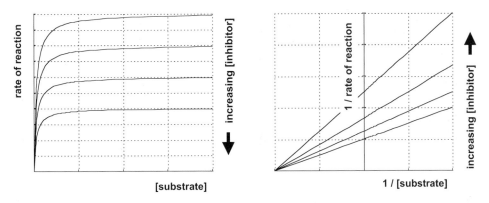

FIGURE 2.13 *Substrate/velocity and Lineweaver–Burk double-reciprocal plots for an enzyme incubated with varying concentrations of a non-competitive inhibitor.*

but not covalently bound are referred to as coenzymes. Like the enzyme itself, the coenzyme or prosthetic group participates in the reaction, but at the end emerges unchanged. Sometimes the coenzyme is chemically modified in the reaction with the first substrate, then restored to its original state by reaction with the second substrate. This would be a ping-pong reaction (section 2.3.3.2); transaminases (section 9.3.1.2) catalyse a ping-pong reaction in which the amino group from the first substrate forms an amino derivative of the coenzyme as an intermediate step in the reaction.

Some compounds that were historically considered as coenzymes do not remain bound to the active site of the enzyme, but bind and leave in the same way as other substrates. Such compounds include the nicotinamide nucleotide coenzymes (NAD and NADP) and coenzyme A. Although they are not really coenzymes, they are present in the cell in very much smaller concentrations than most substrates, and are involved in a relatively large number of reactions, so that they turn over rapidly.

Table 2.1 shows the major coenzymes, the vitamins they are derived from and their principal metabolic functions.

2.4.1 Coenzymes and metals in oxidation and reduction reactions

In its simplest form, oxidation is the combination of a molecule with oxygen. Thus, if a carbohydrate, such as glucose ($C_6H_{12}O_6$), is burned in air (or metabolized in the body), it is oxidized to carbon dioxide and at the same time oxygen is reduced to water:

$$C_6H_{12}O_6 + 6 \times O_2 \rightarrow 6 \times CO_2 + 6 \times H_2O$$

Oxidation reactions need not involve the addition of oxygen; oxidation is the removal of electrons from a molecule. Thus, the conversion of the iron Fe^{2+} ion to Fe^{3+} is also an oxidation, although in this case there is no direct involvement of oxygen.

TABLE 2.1 *The major coenzymes*

		Source	Functions
CoA	Coenzyme A	Pantothenic acid	Acyl transfer reactions
FAD	Flavin adenine dinucleotide	Vitamin B_2	Oxidation reactions
FMN	Flavin mononucleotide	Vitamin B_2	Oxidation reactions
NAD	Nicotinamide adenine dinucleotide	Niacin	Oxidation and reduction reactions
NADP	Nicotinamide adenine dinucleotide phosphate	Niacin	Oxidation and reduction reactions
PLP	Pyridoxal phosphate	Vitamin B_6	Amino acid metabolism

There are a number of other coenzymes, which are discussed as they are relevant to specific metabolic pathways. In addition to those shown in this table, most of the other vitamins also function as coenzymes (see Chapter 11).

In many reactions, the removal of electrons in an oxidation reaction does not result in the formation of a positive ion – hydrogen ions (H^+) are removed together with the electrons. This means that the removal of hydrogen from a compound is also oxidation. For example, a hydrocarbon such as ethane (C_2H_6) is oxidized to ethene (C_2H_4) by removing two hydrogen atoms onto a carrier:

$$CH_3\text{-}CH_3 + \text{carrier} \rightleftharpoons CH_2{=}CH_2 + \text{carrier-}H_2$$

Reduction is the reverse of oxidation – the addition of hydrogen, or electrons, or the removal of oxygen are all reduction reactions. In the reaction above, ethane was oxidized to ethene at the expense of a carrier, which was reduced in the process. The addition of hydrogen to the carrier is a reduction reaction. Similarly, the addition of electrons to a molecule is a reduction, so, just as the conversion of Fe^{2+} to Fe^{3+} is an oxidation reaction, the reverse reaction, the conversion of Fe^{3+} to Fe^{2+}, is a reduction.

Most of the reactions involved in energy metabolism involve the oxidation of metabolic fuels, while many of the biosynthetic reactions involved in the formation of metabolic fuel reserves and the synthesis of body components are reductions.

In some metabolic oxidation and reduction reactions the hydrogen acceptor or donor is a prosthetic group, e.g. haem (section 2.4.1.1) or riboflavin (section 2.4.1.2). In other cases, the hydrogen acceptor or donor acts as a substrate of the enzyme (e.g. the nicotinamide nucleotide coenzymes; section 2.4.1.3).

2.4.1.1 Metal ions

The electron acceptor or donor may be a metal ion that can have two different stable electron configurations. Commonly, iron (which can form Fe^{2+} or Fe^{3+} ions) and copper (which can form Cu^+ or Cu^{2+} ions) are involved.

In some enzymes, the metal ion is bound to the enzyme protein; in others, it is incorporated in an organic molecule, which in turn is attached to the enzyme. For example, haem is an organic compound containing iron that is the coenzyme for a variety of enzymes, collectively known as the cytochromes (section 3.3.1.2). Haem is also the prosthetic group of haemoglobin, the protein in red blood cells that binds and transports oxygen between the lungs and other tissues, and myoglobin in muscle. However, in haemoglobin and myoglobin the iron of haem does not undergo oxidation; it binds oxygen but does not react with it.

2.4.1.2 Riboflavin and flavoproteins

Vitamin B_2 (riboflavin; section 11.7) is important in a wide variety of oxidation and reduction reactions. A few enzymes contain riboflavin itself, while others contain a riboflavin derivative: either riboflavin phosphate (sometimes called flavin mononucleotide) or flavin adenine dinucleotide (FAD; Figure 2.14). When an enzyme contains riboflavin, it is usually covalently bound at the active site. Although riboflavin phosphate and FAD are not normally covalently bound to the enzyme, they are very tightly bound, and can be regarded as prosthetic groups. The resultant enzymes with attached riboflavin are collectively known as flavoproteins.

As shown in Figure 2.15, the riboflavin moiety of flavoproteins can undergo two reduction reactions. It can accept one hydrogen, to form the flavin radical (generally written as flavin-H$^{\bullet}$), followed by a second hydrogen, forming fully reduced flavin-H_2.

Some reactions involve transfer of a single hydrogen to a flavin, forming flavin-H$^{\bullet}$, which is then recycled in a separate reaction. Sometimes two molecules of flavin each accept one hydrogen atom from the substrate to be oxidized. Other reactions involve the sequential transfer of two hydrogens onto the flavin, forming first the flavin-H$^{\bullet}$ radical, then fully reduced flavin-H_2.

As discussed in section 7.4.2.1, the reoxidation of reduced flavins in enzymes that react with oxygen is a major source of potentially damaging oxygen radicals.

2.4.1.3 The nicotinamide nucleotide coenzymes: NAD and NADP

The vitamin niacin (section 11.8) is important for the formation of two closely related compounds, the nicotinamide nucleotide coenzymes – nicotinamide adenine dinucleotide (NAD) and nicotinamide adenine dinucleotide phosphate (NADP). As shown in Figure 2.16, they differ only in that NADP has an additional phosphate group attached to the ribose. The whole of the coenzyme molecule is essential for binding to enzymes, and most enzymes can bind and use only one of these two coenzymes, either NAD or NADP, despite the overall similarity in their structures.

The functionally important part of these coenzymes is the nicotinamide ring, which undergoes a two-electron reduction. In the oxidized coenzymes there is a positive charge associated with the nitrogen atom in the nicotinamide ring, and the oxidized forms of the coenzymes are usually shown as NAD^+ and $NADP^+$. Reduction involves the transfer of two electrons and two hydrogen ions (H^+) from the substrate to the

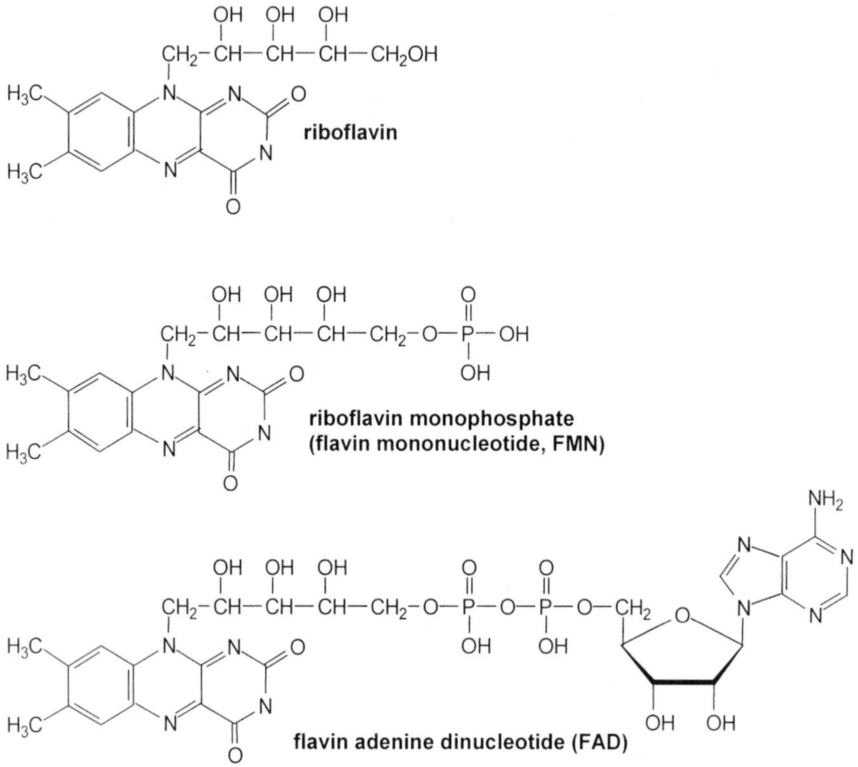

FIGURE 2.14 *Riboflavin and the flavin coenzymes, riboflavin monophosphate and flavin adenine dinucleotide.*

coenzyme. One electron neutralizes the positive charge on the nitrogen atom. The other, with its associated H^+ ion, is incorporated into the ring as a second hydrogen at carbon-2.

The second H^+ ion removed from the substrate remains associated with the coenzyme. This means that the reaction can be shown as

$$X\text{-}H_2 + NAD^+ \rightleftharpoons X + NADH + H^+$$

where $X\text{-}H_2$ is the substrate and X is the product (the oxidized form of the substrate).

Note that the reaction is reversible, and NADH can act as a reducing agent:

$$X + NADH + H^+ \rightleftharpoons X\text{-}H_2 + NAD^+$$

where X is now the substrate and $X\text{-}H_2$ is the product (the reduced form of the substrate).

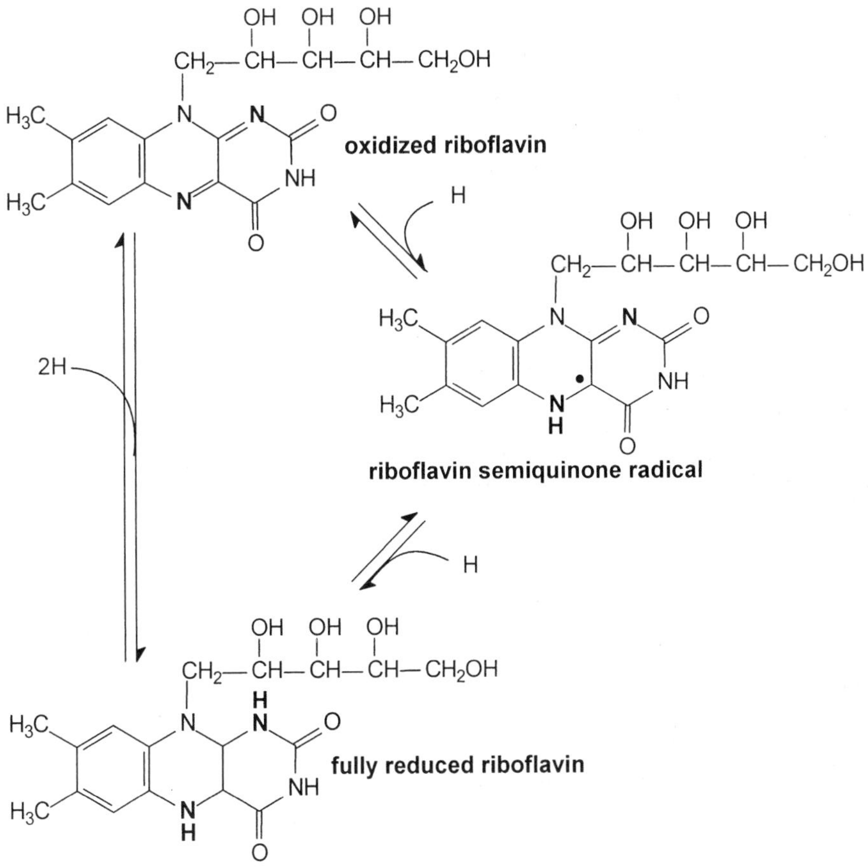

FIGURE 2.15 *Oxidation and reduction of the flavin coenzymes. The reaction may proceed as either a single two-electron reaction or as two single-electron steps by way of intermediate formation of the riboflavin semiquinone radical.*

The usual notation is that NAD and NADP are used when the oxidation state is not relevant, and NAD(P) when either NAD or NADP is being discussed. The oxidized coenzymes are shown as NAD(P)$^+$ and the reduced forms as NAD(P)H.

Unlike flavins and metal coenzymes, the nicotinamide nucleotide coenzymes do not remain bound to the enzyme, but act as substrates, binding to the enzyme, undergoing reduction and then leaving. The reduced coenzyme is then reoxidized either by reaction with another enzyme, for which it acts as a hydrogen donor, or by way of the mitochondrial electron transport chain (section 3.3.1.2). Cells contain only a small amount of NAD(P) (of the order of 400 nmol/g in liver), which is rapidly cycled between the oxidized and reduced forms by different enzymes.

In general, NAD$^+$ is the coenzyme for oxidation reactions, with most of the resultant NADH being reoxidized by the mitochondrial electron transport chain, while NADPH

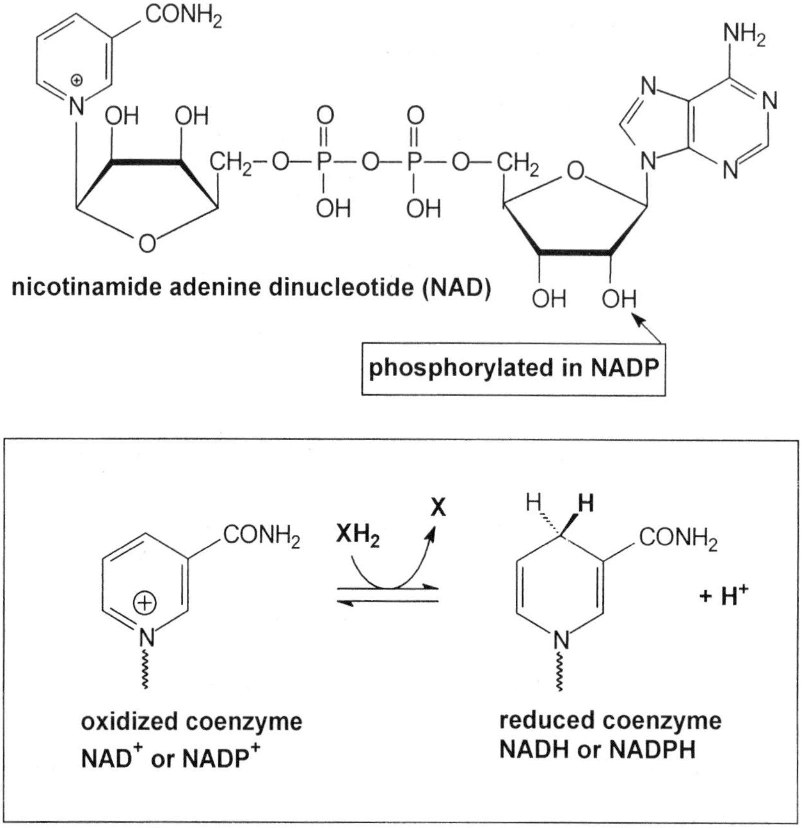

nicotinamide adenine dinucleotide (NAD)

phosphorylated in NADP

oxidized coenzyme
NAD⁺ or NADP⁺

reduced coenzyme
NADH or NADPH

FIGURE 2.16 *The nicotinamide nucleotide coenzymes, NAD and NADP. In the oxidized coenzyme there was one hydrogen at carbon-4, but this is not shown when the ring is drawn. In the reduced coenzymes both hydrogens are shown, with a dotted bond to one hydrogen and a bold bond to the other, to show that the ring as a whole is flat, with one hydrogen at carbon-4 above the plane of the ring and the other below.*

is the main coenzyme for reduction reactions (e.g. the synthesis of fatty acids; section 5.6.1).

2.5 *Classification and naming of enzymes*

There is a formal system of enzyme nomenclature, in which each enzyme has a number, and the various enzymes are classified according to the type of reaction catalysed and the substrates, products and coenzymes of the reaction. This is used in research publications, when there is a need to identify an enzyme unambiguously, but for general use there is a less formal system of naming enzymes. Almost all enzyme names end in -ase, and many are derived simply from the name of the substrate acted on, with the suffix -ase. In some cases, the type of reaction catalysed is also included.

TABLE 2.2 *Classification of enzyme-catalysed reactions*

1	Oxidoreductases	Oxidation and reduction reactions
	Dehydrogenases	Addition or removal of H
	Oxidases	Two-electron transfer to O_2, forming H_2O_2
		Two-electron transfer to $1/2O_2$, forming H_2O
	Oxygenases	Incorporate O_2 into product
	Hydroxylases	Incorporate $1/2O_2$ into product as –OH and form H_2O
	Peroxidases	Use as H_2O_2 as oxygen donor, forming H_2O
2	Transferases	Transfer a chemical group from one substrate to the other
	Kinases	Transfer phosphate from ATP onto substrate
3	Hydrolases	Hydrolysis of C–O, C–N, O–P and C–S bonds
		(e.g. esterases, proteases, phosphatases, deamidases)
4	Lyases	Addition across a C–C double bond
		(e.g. dehydratases, hydratases, decarboxylases)
5	Isomerases	Intramolecular rearrangements
6	Ligases (synthetases)	Formation of bonds between two substrates
		Frequently linked to utilization of ATP, with intermediate
		formation of phosphorylated enzyme or substrate

Altogether there are some 5–10,000 enzymes in human tissues. However, they can be classified into only six groups, depending on the types of chemical reaction they catalyse:

1 oxidation and reduction reactions;
2 transfer of a reactive group from one substrate onto another;
3 hydrolysis of bonds;
4 addition across carbon–carbon double bonds;
5 rearrangement of groups within a single molecule of substrate;
6 formation of bonds between two substrates, frequently linked to the hydrolysis of ATP $\rightarrow$ ADP + phosphate.

This classification of enzymes is expanded in Table 2.2, to give some examples of the types of reactions catalysed.

2.6 *Metabolic pathways*

A simple reaction, such as the oxidation of ethanol (alcohol) to carbon dioxide and water, can proceed in a single step – for example, simply by setting fire to the alcohol in air. The reaction is exothermic, and the oxidation of ethanol to carbon dioxide and water yields an output of 29 kJ/g.

When alcohol is metabolized in the body, although the overall reaction is the same, it does not proceed in a single step, but as a series of linked reactions, each resulting in a small change in the substrate. As shown in Figure 2.17, the metabolic oxidation of ethanol involves 11 enzyme-catalysed reactions, as well as the mitochondrial electron transport chain (section 3.3.1.2). The energy yield is still 29 kJ/g, as the starting material (ethanol) and the end products (carbon dioxide and water) are the same, and hence the change in energy level is the same overall, regardless of the route taken. Such a sequence of linked enzyme-catalysed reactions is a metabolic pathway.

Metabolic pathways can be divided into three broad groups:

- *Catabolic pathways*, involved in the breakdown of relatively large molecules and oxidation, ultimately to carbon dioxide and water. These are the main energy-yielding metabolic pathways.
- *Anabolic pathways*, involved in the synthesis of compounds from simpler precursors. These are the main energy-requiring metabolic pathways. Many are reduction reactions, and many involve condensation reactions. Similar reactions are also involved in the metabolism of drugs and other foreign compounds, and hormones and neurotransmitters, to yield products that are excreted in the urine or bile.
- *Central pathways*, involved in interconversions of substrates, that can be regarded as being both catabolic and anabolic. The principal such pathway is the citric acid cycle (section 5.4.4).

In some metabolic pathways all the enzymes are free in solution, and intermediate products are released from one enzyme, equilibrate with the pool of intermediate in the cell, and then bind to the next enzyme.

In some cases, two or more enzymes catalysing consecutive steps in a pathway may be physically adjacent, either bound to a membrane or in a multienzyme complex, so that the product of one enzyme is passed directly to the active site of the next, without equilibrating with the pool of intermediate in the cell.

2.6.1 LINEAR AND BRANCHED PATHWAYS

The simplest type of metabolic pathway is a single sequence of reactions in which the starting material is converted to the end product with no possibility of alternative reactions or branches in the pathway.

Simple linear pathways are rare, as many of the intermediate compounds in metabolism can be used in a variety of different pathways, depending on the body's need for various end-products. Many metabolic pathways involve branch points, as

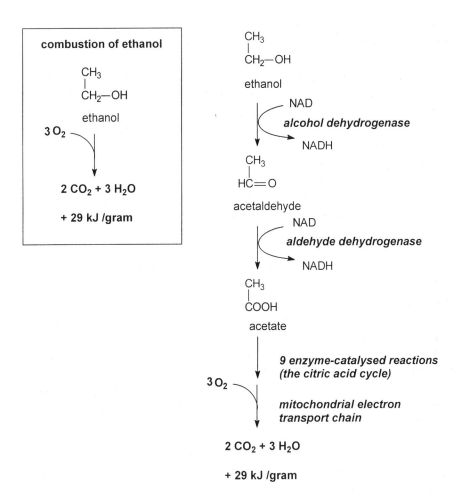

FIGURE 2.17 *The oxidation of ethanol. The box shows the rapid non-enzymic reaction when ethanol is burned in air; metabolic oxidation of ethanol involves 11 separate enzyme-catalysed steps, as well as the mitochondrial electron transport chain.*

shown in Figure 2.18, in which an intermediate may proceed down one branch or another. The fate of an intermediate at a branch point will depend on the relative activities of the two enzymes that are competing for the same substrate. As discussed above (section 2.3.3), if the enzymes catalysing the reactions from D → P and from D → X have different values of K_m, then it is possible to predict which branch will predominate at any given intracellular concentration of D.

Enzymes catalysing reactions at branch points are usually subject to regulation (section 10.1), so as to direct substrates through one branch or the other, depending on the body's requirements at the time.

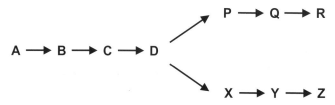

FIGURE 2.18 *Linear and branched metabolic pathways.*

2.6.2 SPIRAL OR LOOPED REACTION SEQUENCES

Sometimes a complete metabolic pathway involves repeating a series of reactions several times over. Thus, the oxidation of fatty acids (section 5.5.2) proceeds by the sequential removal of two-carbon units. The removal of each two-carbon unit involves a repeated sequence of four reactions, and the end-product of each loop of the pathway is a fatty acid that is two carbons shorter than the one that entered the loop. It then undergoes the same sequence of reactions. This is shown in cartoon form in Figure 2.19.

Similarly, the synthesis of fatty acids (section 5.6.1) involves the repeated addition of two-carbon units until the final chain length (commonly 14, 16 or 18 carbon units) has been achieved. The addition of each two-carbon unit involves four separate reaction steps, which are repeated in each loop of the pathway. The synthesis of fatty acids is catalysed by a large multienzyme complex in which the enzymes catalysing each step of the sequence are arranged in a series of concentric rings; the innermost ring catalyses the reaction sequence until the growing fatty acid chain is long enough to reach to the next ring of enzymes outwards from the centre.

2.6.3 CYCLIC PATHWAYS

The third type of metabolic pathway is cyclic; a product is assembled, or a substrate is catabolized, attached to a carrier molecule that is reformed at the end of each cycle of reactions.

Figure 2.20 shows a cyclic biosynthetic pathway in cartoon form; the product is built up in a series of reactions, then released, regenerating the carrier molecule. An example of such a pathway is the urea synthesis cycle (section 9.3.1.4).

Figure 2.21 shows a cyclic catabolic pathway in cartoon form; the substrate is bound to the carrier molecule, then undergoes a series of reactions in which parts are removed, until at the end of the reaction sequence the original carrier molecule is left. An example of such a pathway is the citric acid cycle (section 5.4.4).

The intermediates in a cyclic pathway can be considered to be catalysts, in that they participate in the reaction sequence, but at the end they emerge unchanged. Until all the enzymes in a cyclic pathway are saturated (and hence acting at V_{max}),

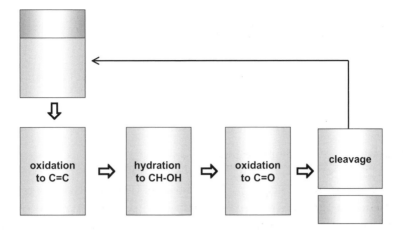

FIGURE 2.19 *A spiral or looped (repeating) metabolic pathway.*

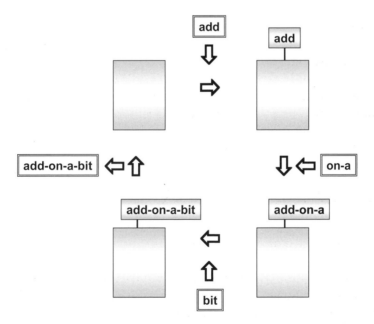

FIGURE 2.20 *A biosynthetic cyclic metabolic pathway.*

addition of any one of the intermediates will result in an increase in the intracellular concentration of all intermediates, and an increase in the rate at which the cycle runs and either substrate is catabolized or product is formed.

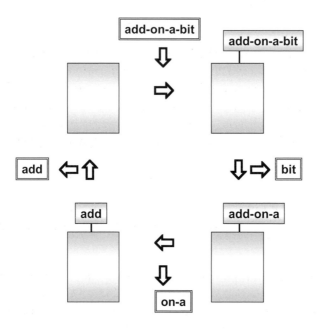

FIGURE 2.21 *A catabolic cyclic metabolic pathway.*

Additional resources

PowerPoint presentation 2 on the CD.
Self-assessment quiz 2 on the CD.

The simulation program Enzyme Assay on the CD will let you simulate experiments with a variety of enzymes to determine the optimum conditions for enzyme assay, investigate their substrate dependence and also study the effects of inhibitors on enzyme activity.

PROBLEM 2.1: *An unusual cause of diabetes*

This problem concerns *a small* number of families with a clear pattern of dominant inheritance of an *unusual* form of diabetes (section 10.7) that can be classified as non-insulin dependent, as those affected secrete significant amounts of insulin (although less than normal subjects), but which develops in early childhood. It is generally referred to as maturity-onset diabetes of the young (MODY).

TISSUE UPTAKE OF GLUCOSE

Glucose enters the cells of most tissues by means of an active transport mechanism (section 3.2.2) that is stimulated by the hormone insulin. This means that insulin promotes the uptake and utilization of glucose in most tissues. After entry, glucose is phosphorylated to glucose 6-phosphate. In the liver, glucose enters cells by facilitated diffusion and is then trapped by phosphorylation to glucose 6-phosphate, which cannot cross cell membranes. Glucose 6-phosphate is then either metabolized as a metabolic fuel (section 5.4.1) or used to synthesize the storage carbohydrate glycogen (section 5.6.3).

Two enzymes catalyse the formation of glucose 6-phosphate from glucose:

- Hexokinase is expressed in all tissues; it has a K_m for glucose of 0.15 mmol/L.
- Glucokinase is expressed only in liver and the β-cells of the pancreas; it has a K_m for glucose of 20 mmol/L.

The normal range of plasma glucose is between 3.5 and 5 mmol/L, rising in peripheral blood to 8–10 mmol/L after a moderately high intake of glucose. The concentration of glucose in the portal blood, coming from the small intestine to the liver (section 4.2.2.3), may be considerably higher than this.

- What effect do you think changes in the plasma concentration of glucose will have on the rate of formation of glucose 6-phosphate catalysed by hexokinase?
- What effect do you think changes in the plasma concentration of glucose will have on the rate of formation of glucose 6-phosphate catalysed by glucokinase?
- What do you think is the importance of glucokinase in the liver?

Froguel and co-workers (1993) reported studies of the glucokinase gene in a number of families affected by MODY, and also in unaffected families. They published a list of 16 variants of the glucokinase gene, shown in Table 2.3. All their patients with MODY had an abnormality of the gene.

- Using the genetic code shown in Table 9.8, fill in the amino acid changes associated with each mutation in the gene.
- Why do you think the mutations affecting codons 4, 10 and 116 had no effect on the people involved?
- What conclusions can you draw from this information?

The same authors also studied the secretion of insulin in response to glucose infusion in patients with MODY and normal control subjects. They were given an intravenous infusion of glucose; the rate of infusion was varied so as to maintain a constant plasma concentration of glucose of 10 mmol/L.

TABLE 2.3 *Known mutations in the glucokinase gene*

Codon	Nucleotide change	Amino acid change	Effect
4	GAC ⇒ AAC	?	None
10	GCC ⇒ GCT	?	None
70	GAA ⇒ AAA	?	MODY
98	CAG ⇒ TAG	?	MODY
116	ACC ⇒ ACT	?	None
175	GGA ⇒ AGA	?	MODY
182	GTG ⇒ ATG	?	MODY
186	CGA ⇒ TGA	?	MODY
203	GTG ⇒ GCG	?	MODY
228	ACG ⇒ ATG	?	MODY
261	GGG ⇒ AGG	?	MODY
279	GAG ⇒ TAG	?	MODY
300	GAG ⇒ AAG	?	MODY
300	GAG ⇒ CAG	?	MODY
309	CTC ⇒ CCC	?	MODY
414	AAG ⇒ GAG	?	MODY

From data reported by Froguel P *et al.* (1993) *New England Journal of Medicine* 328: 697–702.

TABLE 2.4 *Plasma glucose and insulin before and after 60 minutes of glucose infusion in control subjects and patients with maturity-onset diabetes of the young (MODY)*

	Plasma glucose (mmol/L)		Insulin (mU/L)	
	Patients	Control subjects	Patients	Control subjects
Fasting	7.0 ± 0.4	5.1 ± 0.3	5 ± 2	6 ± 2
Glucose infusion	Maintained at 10 mmol/L by varying rate of infusion		12 ± 7	40 ± 11

From data reported by Froguel P *et al.* (1993) *New England Journal of Medicine* 328: 697–702.

Their plasma concentrations of glucose and insulin were measured before and after 60 min of glucose infusion; the results are shown in Table 2.4.

- What conclusions can you draw from this information about the probable role of glucokinase in the β-cells of the pancreas?
- Can you deduce the way in which the β-cells of the pancreas sense an increase in plasma glucose and signal the secretion of insulin?

PROBLEM 2.2: *Studies of a novel endopeptidase*

What reaction is catalysed by an endopeptidase, as opposed to an exopeptidase?

A new enzyme, of bacterial origin, is being studied for its potential use in a washing powder preparation. The enzyme is an endopeptidase, and has been purified by a variety of chromatographic techniques.

The activity of the enzyme has been determined using an assay based on the hydrolysis of a synthetic substrate, *p*-nitrophenyl acetate. On hydrolysis this (colourless) substrate yields 1 mol of *p*-nitrophenol (which is yellow) for each mole of substrate hydrolysed.

In the following experiments, 0.1 mL of a solution containing 1 mg of the purified protein per litre was used in each incubation. The enzyme was incubated at 30 °C and pH 7.5, for 10 min; the formation of *p*-nitrophenol was followed spectro-photometrically. The results are shown in Table 2.5.

Using these results, determine the V_{max} of the enzyme under these incubation conditions.

Given the relative molecular mass of the enzyme (= 50,000), calculate the catalytic rate constant, k_{cat} (the maximum rate of reaction expressed in mole of product formed per mole of enzyme per second).

TABLE 2.5 *The rate of reaction of a novel endopeptidase incubated with p-nitrophenyl acetate as a model substrate*

Concentration of *p*-nitrophenyl acetate added (mol/L)	Nitrophenol formed (μmol/10 min)
1.4×10^{-4}	2.22
2.0×10^{-4}	2.94
3.3×10^{-4}	4.44
5.0×10^{-4}	5.88
1.0×10^{-3}	9.08

PROBLEM 2.3: *Clinical chemistry – determination of serum alkaline phosphatase activity*

The activity of alkaline phosphatase in serum is elevated above normal in a variety of different bone diseases, as well as biliary obstruction and some other liver diseases. Measurement of alkaline phosphatase activity in serum can thus give useful information about these conditions. It is especially useful for diagnosis of preclinical rickets and osteomalacia (section 11.3.4).

According to the literature, the range of alkaline phosphatase activity in serum from healthy adults is (mean ± SD) 75 ± 12 units/L. The reference range (that which

TABLE 2.6 *The absorbance of* p-*nitrophenylate at pH 12*

p-Nitrophenylate (mmol/L)	Absorbance at 405 nm
0.1	1.830
0.05	0.915
0.025	0.458
0.0125	0.229
0.00625	0.114

is considered 'normal') is ± 2 SD around the mean; values outside this range are considered abnormal.

The activity of alkaline phosphatase is measured by hydrolysis of *p*-nitrophenyl phosphate to yield *p*-nitrophenol and free phosphate. At alkaline pH, *p*-nitrophenol dissociates; the *p*-nitrophenylate ion has a strong yellow colour, with maximum absorbance at 405 nm.

The activity of alkaline phosphatase in a serum sample was determined by incubating 0.1 mL of serum with 0.2 mL of *p*-nitrophenyl phosphate at 14 mmol/L in 2.7 mL of buffer at pH 10.4 at 30 °C for 10 min. The reaction was stopped by addition of 3 mL of 0.2 mol/L sodium hydroxide, which both denatures the enzyme and also raises the pH of the incubation mixture to 12. The absorbance of the final reaction mixture was then determined at 405 nm, using a cuvette with a 1-cm light path. The result was a reading of 0.95 absorbance units.

Table 2.6 shows the absorbance at 405 nm of *p*-nitrophenylate in buffer at pH 12, using a cuvette with a 1-cm light path.

Was the activity of alkaline phosphatase in the serum sample within the reference range?

The role of ATP in metabolism

The coenzyme adenosine triphosphate (ATP) acts as the central link between energy-yielding metabolic pathways and energy expenditure on physical and chemical work. The oxidation of metabolic fuels is linked to the phosphorylation of adenosine diphosphate (ADP) to adenosine triphosphate (ATP), while the expenditure of metabolic energy for the synthesis of body constituents, transport of compounds across cell membranes and the contraction of muscle results overall in the hydrolysis of ATP to yield ADP and phosphate ions. The total body content of ATP + ADP is under 350 mmol (about 10 g), but the amount of ATP synthesized and used each day is about 100 mol – about 70 kg, an amount equal to body weight.

Objectives

After reading this chapter you should be able to:

- explain how endothermic reactions can be linked to the overall hydrolysis of ATP to ADP and phosphate;
- describe how compounds can be transported across cell membranes against a concentration gradient and explain the roles of ATP and proton gradients in active transport;
- describe the role of ATP in muscle contraction and the role of creatine phosphate as a phosphagen;

- describe the structure and functions of the mitochondrion and explain the processes involved in the mitochondrial electron transport chain and oxidative phosphorylation, explain how substrate oxidation is regulated by the availability of ADP and explain how respiratory poisons and uncouplers act.

3.1 *The adenine nucleotides*

Nucleotides consist of a purine or pyrimidine base linked to the five-carbon sugar ribose. The base plus sugar is a nucleoside; in a nucleotide the sugar is phosphorylated. Nucleotides may be mono-, di- or triphosphates.

Figure 3.1 shows the nucleotides formed from the purine adenine – the adenine nucleotides, adenosine monophosphate (AMP), adenosine diphosphate (ADP) and adenosine triphosphate (ATP) – as well as the nucleotide triphosphates formed from the purine guanine and the pyrimidine uracil (see also section 10.3.2 for a discussion of the role of cyclic AMP in metabolic regulation and hormone action).

In the nucleic acids (DNA and RNA; sections 9.2.1 and 9.2.2 respectively) it is the purine or pyrimidine that is important, carrying the genetic information. However, in the link between energy-yielding metabolism and the performance of physical and chemical work, what is important is the phosphorylation of the ribose. Although most reactions are linked to adenosine triphosphate, a small number are linked to guanosine triphosphate (GTP; see, for example, sections 5.7 and 9.2.3.2) or uridine triphosphate (UTP; section 5.5.3).

3.2 *Functions of ATP*

Under normal conditions, the processes shown in Figure 3.2 are tightly coupled, so that the oxidation of metabolic fuels is controlled by the availability of ADP, which, in turn is controlled by the rate at which ATP is being utilized in performing physical and chemical work. Work output, or energy expenditure, thus controls the rate at which metabolic fuels are oxidized, and hence the amount of food that must be eaten to meet energy requirements. As discussed in section 5.3.1, metabolic fuels in excess of immediate requirements are stored as reserves of glycogen in muscle and liver and as fat in adipose tissue.

In all of the reactions in which ATP is utilized, what is observed overall is hydrolysis of ATP to ADP and phosphate. However, as discussed below, although this is the overall reaction, simple hydrolysis of ATP does not achieve any useful result; it is the intermediate steps in the reaction of ATP + $H_2O \rightarrow$ ADP + phosphate that are important.

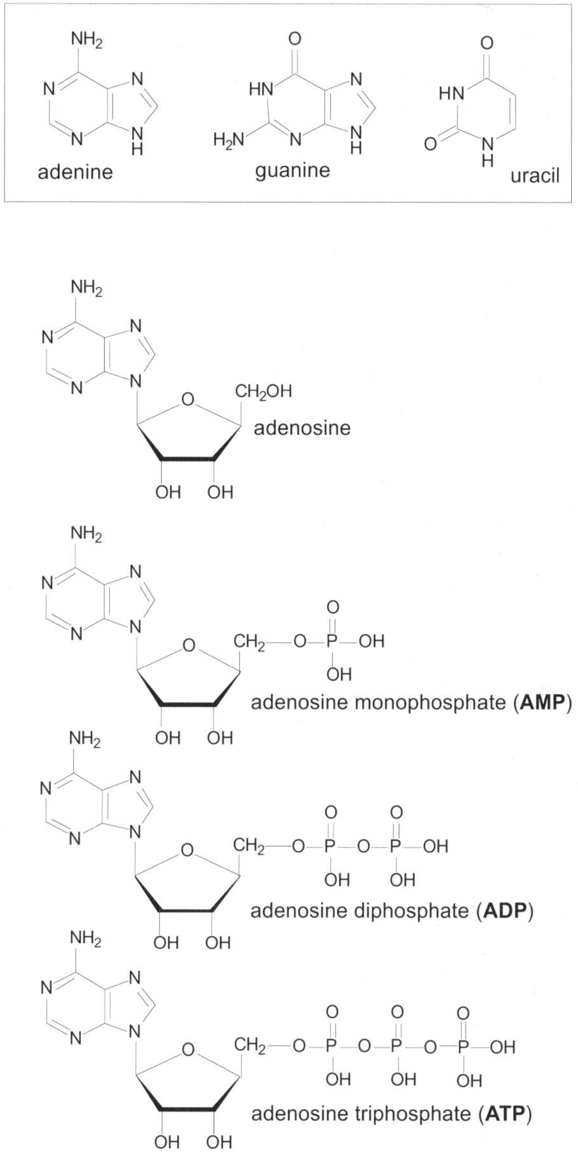

FIGURE 3.1 *The adenine nucleotides (the box shows the structures of adenine, guanine and uracil; guanine and uracil form a similar series of nucleotides).*

3.2.1 THE ROLE OF ATP IN ENDOTHERMIC REACTIONS

As discussed in section 2.1.1, the equilibrium of an endothermic reaction A + B $\rightleftharpoons$ C + D lies well to the left unless there is an input of energy. The hydrolysis of ATP is

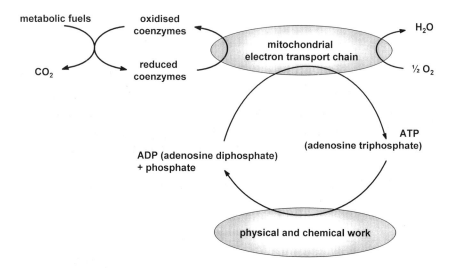

FIGURE 3.2 *Linkage between ATP utilization in physical and chemical work and the oxidation of metabolic fuels.*

exothermic, and the equilibrium of the reaction $ATP + H_2O \rightleftharpoons ADP + phosphate$ lies well to the right. Linkage between the two reactions could thus ensure that the (unfavoured) endothermic reaction could proceed together with overall hydrolysis of ATP to ADP + phosphate.

Such linkage between two apparently unrelated reactions can easily be achieved in enzyme-catalysed reactions; there are three possible mechanisms:

1 Phosphorylation of the hydroxyl group of a serine, threonine or tyrosine residue in the enzyme (Figure 3.3), thus altering the chemical nature of its catalytic site. As discussed in section 10.3, phosphorylation of the enzyme is also important in regulating metabolic pathways, especially in response to hormone action.
2 Phosphorylation of one of the substrates; as shown in Figure 3.4, the synthesis of glutamine from glutamate and ammonia (section 9.3.1.3) involves the formation of a phosphorylated intermediate.
3 Transfer of the adenosyl group of ATP onto one of the substrates, as shown in Figure 3.5. The activation of the methyl group of the amino acid methionine in methyltransfer reactions involves formation of S-adenosyl methionine (see also Figure 11.22).

Not only is the hydrolysis of ATP to ADP and phosphate an exothermic reaction, but the concentration of ATP in cells is always very much higher than that of ADP (the ratio of ATP to ADP is about 500:1), again ensuring that the reaction will indeed proceed in the direction of ATP hydrolysis. Furthermore, the concentration of ADP

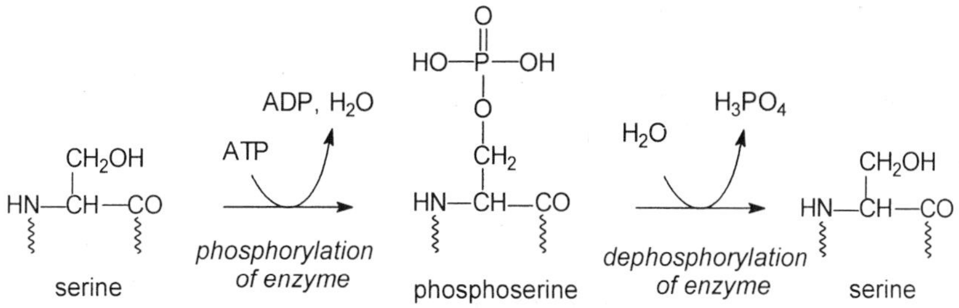

FIGURE 3.3 *The role of ATP in endothermic reactions – phosphorylation of the enzyme.*

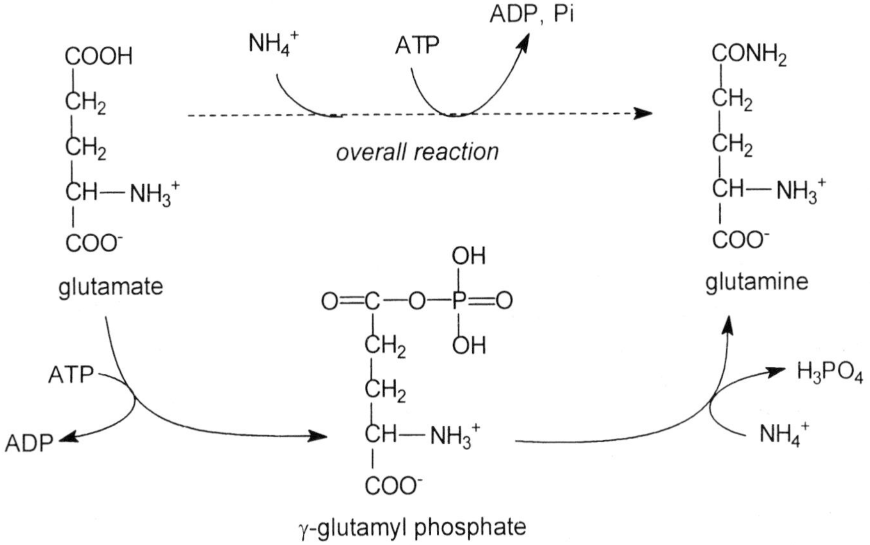

FIGURE 3.4 *The role of ATP in endothermic reactions – phosphorylation of the substrate.*

in cells is kept extremely low by rephosphorylation to ATP, linked to the oxidation of metabolic fuels (section 3.3). Again, this serves to ensure that the equilibrium of the reaction ATP + H$_2$O $\rightarrow$ ADP + phosphate lies well to the right.

In a number of cases, there is a further mechanism to ensure that the equilibrium of an ATP-linked reaction is kept well to the right, to such an extent that the reaction is essentially irreversible. The reaction shown in Figure 3.6 results in the hydrolysis of ATP to AMP and pyrophosphate. There is an active pyrophosphatase in cells, which catalyses the hydrolysis of pyrophosphate to yield 2 mol of phosphate, so removing one of the products of the reaction, and ensuring that it is essentially irreversible.

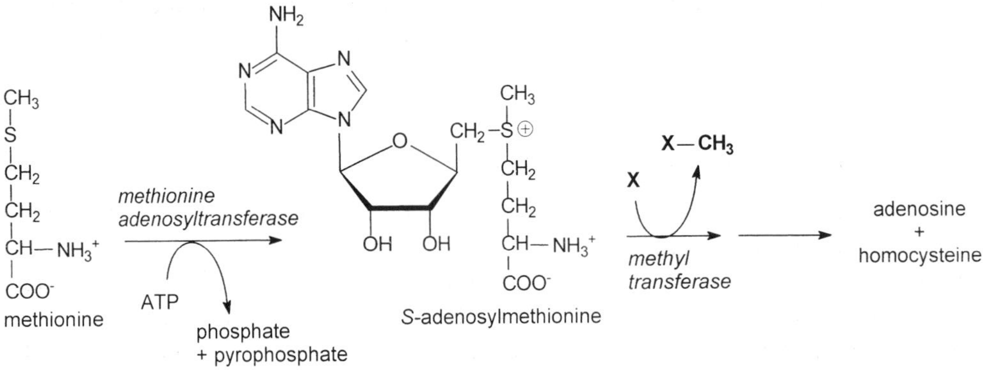

FIGURE 3.5   *The role of ATP in endothermic reactions – adenylation of the substrate (see also Figure 11.22).*

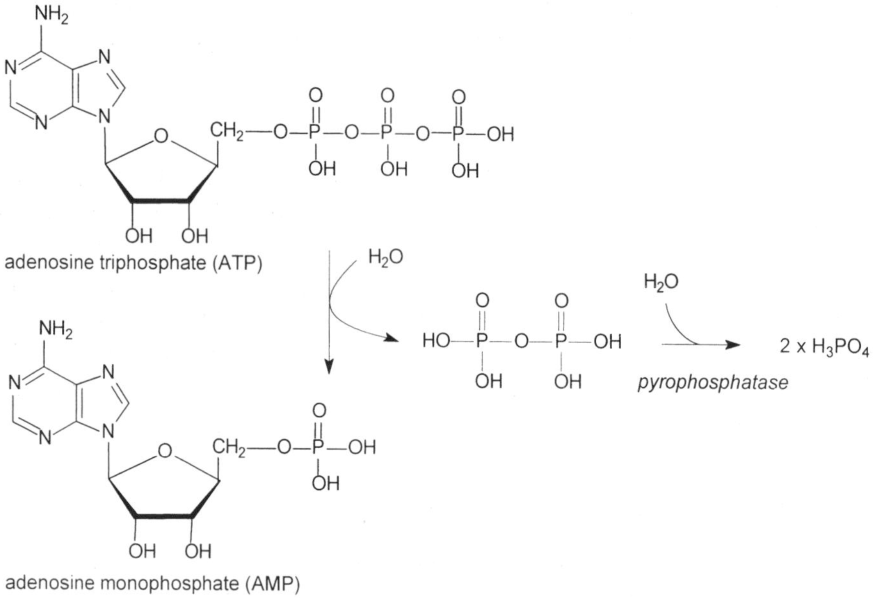

FIGURE 3.6   *Hydrolysis of ATP to AMP and pyrophosphate.*

3.2.2 TRANSPORT OF MATERIALS ACROSS CELL MEMBRANES

Compounds that are lipid soluble will diffuse freely across cell membranes, as they can dissolve in the lipid of the membrane – this is passive diffusion. Hydrophilic compounds require a transport protein in order to cross the lipid membrane – this is facilitated or carrier-mediated diffusion. Neither passive nor facilitated diffusion alone can lead to the concentration of the transported material being greater inside the cell than outside.

Concentrative uptake of the material being transported may be achieved in three main ways: protein binding, metabolic trapping and active transport. These last two mechanisms are both ATP dependent.

3.2.2.1 Protein binding for concentrative uptake

In the case of a hydrophilic compound that enters the cell by carrier-mediated diffusion, a net increase in concentration inside the cell can sometimes be achieved by binding it to an intracellular protein. Only material in free solution can equilibrate across the membrane, not that which is protein bound. Such binding proteins are important, for example, in the intestinal absorption of calcium (section 4.6.1) and iron (section 4.6.2).

Hydrophobic compounds are transported in plasma bound to transport proteins (e.g. the plasma retinol binding protein; section 11.2.2.2) or dissolved in the lipid core of plasma lipoproteins (section 5.6.2), and net intracellular accumulation to a higher concentration than in plasma depends on an intracellular binding protein that has a greater affinity for the ligand than does the plasma transport protein.

3.2.2.2 Metabolic trapping

Glucose enters cells by carrier-mediated diffusion. Once inside the cell, it is phosphorylated to glucose 6-phosphate, a reaction catalysed by the enzyme hexokinase, using ATP as the phosphate donor (section 5.4.1 and Problem 2.1). Glucose 6-phosphate does not cross cell membranes, and therefore there is a net accumulation of [glucose plus glucose 6-phosphate] inside the cell, at the expense of 1 mol of ATP utilized per mole of glucose trapped in this way. Vitamins B_2 (riboflavin; section 11.7.1) and B_6 (section 11.9.1) are similarly accumulated inside cells by phosphorylation at the expense of ATP.

3.2.2.3 Ion pumps and active transport

Active transport is the accumulation of a higher concentration of a compound on one side of a cell membrane than on the other, without chemical modification such as phosphorylation. The process is dependent on hydrolysis of ATP to ADP and phosphate, either directly, as in the case of ion pumps, or indirectly, as is the case when metabolites are transported by sodium-dependent transporters.

In some ion pumps the role of ATP is simple. As shown in Figure 3.7, when the membrane transport protein is phosphorylated it undergoes a conformational change that opens the transmembrane pore and permits it to transport an ion across the membrane. Before the ion can be released at the membrane surface, the transport protein has to be dephosphorylated.

The key to understanding the role of ATP in the sodium pump lies in the fact that the hydrolysis is effected not by H_2O, but by H^+ and OH^- ions. As shown in Figure 3.8, the ATPase that catalyses the hydrolysis of ATP to ADP and phosphate is within

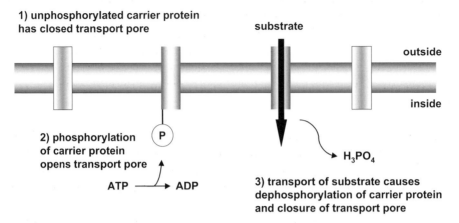

1) unphosphorylated carrier protein has closed transport pore

substrate

outside

inside

2) phosphorylation of carrier protein opens transport pore

P

H_3PO_4

ATP $\longrightarrow$ ADP

3) transport of substrate causes dephosphorylation of carrier protein and closure of transport pore

FIGURE 3.7 *The role of ATP in active transport – P-type transporters which have to be phosphorylated in order to permit transport across the cell membrane.*

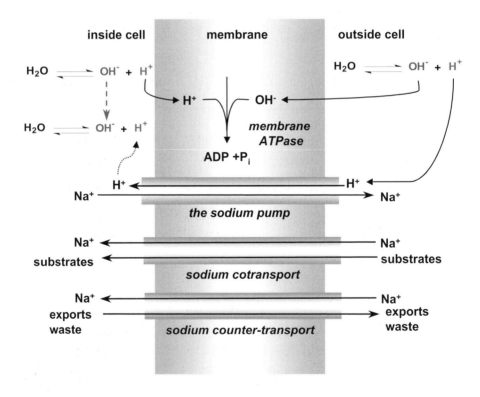

inside cell   membrane   outside cell

$H_2O \longrightarrow OH^- + H^+$

$H_2O \longrightarrow OH^- + H^+$

H^+ OH^-

membrane ATPase

$ADP + P_i$

$H_2O \longrightarrow OH^- + H^+$

H^+ H^+

Na^+ Na^+

the sodium pump

Na^+ Na^+

substrates   substrates

sodium cotransport

Na^+ Na^+

exports waste   exports waste

sodium counter-transport

FIGURE 3.8 *The role of ATP in active transport – generation of a proton gradient linked to the sodium pump and sodium-dependent transporters.*

the membrane, and takes an H^+ ion from inside the cell and an OH^- ion from the extracellular fluid, so creating a pH gradient across the membrane.

The protons in the extracellular fluid then enter the cell on a transmembrane carrier protein, and react with the hydroxyl ions within the cell, so discharging the pH gradient. The carrier protein that transports the protons across the cell membrane does so only in exchange for sodium ions. The sodium ions in turn re-enter the cell either:

* Together with substrates such as glucose and amino acids, thus providing a mechanism for net accumulation of these substrates, driven by the sodium gradient, which in turn has been created by the proton gradient produced by the hydrolysis of ATP. This is a co-transport mechanism as the sodium ions and substrates travel in the same direction across the cell membrane;
* In exchange for compounds being exported or excreted from the cell. This is a counter-transport mechanism, since the sodium ions and the compounds being transported move in opposite directions across the membrane.

3.2.3 THE ROLE OF ATP IN MUSCLE CONTRACTION

The important proteins of muscle are actin and myosin. As shown in Figure 3.9, myosin is a filamentous protein, consisting of several subunits, and with ATPase activity

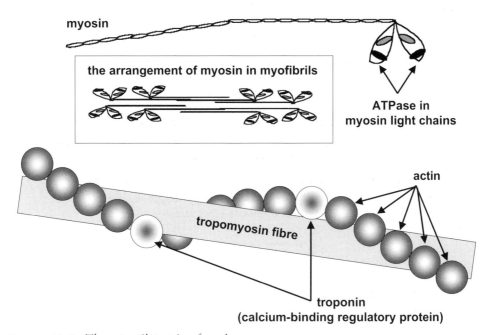

FIGURE 3.9 *The contractile proteins of muscle.*

in the head region. In myofibrils, myosin molecules are arranged in clusters with the tail regions overlapping. Actin is a smaller, globular protein, and actin molecules are arranged around a fibrous protein, tropomyosin, so creating a chain of actin molecules, interspersed with molecules of a calcium-binding regulatory protein, troponin.

In resting muscle, each myosin head unit binds ADP, and is bound to an actin molecule, as shown in Figure 3.10. The binding of ATP to myosin displaces the bound ADP and causes a conformation change in the molecule, so that, while it remains associated with the actin molecule, it is no longer tightly bound. Hydrolysis of the bound ATP to ADP and phosphate causes a further conformational change in the myosin molecule, this time affecting the tail region, so that the head region becomes associated with an actin molecule further along. This is the power stroke which causes the actin and myosin filaments to slide over one another, contracting the muscle filament. When the phosphate is released, the head region of myosin undergoes the reverse conformational change, so that it now becomes tightly bound to the new actin molecule, and is ready to undergo a further cycle of ATP binding, hydrolysis and movement.

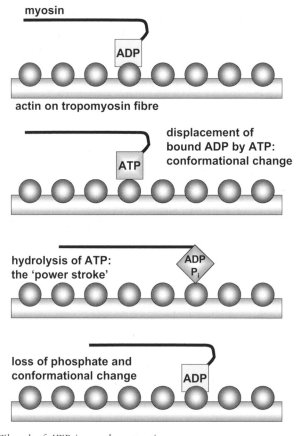

FIGURE 3.10 *The role of ATP in muscle contraction.*

3.2.3.1 Creatine phosphate in muscle

It was noted above that the small amount of ATP in the body turns over rapidly, and ADP is rapidly rephosphorylated to ATP. However, neither the small amount of ATP in muscle nor the speed with which metabolic activity can be increased, and hence ADP can be rephosphorylated, matches the demand for ATP for rapid or sustained muscle contraction. Muscle contains about four times more creatine phosphate than ATP; as shown in Figure 3.11, this acts as a reservoir or buffer to maintain a supply of ATP for muscle contraction until metabolic activity increases. Creatine phosphate is sometimes called a phosphagen because it can be used to rephosphorylate ADP to ADP.

Creatine is not a dietary essential; as shown in Figure 3.12, it is synthesized from the amino acids glycine, arginine and methionine. However, a single serving of meat will provide about 1 g of preformed creatine, whereas the average daily rate of *de novo* synthesis is 1–2 g. Both creatine and creatine phosphate undergo a non-enzymic reaction to yield creatinine, which is metabolically useless and is excreted in the urine. Because the formation of creatinine is a non-enzymic reaction, the rate at which it is formed, and hence the amount excreted each day, depends mainly on muscle mass, and is therefore relatively constant from day to day in any one individual. This is commonly exploited in clinical chemistry; urinary metabolites are commonly expressed per mole of creatinine, or the excretion of creatinine is measured to assess the completeness of a 24-hour urine collection. Obviously, simple concentration of urinary metabolites is not a useful measurement, as the concentration will depend on the volume of urine excreted, and in turn this depends on fluid intake and fluid losses from the body. There is normally little or no excretion of creatine in urine; significant amounts are excreted only when there is breakdown of muscle tissue.

Because of its role as a phosphagen in muscle, creatine supplements are often used as a so-called ergogenic aid, to enhance athletic performance and muscle work output. In subjects who have an initially low concentration of creatine in muscle, supplements of 2–5 g of creatine per day do increase muscle creatine; however, in people whose muscle creatine is within the normal range, additional creatine has little or no effect.

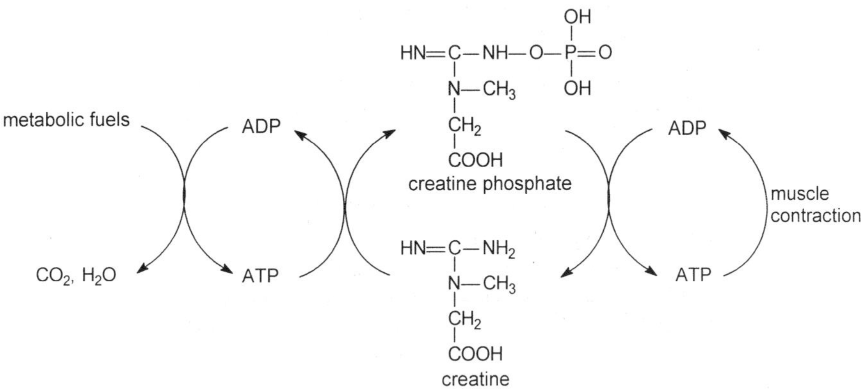

FIGURE 3.11 *The role of creatine phosphate in muscle.*

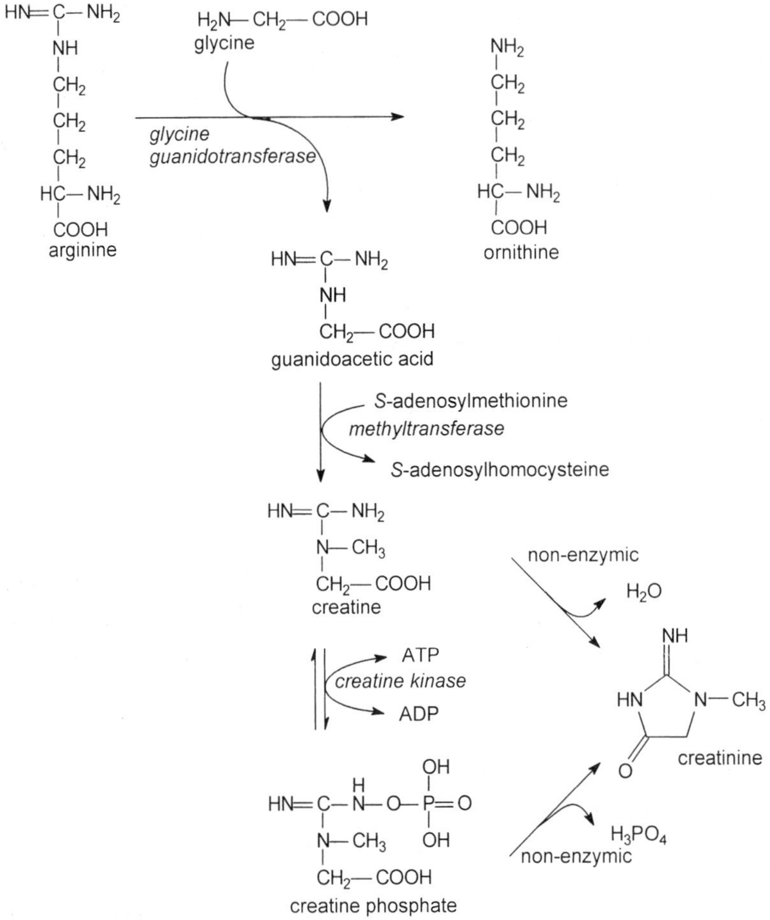

FIGURE 3.12 *The synthesis of creatine and non-enzymic formation of creatinine.*

There is control over the uptake and retention of creatine in muscle cells. There is little or no evidence that supplements of creatine have any beneficial effect on muscle work output or athletic performance, although obviously people whose muscle creatine was initially low will benefit.

3.3 *The phosphorylation of ADP to ATP*

A small number of metabolic reactions involve direct transfer of phosphate from a phosphorylated substrate onto ADP, forming ATP – substrate-level phosphorylation. Two such reactions are shown in Figure 3.13 – both are reactions in the glycolytic pathway of glucose metabolism (section 5.4.1). Substrate-level phosphorylation is of

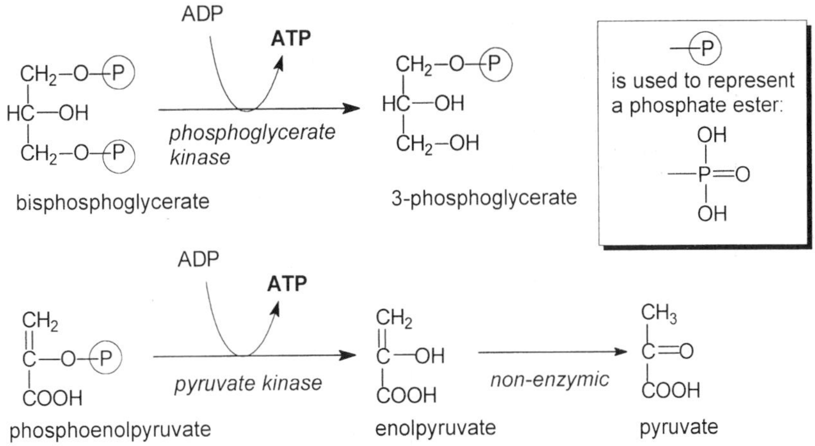

FIGURE 3.13 *Formation of ATP by substrate level phosphorylation (see also Figure 5.10).*

relatively minor importance in ensuring a supply of ATP, although, as discussed in section 5.4.1.2, it becomes important in muscle under conditions of maximum exertion. Normally almost all of the phosphorylation of ADP to ATP occurs in the mitochondria, by the process of oxidative phosphorylation.

3.3.1 OXIDATIVE PHOSPHORYLATION: THE PHOSPHORYLATION OF ADP TO ATP LINKED TO THE OXIDATION OF METABOLIC FUELS

With the exception of glycolysis (section 5.4.1), which is a cytosolic pathway, most of the reactions in the oxidation of metabolic fuels occur inside the mitochondria, and lead to the reduction of nicotinamide nucleotide and flavin coenzymes (section 2.4.1). The reduced coenzymes are then reoxidized, ultimately leading to the reduction of oxygen to water. Within the inner membrane of the mitochondrion (section 3.3.1.2) there is a series of coenzymes that are able to undergo reduction and oxidation. The first coenzyme in the chain is reduced by reaction with NADH, and is then reoxidized by reducing the next coenzyme. In turn, each coenzyme in the chain is reduced by the preceding coenzyme, and then reoxidized by reducing the next one. The final step is the oxidation of a reduced coenzyme by oxygen, resulting in the formation of water.

Experimentally, mitochondrial metabolism is measured using the oxygen electrode, in which the percentage saturation of the buffer with oxygen is measured electrochemically as the mitochondria oxidize substrates and reduce oxygen to water. Figure 3.14 shows the oxygen electrode traces for mitochondria incubated with varying amounts of ADP, and a super-abundant amount of malate. As more ADP is provided, so there is more oxidation of substrate, and hence more consumption of

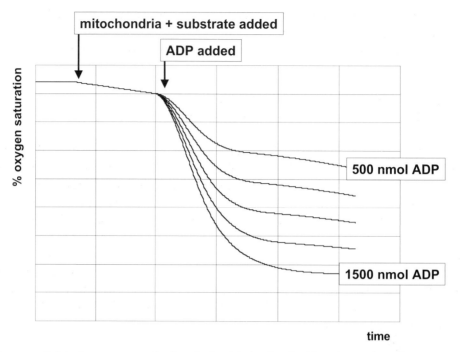

FIGURE 3.14 *Oxygen consumption by mitochondria incubated with malate and varying amounts of ADP.*

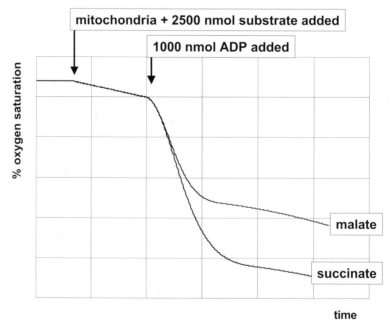

FIGURE 3.15 *Oxygen consumption by mitochondria incubated with malate or succinate and a constant amount of ADP.*

oxygen. This illustrates the tight coupling between the oxidation of metabolic fuels and availability of ADP shown in Figure 3.2.

Figure 3.15 shows the oxygen electrode traces for incubation of mitochondria with a limiting amount of ADP and:

1 malate, which reduces NAD^+ to NADH;
2 succinate, which reduces a flavin coenzyme, then ubiquinone.

The stepwise oxidation of NADH and reduction of oxygen to water is obligatorily linked to the phosphorylation of ADP to ATP. Approximately 3 mol of ATP is formed for each mole of NADH that is oxidized. Flavoproteins reduce ubiquinone, which is an intermediate coenzyme in the chain, and approximately 2 mol of ADP is phosphorylated to ATP for each mole of reduced flavoprotein that is oxidized.

This means that 2 mol of ADP is required for the oxidation of a substrate such as succinate, but 3 mol of ADP is required for the oxidation of malate. Therefore, the oxidation of succinate will consume more oxygen when ADP is limiting than does the oxidation of malate. This is usually expressed as the ratio of phosphate to oxygen consumed in the reaction; the P/O ratio is approximately 3 for malate and approximately 2 for succinate.

3.3.1.1 The mitochondrion

Mitochondria are intracellular organelles with a double-membrane structure. Both the number and size of mitochondria vary in different cells – for example, a liver cell contains some 800 mitochondria, a renal tubule cell some 300 and a sperm about 20. The outer mitochondrial membrane is permeable to a great many substrates, while the inner membrane provides a barrier to regulate the uptake of substrates and output of products (see, for example, the regulation of palmitoyl CoA uptake into the mitochondrion for oxidation in section 5.5.1).

The inner mitochondrial membrane forms the cristae, which are paddle-shaped, double-membrane structures that protrude from the inner membrane into the matrix, as shown in Figure 3.16. The crista membrane is continuous with the inner mitochondrial membrane, and the internal space of the crista is contiguous with the inter-membrane space. However, there is only a relatively narrow stalk connecting the crista to the inter-membrane space, so that the crista space is effectively separate from, albeit communicating with, the inter-membrane space.

The five compartments of the mitochondrion have a range of specialized functions:

1 The outer membrane contains the enzymes that are responsible for the desaturation and elongation of fatty acids synthesized in the cytosol (section 5.6.1.1), the enzymes for triacylglycerol synthesis from fatty acids (section 5.6.1.2) and phospholipases that catalyse the hydrolysis of phospholipids (section 4.3.1.2).
2 The inter-membrane space contains enzymes involved in nucleotide metabolism, transamination of amino acids (section 9.3.1.2) and a variety of kinases.

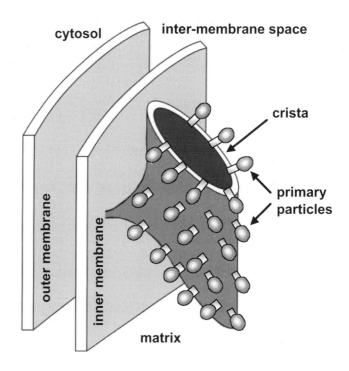

FIGURE 3.16 *The membranes of the mitochondrion and infolding to form mitochondrial cristae.*

3 The inner membrane regulates the uptake of substrates into the matrix for oxidation. There is also a transport protein in the mitochondrial inner membrane that transports ADP into the matrix to undergo phosphorylation only in exchange for ATP being transported out to the cytosol.

4 The membrane of the cristae contains the coenzymes associated with electron transport, the oxidation of reduced coenzymes, and the reduction of oxygen to water (section 3.3.1.2). The primary particles on the matrix surface of the cristae contain the enzyme that catalyses the phosphorylation of ADP to ATP (section 3.3.1.3).

5 The mitochondrial matrix contains the enzymes concerned with the oxidation of fatty acids (section 5.5.2), the citric acid cycle (section 5.4.4), a variety of other oxidases and dehydrogenases, the enzymes for mitochondrial replication and the DNA that codes for some of the mitochondrial proteins.

The overall process of oxidation of reduced coenzymes, reduction of oxygen to water, and phosphorylation of ADP to ATP requires intact mitochondria, or intact sealed vesicles of mitochondrial inner membrane prepared by disruption of mitochondria; it will not occur with solubilized preparations from mitochondria, or with open fragments of mitochondrial inner membrane. Under normal conditions, these three processes are linked, and none can occur without the others.

3.3.1.2 The mitochondrial electron transport chain

The mitochondrial electron transport chain is a series of enzymes and coenzymes in the crista membrane, each of which is reduced by the preceding coenzyme, and in turn reduces the next, until finally the protons and electrons that have entered the chain from either NADH or reduced flavin reduce oxygen to water. The sequence of the electron carriers shown in Figure 3.17 has been determined in two ways:

- By consideration of their electrochemical redox potentials, which permits determination of which carrier is likely to reduce another, and which is likely to be reduced. There is a gradual fall in redox potential between the enzyme that oxidizes NADH and that which reduces oxygen to water.
- By incubation of mitochondria with substrates, in the absence of oxygen, when all of the carriers become reduced, then introducing a limited amount of oxygen, and following the sequence in which the carriers become oxidized. The oxidation state of the carriers is determined by following changes in their absorption spectra.

Studies with inhibitors of specific electron carriers, and with artificial substrates that oxidize or reduce one specific carrier, permit dissection of the electron transport chain into four complexes of electron carriers:

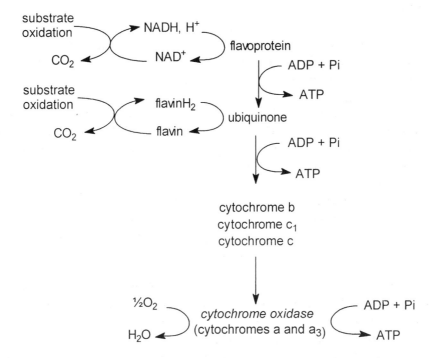

FIGURE 3.17 *An overview of the mitochondrial electron transport chain.*

- Complex I catalyses the oxidation of NADH and the reduction of ubiquinone, and is associated with the phosphorylation of ADP to ATP.
- Complex II catalyses the oxidation of reduced flavins and the reduction of ubiquinone. This complex is not associated with phosphorylation of ADP to ATP.
- Complex III catalyses the oxidation of reduced ubiquinone and the reduction of cytochrome c, and is associated with the phosphorylation of ADP to ATP;
- Complex IV catalyses the oxidation of reduced cytochrome c and the reduction of oxygen to water, and is associated with the phosphorylation of ADP to ATP.

In order to understand how the transfer of electrons through the electron transport chain can be linked to the phosphorylation of ADP to ATP, it is necessary to consider the chemistry of the various electron carriers. They can be classified into two groups:

- *Hydrogen carriers*, which undergo reduction and oxidation reactions involving both protons and electrons – these are NAD, flavins, and ubiquinone. As shown in Figure 2.17, NAD undergoes a two-electron oxidation/reduction reaction, while both the flavins (Figure 2.16) and ubiquinone (Figure 3.18) undergo two single-electron reactions to form a half-reduced radical, then the fully reduced coenzyme. Flavins can also undergo a two-electron reaction in a single step.

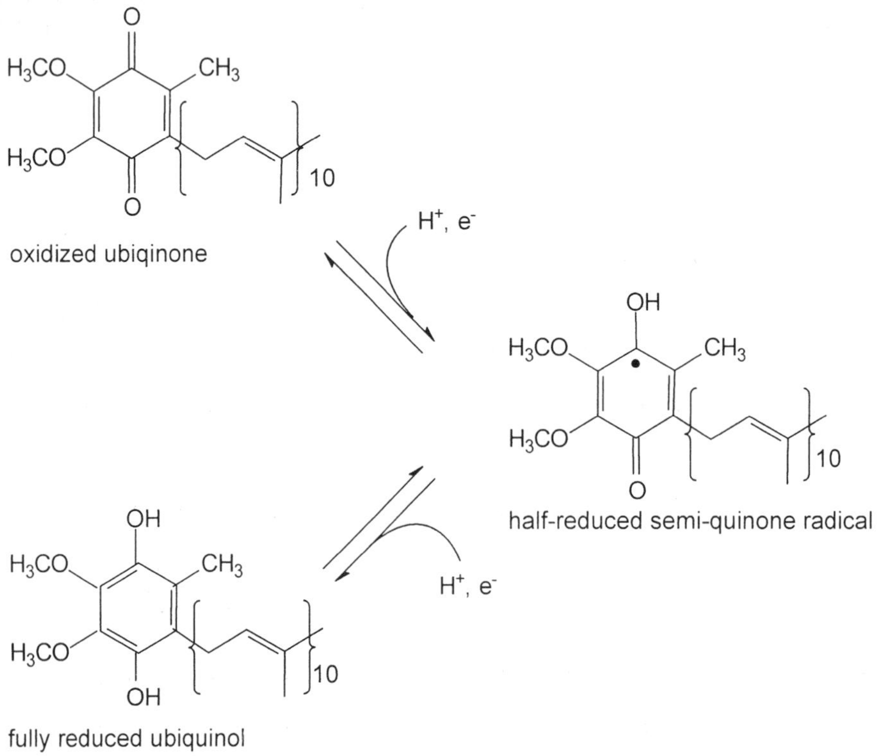

FIGURE 3.18 *Oxidation and reduction of ubiquinone (coenzyme Q).*

- *Electron carriers*, which contain iron (and in the case of cytochrome oxidase also copper); they undergo oxidation and reduction by electron transfer alone. These are the cytochromes, in which the iron is present in a haem molecule, and non-haem iron proteins, sometimes called iron–sulphur proteins, because the iron is bound to the protein through the sulphur of the amino acid cysteine. Figure 3.19 shows the arrangement of the iron in non-haem iron proteins and the three different types of haem that occur in cytochromes:
  - haem (protoporphyrin IX), which is tightly but non-covalently bound to proteins, including cytochromes b and b_1, as well as enzymes such as catalase and the oxygen transport proteins haemoglobin and myoglobin;
  - haem C, which is covalently bound to protein in cytochromes c and c_1;
  - haem A, which is anchored in the membrane by its hydrophobic side-chain, in cytochromes a and a_3 (which together form cytochrome oxidase).

The hydrogen and electron carriers of the electron transport chain are arranged in sequence in the crista membrane, as shown in Figure 3.20. Some carriers are entirely within the membrane, while others are located at the inner or outer face of the membrane.

There are two steps in which a hydrogen carrier reduces an electron carrier: the reaction between the flavin and non-haem iron protein in complex I and the reaction between ubiquinol and cytochrome b plus a non-haem iron protein in complex II.

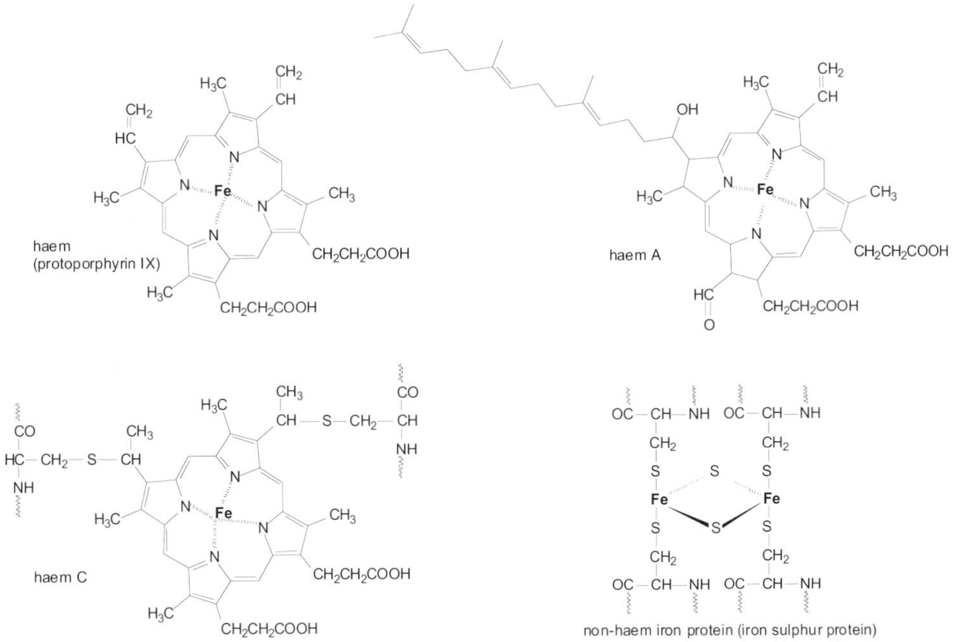

FIGURE 3.19 *Iron-containing carriers of the electron transport chain – haem and non-haem iron.*

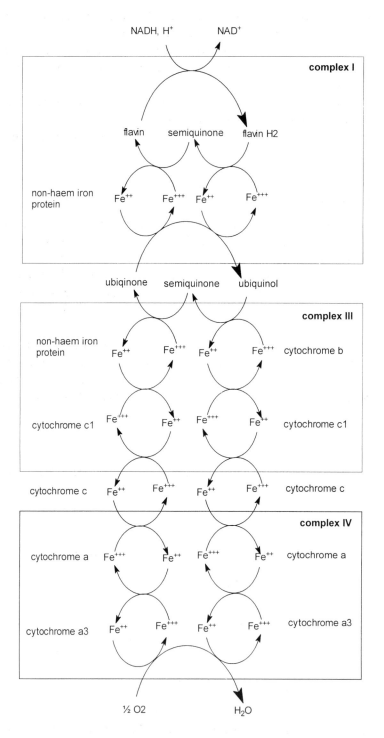

FIGURE 3.20 *Complexes of the mitochondrial electron transport chain.*

The reaction between non-haem iron protein and ubiquinone in complex I is the reverse – a hydrogen carrier is reduced by an electron carrier.

When a hydrogen carrier reduces an electron carrier, there is a proton that is not transferred onto the electron carrier but is extruded from the membrane, into the crista space, as shown in Figure 3.21.

When an electron carrier reduces a hydrogen carrier, there is a need for a proton to accompany the electron that is transferred. This is acquired from the mitochondrial matrix, thus shifting the equilibrium between $H_2O \rightleftharpoons H^+ + OH^-$, resulting in an accumulation of hydroxyl ions in the matrix.

3.3.1.3 Phosphorylation of ADP linked to electron transport

The result of electron transport through the sequence of carriers shown in Figure 3.20, and the alternation between hydrogen carriers and electron carriers, is a separation of protons and hydroxyl ions across the crista membrane, with an accumulation of protons in the crista space and an accumulation of hydroxyl ions in the matrix – i.e. creation of a pH gradient across the inner membrane. This proton gradient provides the driving force for the phosphorylation of ADP to ATP, shown in Figure 3.22 – a highly endothermic reaction.

ATP synthase acts as a molecular motor, driven by the flow of protons down the concentration gradient from the crista space into the matrix, through the transmembrane stalk of the primary particle. As protons flow through the stalk, so they cause rotation of the core of the multienzyme complex that makes up the primary particle containing ATP synthase.

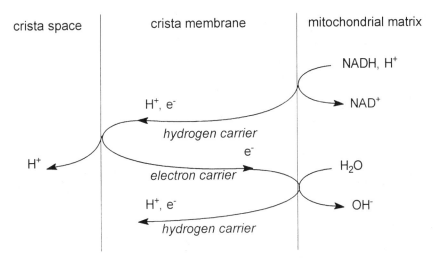

FIGURE 3.21 *Hydrogen and electron carriers in the mitochondrial electron transport chain – generation of a transmembrane proton gradient.*

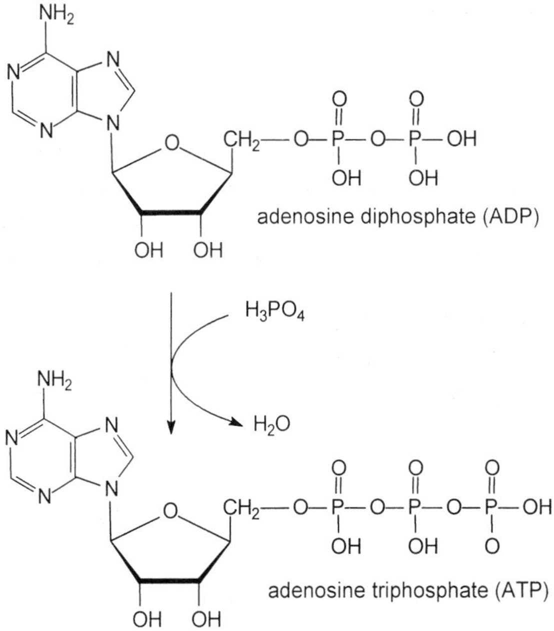

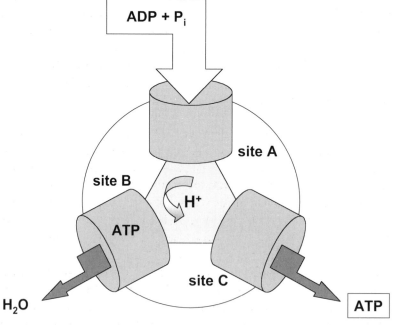

NH₂ structure — adenosine diphosphate (ADP)

$$H_3PO_4$$

$$H_2O$$

adenosine triphosphate (ATP)

FIGURE 3.22 *Condensation of ADP + phosphate → ATP.*

ADP + P$_i$

site A

site B

site C

ATP

H⁺

H₂O

ATP

FIGURE 3.23 *The mitochondrial ATP synthase – a molecular motor. As the central core rotates, so each site in turn undergoes a conformational change, A becoming equivalent to B, B to C and C to A.*

As shown in Figure 3.23, there are three ATP synthase catalytic sites in the primary particle, and each one-third turn of the central core causes a conformational change at each active site:

- At one site the conformational change permits binding of ADP and phosphate.
- At the next site the conformational change brings ADP and phosphate close enough together to undergo condensation and expel a proton and a hydroxyl ion.
- At the third site the conformational change causes expulsion of ATP from the site, leaving it free to accept ADP and phosphate at the next part-turn.

At any time, one site is binding ADP and phosphate, one is undergoing condensation and the third is expelling ATP. If ADP is not available to bind, then rotation cannot occur – and if rotation cannot occur, then protons cannot flow through the stalk from the crista space into the matrix.

3.3.1.4 The coupling of electron transport, oxidative phosphorylation and fuel oxidation

The processes of oxidation of reduced coenzymes and the phosphorylation of ADP to ATP are normally tightly coupled:

- ADP phosphorylation cannot occur unless there is a proton gradient across the crista membrane resulting from the oxidation of NADH or reduced flavins.
- If there is little or no ADP available, the oxidation of NADH and reduced flavins is inhibited, because the protons cannot cross the stalk of the primary particle, and so the proton gradient becomes large enough to inhibit further transport of protons into the crista space. Indeed, experimentally it is possible to force reverse electron transport and reduction of NAD^+ and flavins by creating a proton gradient across the crista membrane.

Metabolic fuels can only be oxidized when NAD^+ and oxidized flavoproteins are available. Therefore, if there is little or no ADP available in the mitochondria (i.e. it has all been phosphorylated to ATP), there will be an accumulation of reduced coenzymes, and hence a slowing of the rate of oxidation of metabolic fuels. This means that substrates are only oxidized when there is a need for the phosphorylation of ADP to ATP and ADP is available. The availability of ADP is dependent on the utilization of ATP in performing physical and chemical work, as shown in Figure 3.2.

It is possible to uncouple electron transport and ADP phosphorylation by adding a weak acid, such as dinitrophenol, that transports protons across the crista membrane. As shown in Figure 3.24, in the presence of such an uncoupler, the protons extruded during electron transport do not accumulate in the crista space but are transported into the mitochondrial matrix, where they react with hydroxyl ions, forming water. Under these conditions, ADP is not phosphorylated to ATP, and the oxidation of

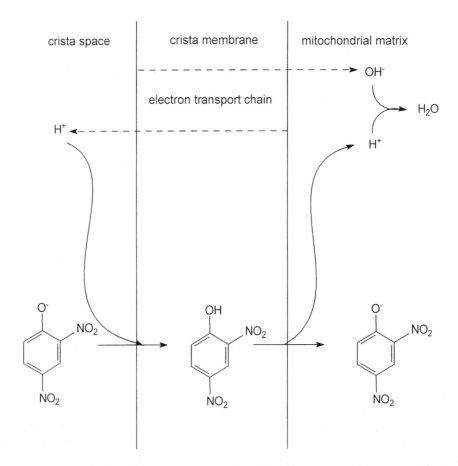

FIGURE 3.24 *Uncoupling of electron transport and oxidative phosphorylation by a weak acid such as 2,4-dinitrophenol.*

NADH and reduced flavins can continue unimpeded until all the available substrate or oxygen has been consumed. Figure 3.25 shows the oxygen electrode trace in the presence of an uncoupler.

The result of uncoupling electron transport from the phosphorylation of ADP is that a great deal of substrate is oxidized, with little production of ATP, although heat is produced. This is one of the physiological mechanisms for heat production to maintain body temperature without performing physical work – non-shivering thermogenesis. There are a number of proteins in the mitochondria of various tissues that act as proton transporters across the crista membrane when they are activated.

The first such uncoupling protein to be identified was in brown adipose tissue, and was called thermogenin because of its role in thermogenesis. Brown adipose tissue is anatomically and functionally distinct from the white adipose tissue that is the main site of fat storage in the body. It has a red–brown colour because it is especially rich in mitochondria. Brown adipose tissue is especially important in the maintenance of

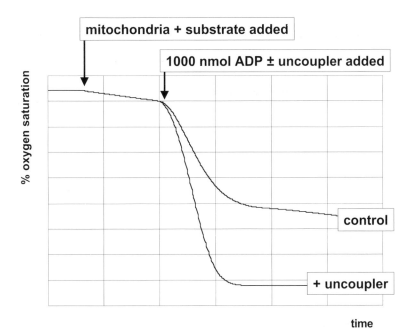

FIGURE 3.25 *Oxygen consumption by mitochondria incubated with malate and ADP, with and without an uncoupler.*

body temperature in infants, but it remains active in adults, although its importance compared with uncoupling proteins in muscle and other tissues is unclear.

In addition to maintenance of body temperature, uncoupling proteins are important in overall energy balance and body weight (section 5.2). It was noted in section 1.3.2 that the hormone leptin secreted by (white) adipose tissue increases expression of uncoupling proteins in muscle and adipose tissue, so increasing energy expenditure and the utilization of adipose tissue fat reserves.

3.3.1.5 Respiratory poisons

Much of our knowledge of the processes involved in electron transport and oxidative phosphorylation has come from studies using inhibitors. Figure 3.26 shows the oxygen electrode traces from mitochondria incubated with malate and an inhibitor of electron transport, with or without the addition of dinitrophenol as an uncoupler. Inhibitors of electron transport include:

1 Rotenone, the active ingredient of derris powder, an insecticide prepared from the roots of the leguminous plant *Lonchocarpus nicou*. It is an inhibitor of complex I (NADH → ubiquinone reduction). The same effect is seen in the presence of amytal (amobarbital), a barbiturate sedative drug, which again inhibits complex I. These two compounds inhibit oxidation of malate, which requires complex I, but not succinate, which reduces ubiquinone directly. The addition of the uncoupler

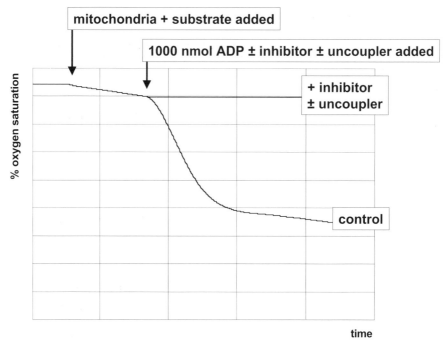

FIGURE 3.26 *Oxygen consumption by mitochondria incubated with malate and ADP, plus an inhibitor of electron transport, with and without an uncoupler.*

has no effect on malate oxidation in the presence of these two inhibitors of electron transport, but leads to uncontrolled oxidation of succinate.

2 Antimycin A, an antibiotic produced by *Streptomyces* spp. that is used as a fungicide against fungi that are parasitic on rice. It inhibits complex III (ubiquinone → cytochrome c reduction). It inhibits the oxidation of both malate and succinate, as both require complex III, and the addition of the uncoupler has no effect.

3 Cyanide, azide or carbon monoxide, all of which bind irreversibly to the iron of cytochrome a_3, and thus inhibit complex IV. Again these compounds inhibit oxidation of malate and succinate, as both rely on cytochrome oxidase, and again the addition of the uncoupler has no effect.

Figure 3.27 shows the oxygen electrode traces from mitochondria incubated with malate and an inhibitor of ATP synthesis, with or without the addition of dinitrophenol as an uncoupler. Oligomycin is a therapeutically useless antibiotic produced by *Streptomyces* spp. that inhibits the transport of protons across the stalk of the primary particle. This results in inhibition of oxidation of both malate and succinate, because, if the protons cannot be transported back into the matrix, they will accumulate and

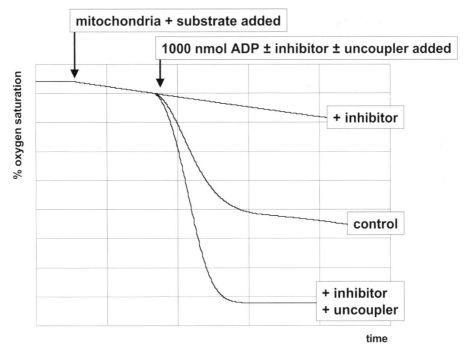

FIGURE 3.27 *Oxygen consumption by mitochondria incubated with malate and ADP, plus an inhibitor of ATP synthesis such as oligomycin, with and without an uncoupler.*

inhibit further electron transport. In this case, addition of the uncoupler permits re-entry of protons across the crista membrane, and hence uncontrolled oxidation of substrates.

Two further compounds also inhibit ATP synthesis not by inhibiting the ATP synthase, but by inhibiting the transport of ADP into, and ATP out of, the mitochondria:

1 Atractyloside is a toxic glycoside from the rhizomes of the Mediterranean thistle *Atractylis gummifera*; it competes with ADP for binding to the carrier.
2 Bongkrekic acid is a toxic antibiotic formed by *Pseudomonas cocovenenans* growing on coconut; it is named after bongkrek, an Indonesian mould-fermented coconut product that becomes highly toxic when *Pseudomonas* outgrows the mould. It fixes the carrier protein at the inner face of the membrane, so that ATP cannot be transported out, nor ADP in.

Both compounds thus inhibit ATP synthesis, and therefore the oxidation of substrates. However, as with oligomycin (see Figure 3.27), addition of an uncoupler permits rapid and complete utilization of oxygen, as electron transport can now continue uncontrolled by the availability of ADP.

Additional resources

PowerPoint presentation 3 on the CD.
Self-assessment quiz 3 on the CD.

The simulation program Oxygen Electrode on the CD permits you to perform experiments on mitochondria incubated with malate or succinate, using varying concentrations of ADP, with and without inhibitors of electron transport, oligomycin and an uncoupler.

PROBLEM 3.1: *Dinitrophenol as a slimming agent*

Dinitrophenol was at one time used as a slimming agent. Explain how it acted, and describe what you would expect to observe in a person who had consumed a modest (non-toxic) amount of dinitrophenol.

PROBLEM 3.2: *ATP in working muscle*

Table 3.1 shows the concentrations of ATP, ADP, creatine phosphate and creatine in rat gastrocnemius muscle (1) at rest and (2) after electrical stimulation (causing contraction) for 3 minutes. What conclusions can you draw from these results?

Table 3.1 ATP, ADP and creatine phosphate in muscle (μmol/g)

	At rest	**After stimulation**
ATP	5.00	4.90
ADP	0.01	0.11
Creatine phosphate	17.00	1.00
Creatine	0.10	16.10

4

Digestion and absorption

The major components of the diet are starches, sugars, fats and proteins. These have to be hydrolysed to their constituent smaller molecules for absorption and metabolism. Starches and sugars are absorbed as monosaccharides; fats are absorbed as free fatty acids and glycerol (plus a small amount of intact triacylglycerol); proteins are absorbed as their constituent amino acids and small peptides.

The fat-soluble vitamins (A, D, E and K) are absorbed dissolved in dietary lipids; there are active transport systems (section 3.2.2) in the small intestinal mucosa for the absorption of the water-soluble vitamins. The absorption of vitamin B_{12} (section 11.10.1) requires a specific binding protein that is secreted in the gastric juice in order to bind to the mucosal transport system.

Minerals generally enter the intestinal mucosal cells by carrier-mediated diffusion and are accumulated intracellularly by binding to specific binding proteins (section 3.2.2.1). They are then transferred into the bloodstream by active transport mechanisms at the serosal side of the epithelial cells, usually onto plasma binding proteins. The absorption of calcium is discussed in section 11.15.3.1, and that of iron in section 4.5.1.

Objectives

After reading this chapter you should be able to:

- describe the major functions of each region of the gastrointestinal tract;

- describe and explain the classification of carbohydrates according to their chemical and nutritional properties and explain what is meant by the glycaemic index;
- describe and explain the digestion and absorption of carbohydrates;
- describe and explain the classification of dietary lipids and the different types of fatty acid;
- describe and explain the digestion and absorption of lipids, the role of bile salts and the formation of chylomicrons;
- describe and explain the classification of amino acids according to their chemical and nutritional properties;
- describe the levels of protein structure and explain what is meant by denaturation;
- describe and explain the digestion and absorption of proteins;
- describe the absorption of minerals, especially iron.

4.1 *The gastrointestinal tract*

The gastrointestinal tract is shown in Figure 4.1. The major functions of each region are:

- Mouth
  - starch hydrolysis catalysed by amylase, secreted by the salivary glands;
  - fat hydrolysis catalysed by lingual lipase, secreted by the tongue;
  - absorption of small amounts of vitamin C and a variety of non-nutrients (including nicotine).
- Stomach
  - denaturation of dietary proteins (section 4.4.2) and the release of vitamin B_{12}, iron and other minerals from protein binding, for which gastric acid is important;
  - protein hydrolysis catalysed by pepsin;
  - fat hydrolysis catalysed by lipase.
  - secretion of intrinsic factor, required for the absorption of vitamin B_{12} (section 11.10.1).
- Small intestine (duodenum, jejunum and ileum)
  - starch hydrolysis catalysed by amylase secreted by the pancreas;
  - hydrolysis of disaccharides within the brush border of the intestinal mucosa;
  - fat hydrolysis catalysed by lipase secreted by the pancreas;
  - protein hydrolysis catalysed by a variety of exo- and endopeptidases (section 4.4.3) secreted by the pancreas and small intestinal mucosa;
  - hydrolysis of di- and tripeptides within the brush border of the intestinal mucosa;
  - absorption of the products of digestion;
  - absorption of water (failure of water absorption, as in diarrhoea, can lead to serious dehydration).

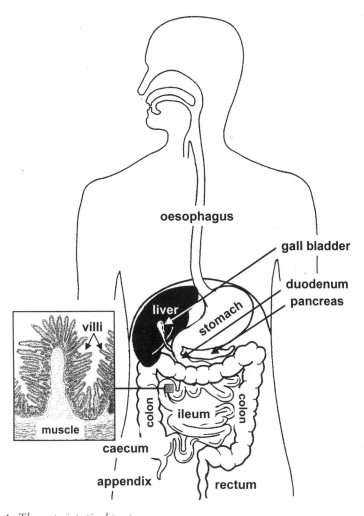

oesophagus

gall bladder

duodenum
pancreas

liver

stomach

villi

colon

ileum

colon

muscle

caecum

appendix

rectum

FIGURE 4.1 *The gastrointestinal tract.*

- Large intestine (caecum and colon)
  - bacterial metabolism of undigested carbohydrates and shed intestinal mucosal cells;
  - absorption of some of the products of bacterial metabolism;
  - absorption of water.
- Rectum
  - storage of undigested gut contents prior to evacuation as faeces;

Throughout the gastrointestinal tract, and especially in the small intestine, the surface area of the mucosa is considerably greater than would appear from its superficial appearance. As shown in the inset in Figure 4.1, the intestinal mucosa is folded longitudinally into the lumen. The surface of these folds is covered with villi: fingerlike projections into the lumen, some 0.5–1.5 mm long. There are some 20– 40 villi per mm^2, giving a total absorptive surface area of some 300 m^2 in the small intestine.

As shown in Figure 4.2, each villus has both blood capillaries, which drain into the hepatic portal vein, and a lacteal, which drains into the lymphatic system. Water-soluble products of digestion (carbohydrates and amino acids) are absorbed into the blood capillaries, and the liver has a major role in controlling the availability of the products of carbohydrate and protein digestion to other tissues in the body. As discussed in section 4.3.3.2, lipids are absorbed into the lacteals; the lymphatic system joins the bloodstream at the thoracic duct, and extrahepatic tissues are exposed to the products of lipid digestion uncontrolled by the liver, which functions to clear the remnants from the circulation.

There is rapid turnover of the cells of the intestinal mucosa; epithelial cells proliferate in the crypts, alongside the cells that secrete digestive enzymes, and migrate to the tip of the villus, where they are shed into the lumen. The average life of an intestinal mucosal epithelial cell is about 48 hours. As discussed in section 4.5, this rapid turnover of epithelial cells is important in controlling the absorption of iron, and possible other minerals.

The rapid turnover of intestinal mucosal cells is also important for protection of the intestine against the digestive enzymes secreted into the lumen. Further protection is afforded by the secretion of mucus, a solution of proteins that are resistant to enzymic

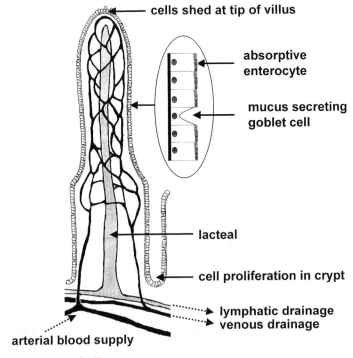

FIGURE 4.2 *An intestinal villus.*

hydrolysis and which coats the intestinal mucosa. The secretion of intestinal mucus explains a considerable part of an adult's continuing requirement for dietary protein (section 9.1.2).

4.2 *Digestion and absorption of carbohydrates*

Carbohydrates are compounds of carbon, hydrogen and oxygen in the ratio $C_n:H_{2n}:O_n$. The basic unit of the carbohydrates is the sugar molecule or monosaccharide. Note that sugar is used here in a chemical sense, and includes a variety of simple carbohydrates that are collectively known as sugars. Ordinary table sugar (cane sugar or beet sugar) is correctly known as sucrose; as discussed in section 4.2.1.3, it is a disaccharide. It is just one of a number of different sugars found in the diet.

4.2.1 THE CLASSIFICATION OF CARBOHYDRATES

Dietary carbohydrates can be considered in two main groups: sugars and polysaccharides. As shown in Figure 4.3, the polysaccharides can be further subdivided into starches and non-starch polysaccharides.

The simplest type of sugar is a monosaccharide – a single sugar unit (section 4.2.1.1). Monosaccharides normally consist of between three and seven carbon atoms (and the corresponding number of hydrogen and oxygen atoms). A few larger monosaccharides also occur, although they are not important in nutrition and metabolism.

Disaccharides (section 4.2.1.3) are formed by condensation between two monosaccharides to form a glycoside bond. The reverse reaction, cleavage of the glycoside bond to release the individual monosaccharides, is a hydrolysis.

Oligosaccharides consist of three or four monosaccharide units (trisaccharides and tetrasaccharides), and occasionally more, linked by glycoside bonds. Nutritionally, they are not particularly important, and indeed they are generally not digested, although they may be fermented by intestinal bacteria and make a significant contribution to the production of intestinal gas.

Nutritionally, it is useful to consider sugars (both monosaccharides and disaccharides) in two groups:

* Sugars contained within plant cell walls in foods. These are known as intrinsic sugars.
* Sugars that are in free solution in foods, and therefore provide a substrate for oral bacteria, leading to the formation of dental plaque and caries. These are known as extrinsic sugars. As discussed in section 7.3.3.1, it is considered desirable to reduce the consumption of extrinsic sugars because excessive amounts are associated with dental decay as well as obesity (section 6.3) and possibly also an increased risk of developing diabetes mellitus (section 10.7).

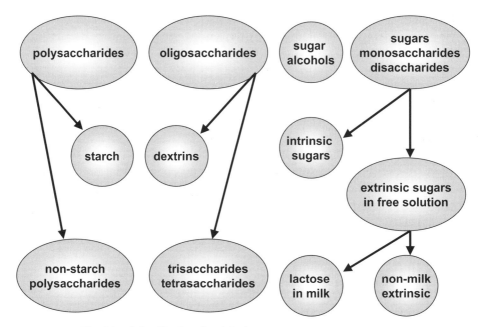

FIGURE 4.3 *Nutritional classification of carbohydrates.*

A complication in the classification of sugars as intrinsic (which are considered desirable in the diet) and extrinsic (which are considered undesirable in the diet) is that lactose (section 4.2.1.3) occurs in free solution in milk, and hence is an extrinsic sugar. However, lactose is not a cause of dental decay, and milk is an important source of calcium (section 11.15.1), protein (see Chapter 9) and vitamin B$_2$ (section 11.7). It is not considered desirable to reduce intakes of milk, which is the only significant source of lactose, and extrinsic sugars are further subdivided into milk sugar and non-milk extrinsic sugars.

Polysaccharides are polymers of many hundreds of monosaccharide units, again linked by glycoside bonds. The most important are starch and glycogen (section 4.2.1.5), both of which are polymers of the monosaccharide glucose. There are also a number of other polysaccharides, composed of other monosaccharides or of glucose units linked differently from the linkages in starch and glycogen. Collectively these are known as non-starch polysaccharides. They are generally not digested but have important roles in nutrition (section 4.2.1.6).

4.2.1.1 Monosaccharides

The classes of monosaccharides are named by the number of carbon atoms in the ring, using the Greek names for the numbers, with the ending '-ose' to show that they are sugars. The names of all sugars end in '-ose'.

- Four-carbon monosaccharides are tetroses.

- Five-carbon monosaccharides are pentoses.
- Six-carbon monosaccharides are hexoses.
- Seven-carbon monosaccharides are heptoses.

In general, trioses, tetroses and heptoses are important as intermediate compounds in the metabolism of pentoses and hexoses. Hexoses are the nutritionally important sugars.

The pentoses and hexoses can either exist as straight-chain compounds or can form heterocyclic rings, as shown in Figure 4.4. By convention, the ring of sugars is drawn with the bonds of one side thicker than on the other. This is to show that the rings are planar and can be considered to lie at right angles to the plane of the paper. The boldly drawn part of the molecule is then coming out of the paper, while the lightly

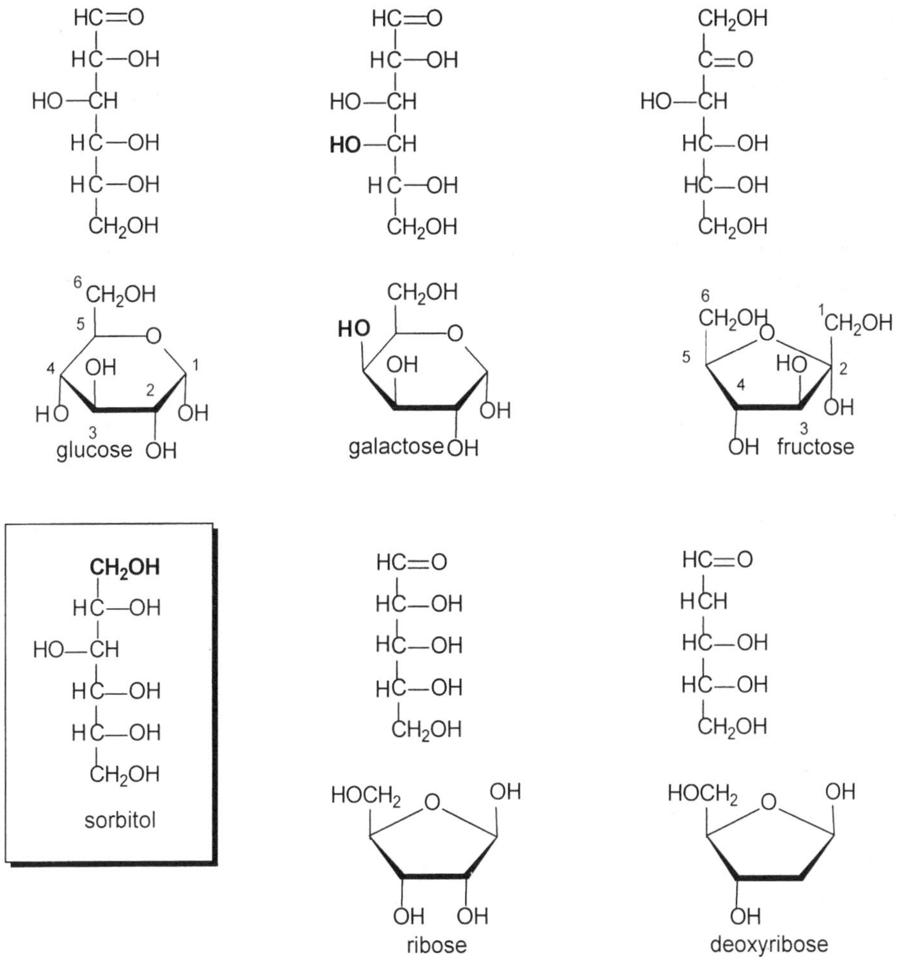

FIGURE 4.4 *The nutritionally important monosaccharides.*

drawn part is going behind the paper. The hydroxyl groups lie above or below the plane of the ring, in the plane of the paper. Each carbon has a hydrogen atom attached as well as a hydroxyl group. For convenience in drawing the structures of sugars, this hydrogen is generally omitted when the structures are drawn as rings.

The nutritionally important hexoses are glucose, galactose and fructose. Glucose and galactose differ from each other only in the arrangement of one hydroxyl group above or below the plane of the ring. Fructose differs from glucose and galactose in that it has a C=O (keto) group at carbon 2, whereas the other two have an H–C=O (aldehyde) group at carbon 1.

There are two important pentose sugars, ribose and deoxyribose. Deoxyribose is unusual, in that it has lost one of its hydroxyl groups. The main role of ribose and deoxyribose is in the nucleotides (see Figure 3.1) and the nucleic acids: RNA, in which the sugar is ribose (section 9.2.2), and DNA, in which the sugar is deoxyribose (section 9.2.1). Although pentoses do occur in the diet, they are also readily synthesized from glucose (section 5.4.2)

4.2.1.2 Sugar alcohols

Sugar alcohols are formed by the reduction of the aldehyde group of a monosaccharide to a hydroxyl (–OH) group. The most important of these is sorbitol, formed by the reduction of glucose. It is absorbed from the intestinal tract and metabolized only slowly, so that it has very much less effect on the concentration of glucose in the bloodstream than other carbohydrates. Because of this, it is widely used in preparation of foods suitable for use by diabetics, as it tastes sweet and can replace sucrose and other sugars in food manufacture. However, sorbitol is metabolized as a metabolic fuel, with an energy yield approximately half that of glucose, because it is poorly absorbed, so that it is not suitable for the replacement of carbohydrates in weight-reducing diets.

Xylitol is the sugar alcohol formed by reduction of the five-carbon sugar xylose, an isomer of ribose. It is of interest because, so far from promoting dental caries, as does sucrose (section 7.3.3.1), xylitol has an anti-cariogenic action. The reasons for this are not well understood, but sucking sweets made from xylitol results in a significant reduction in the incidence of caries – such sweets are sometimes called 'tooth-friendly' because of this.

4.2.1.3 Disaccharides

The major dietary disaccharides, shown in Figure 4.5, are:

- sucrose, cane or beet sugar, which is glucosyl-fructose;
- lactose, the sugar of milk, which is galactosyl-glucose;
- maltose, the sugar originally isolated from malt, which is is glucosyl-glucose;
- isomaltose, which is glucosyl-glucose linked 1→6;

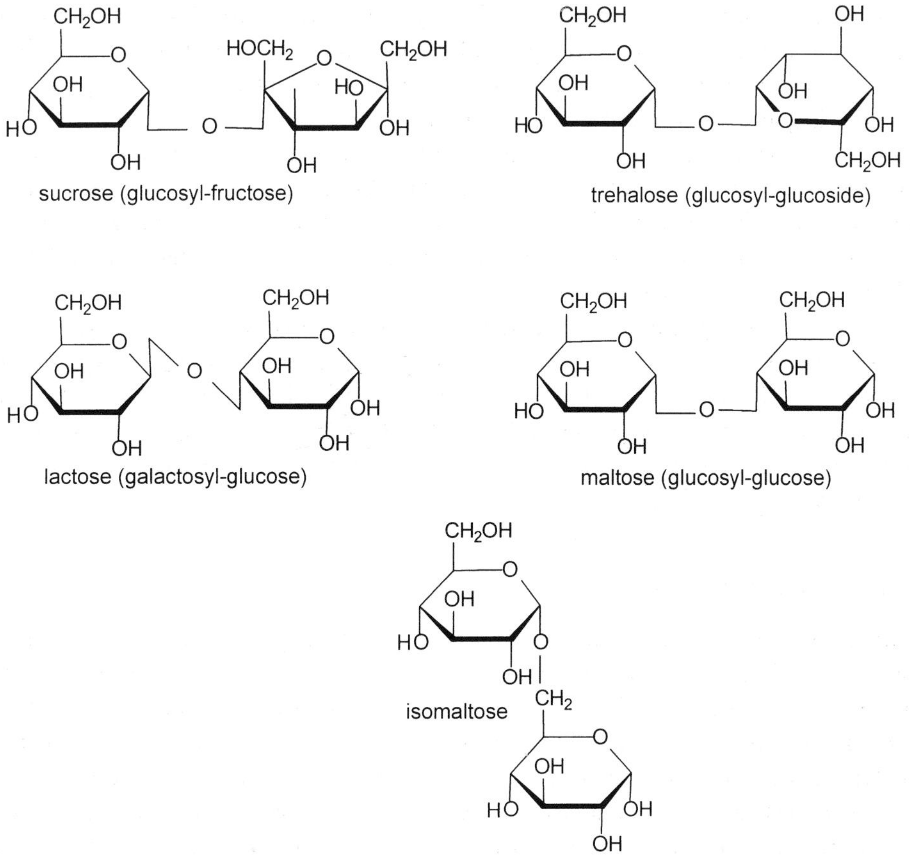

FIGURE 4.5 *The nutritionally important disaccharides.*

- trehalose, the sugar found especially in mushrooms, but also as the blood sugar of some insects, which is glucosyl-glucoside.

Both maltose and isomaltose arise from the digestion of starch.

4.2.1.4 Reducing and non-reducing sugars

Chemically, the aldehyde group of glucose is a reducing agent. As shown in Figure 4.6, this provides a simple test for glucose in urine. Glucose reacts with copper (Cu^{2+}) ions in alkaline solution, reducing them to Cu^+ oxide, and itself being oxidized. The original solution of Cu^{2+} ions has a blue colour; the copper oxide forms a yellow–brown precipitate.

This reaction is not specific for glucose. Other sugars with a free aldehyde group at carbon-1, including vitamin C (section 11.14) and a number of pentose sugars that occur in foods, can undergo the same reaction, giving a false-positive result.

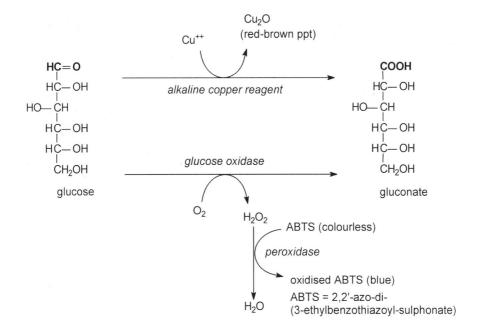

FIGURE 4.6 *Measurement of glucose using alkaline copper reagents and glucose oxidase.*

While alkaline copper reagents are sometimes used to measure urine glucose in monitoring diabetic control (section 10.7), a test using the enzyme glucose oxidase measures only glucose. As shown in Figure 4.6, glucose oxidase reduces oxygen to hydrogen peroxide; in turn, this reacts with a colourless compound to yield a coloured dyestuff that can readily be measured. High concentrations of vitamin C (section 11.14), as may occur in the urine of people taking supplements of the vitamin, can react with hydrogen peroxide before it oxidizes the colourless precursor, or can reduce the dyestuff back to its colourless form. This means that tests using glucose oxidase can yield a false-negative result in the presence of high concentrations of vitamin C (see Problem 4.1 at the end of this chapter).

It is important to realize that the term 'reducing sugars' reflects a chemical reaction of the sugars – the ability to reduce a suitable acceptor such as copper ions. It has nothing to do with weight reduction and slimming, although some people erroneously believe that reducing sugars somehow help one to reduce excessive weight. This is not correct – the energy yield from reducing sugars and non-reducing sugars is exactly the same, and excess of either will contribute to obesity.

4.2.1.5 Polysaccharides: starches and glycogen

Starch is a polymer of glucose, containing a large, but variable, number of glucose units. It is thus impossible to quote a relative molecular mass for starch, or to discuss amounts of starch in terms of moles. It can, however, be hydrolysed to glucose, and the result expressed as moles of glucose.

The simplest type of starch is amylose, a straight chain of glucose molecules, with glycoside links between carbon-1 of one glucose unit and carbon-4 of the next. Some types of starch have a branched structure, in which every 30th glucose molecule has glycoside links to three others instead of just two. The branch is formed by linkage between carbon-1 of one glucose unit and carbon-6 of the next, as shown in Figure 4.7. This is amylopectin.

Starches are the storage carbohydrates of plants, and the relative amounts of amylose and amylopectin differ in starches from different sources, as indeed does the size of the overall starch molecule. On average, about 20–25% of starch in foods is amylose, and the remaining 75–80% is amylopectin.

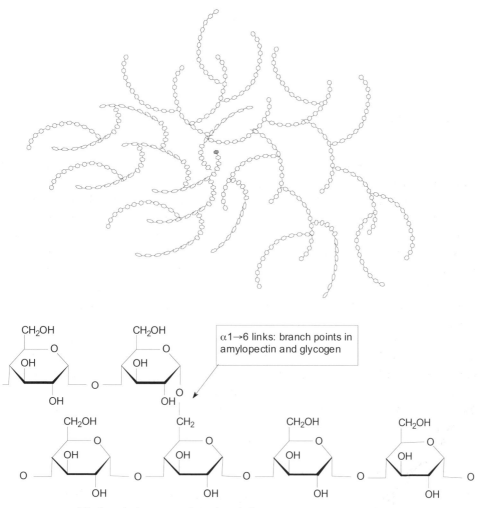

FIGURE 4.7 *The branched structure of starch and glycogen.*

Glycogen is the storage carbohydrate of mammalian muscle and liver. It is synthesized from glucose in the fed state (section 5.6.3), and its constituent glucose units are used as a metabolic fuel in the fasting state. Glycogen is a branched polymer, with essentially the same structure as amylopectin, except that it is more highly branched, with a 1→6 bond about every 10th glucose.

4.2.1.6 Non-starch polysaccharides (dietary fibre)

There are a number of other polysaccharides in foods. Collectively they are known as non-starch polysaccharides, the major components of dietary fibre (section 7.3.3.2). Non-starch polysaccharides are not digested by human enzymes, although all can be fermented to some extent by intestinal bacteria, and the products of bacterial fermentation may be absorbed and metabolized as metabolic fuels. The major non-starch polysaccharides (shown in Figure 4.8) are:

- cellulose, a polymer of glucose in which the configuration of the glycoside bond between the glucose units is in the opposite configuration (β1→4) from that in starch (α1→4) and cannot be hydrolysed by human enzymes;
- hemicelluloses, branched polymers of pentose (five-carbon) and hexose (six-carbon) sugars;
- inulin, a polymer of fructose that is the storage carbohydrate of Jerusalem artichoke and some other root vegetables;
- pectin, a complex polymer of a variety of monosaccharides, including some methylated sugars;
- plant gums such as gum Arabic, gum tragacanth, acacia, carob and guar gums – complex polymers of mixed monosaccharides;
- mucilages such as alginates, agar and carrageen, complex polymers of mixed monosaccharides found in seaweeds and other algae.

Cellulose, hemicelluloses and inulin are insoluble non-starch polysaccharides, whereas pectin and the plant gums and mucilages are soluble. The other major constituent of dietary fibre, lignin, is not a carbohydrate at all but a complex polymer of a variety of aromatic alcohols.

4.2.2 CARBOHYDRATE DIGESTION AND ABSORPTION

The digestion of carbohydrates is by hydrolysis to liberate small oligosaccharides, then free mono- and disaccharides. The extent and speed with which a carbohydrate is hydrolysed and the resultant monosaccharides absorbed is measured as the glycaemic index – the increase in blood glucose after a test dose of the carbohydrate compared with that after an equivalent amount of glucose.

Glucose and galactose have a glycaemic index of 1, as do lactose, maltose, isomaltose and trehalose, which give rise to these monosaccharides on hydrolysis. However, because

inulin - fructose polymer linked β2→1

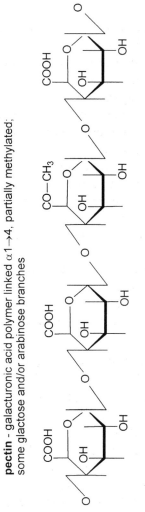

cellulose - glucose polymer linked β1→4

chitin - *N*-acetylglucosamine polymer linked β1→4

pectin - galacturonic acid polymer linked α1→4, partially methylated; some glactose and/or arabinose branches

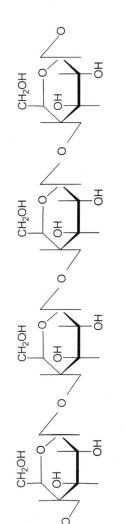

FIGURE 4.8 *The major types of dietary non-starch polysaccharide.*

plant cell walls are largely cellulose, which is not digested, intrinsic sugars in fruits and vegetables have a lower glycaemic index. Other monosaccharides (e.g. fructose) and the sugar alcohols are absorbed less rapidly (section 4.4.2.3) and have a lower glycaemic index, as does sucrose, which yields glucose and fructose on hydrolysis. As discussed in section 4.4.2.1, the glycaemic index of starch is variable, and that of non-starch polysaccharides is zero.

Carbohydrates with a high glycaemic index lead to a greater secretion of insulin after a meal than do those with a lower glycaemic index; this results in increased synthesis of fatty acids and triacylglycerol (section 5.6.1), and is therefore a factor in the development of obesity (see Chapter 6). There is also some evidence that habitual consumption of carbohydrates with a high glycaemic index may be a factor in the development of non-insulin-dependent diabetes (section 10.7).

4.2.2.1 Starch digestion

The enzymes that catalyse the hydrolysis of starch are amylases, which are secreted in both the saliva and the pancreatic juice. (Salivary amylase is sometimes known by its old name of ptyalin.) Both salivary and pancreatic amylases catalyse random hydrolysis of glycoside bonds, yielding initially dextrins and other oligosaccharides, then a mixture of glucose, maltose and isomaltose (from the branch points in amylopectin).

The digestion of starch begins when food is chewed, and continues for a time in the stomach. As discussed in section 1.3.3.1, hydrolysis of starch to sweet sugars in the mouth may be a factor in determining food and nutrient intake.

The gastric juice is very acid (about pH 1.5–2), and amylase is inactive at this pH; as the food bolus is mixed with gastric juice, so starch digestion ceases. When the food leaves the stomach and enters the small intestine, it is neutralized by the alkaline pancreatic juice (pH 8.8) and bile (pH 8). Amylase secreted by the pancreas continues the digestion of starch begun by salivary amylase.

Starches can be classified as:

- rapidly hydrolysed, with a glycaemic index near 1 – these are more or less completely hydrolysed in the small intestine;
- slowly hydrolysed, with a glycaemic index significantly less than 1, so that a significant proportion remains in the gut lumen and is a substrate for bacterial fermentation in the colon;
- resistant to hydrolysis, with a glycaemic index near to zero, so that most remains in the gut lumen and is a substrate for bacterial fermentation in the colon.

A proportion of the starch in foods is still enclosed by plant cell walls, which are mainly composed of cellulose. Cellulose is not digested by human enzymes, and therefore this starch is protected against digestion. Similarly, intrinsic sugars (section 4.4.2.1) have a lower glycaemic index than would be expected, because they are within intact cells.

Uncooked starch is resistant to amylase action, because it is present as small insoluble granules. The process of cooking swells the starch granules, resulting in a gel on which amylase can act. However, as cooked starch cools, a proportion undergoes crystallization to a form that is again resistant to amylase action – this is part of the process of staling of starchy foods.

Much of the resistant and slowly hydrolysed starch is fermented by bacteria in the colon, and a proportion of the products of bacterial metabolism, including short-chain fatty acids, may be absorbed and metabolized. As discussed in section 7.3.3.2, butyrate produced by bacterial fermentation of resistant starch and non-starch polysaccharides has an antiproliferative action against tumour cells in culture, and may provide protection against the development of colorectal cancer.

4.2.2.2 Digestion of disaccharides

The enzymes that catalyse the hydrolysis of disaccharides (the disaccharidases) are located on the brush border of the intestinal mucosal cells; the resultant monosaccharides return to the lumen of the small intestine, and are absorbed together with dietary monosaccharides and glucose arising from the digestion of starch (section 4.2.2.1). There are four disaccharidases:

- Maltase catalyses the hydrolysis of maltose to two molecules of glucose.
- Sucrase–isomaltase is a bifunctional enzyme that catalyses the hydrolysis of sucrose to glucose and fructose, and of isomaltose to two molecules of glucose.
- Lactase catalyses the hydrolysis of lactose to glucose and galactose.
- Trehalase catalyses the hydrolysis of trehalose to two molecules of glucose.

Deficiency of the enzyme lactase is common. Indeed, it is only in people of north European origin that lactase persists after childhood. In most other people, and in a number of Europeans, lactase is gradually lost through adolescence – alactasia (see Problem 4.2). In the absence of lactase, lactose cannot be absorbed. It remains in the intestinal lumen, where it is a substrate for bacterial fermentation to lactate (section 5.4.1.2). This results in a considerable increase in the osmolality of the gut contents, as 1 mol of lactose yields 4 mol of lactate and 4 mol of protons. In addition, bacterial fermentation produces carbon dioxide, methane and hydrogen, and the result of consuming a moderate amount of lactose is an explosive watery diarrhoea and severe abdominal pain. Even the relatively small amounts of lactose in milk may upset people with a complete deficiency of lactase. Such people can normally tolerate yoghurt and other fermented milk products, as much of the lactose has been converted to lactic acid. Fortunately for people who suffer from alactasia, milk is the only significant source of lactose in the diet, so it is relatively easy to avoid consuming lactose.

Rarely, people may lack sucrase–isomaltase, maltase and/or trehalase. This may be either a genetic lack of the enzyme or an acquired loss as a result of intestinal infection, when all four disaccharidases are lost. These people are intolerant of the sugar(s) that cannot be hydrolysed and suffer in the same way as alactasic subjects given lactose. It is relatively easy to avoid maltose and trehalose, as there are few sources in the diet. People who lack sucrase have a more serious problem because, as well as the obvious sugar in cakes and biscuits and jams, many manufactured foods contain added sucrose.

Genetic lack of sucrase–isomaltase is very common among the Inuit of North America. On their traditional diet this caused no problems, as they had no significant sources of sucrose or isomaltose. With the adoption of a more Western diet, sucrose-induced diarrhoea has become a significant cause of undernutrition among infants and children.

4.2.2.3 The absorption of monosaccharides

As shown in Figure 4.9, there are two separate mechanisms for the absorption of monosaccharides in the small intestine.

Glucose and galactose are absorbed by a sodium-dependent active process (section 3.2.2.3). The sodium pump and the sodium/potassium ATPase create a sodium gradient across the membrane; the sodium ions then re-enter the cell together with glucose or galactose. These two monosaccharides are carried by the same transport protein, and compete with each other for intestinal absorption.

Other monosaccharides are absorbed by carrier-mediated diffusion; there are at least three distinct carrier proteins: one for fructose, one for other monosaccharides and one for sugar alcohols. Because they are not actively transported, fructose and sugar alcohols are absorbed only to a limited extent, and after a moderately high intake a significant amount will avoid absorption and remain in the intestinal lumen, acting as a substrate for colon bacteria and, like unabsorbed disaccharides in people with disaccharidase deficiency, causing abdominal pain and diarrhoea.

4.3 *Digestion and absorption of fats*

The major fats in the diet are triacylglycerols and, to a lesser extent, phospholipids. These are hydrophobic molecules and have to be emulsified to very small droplets (micelles; section 4.3.2.2) before they can be absorbed. This emulsification is achieved by hydrolysis to monoacyl- and diacylglycerols and free fatty acids, and also by the action of the bile salts (section 4.3.2.1).

4.3.1 THE CLASSIFICATION OF DIETARY LIPIDS

Four groups of compounds that are metabolically important can be considered under the heading of lipids:

• Triacylglycerols (sometimes also known as triglycerides), in which glycerol is esterified to three fatty acids (Figure 4.10). These are the oils and fats of the diet,

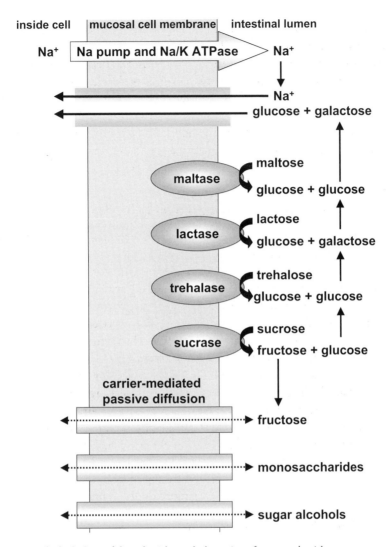

FIGURE 4.9 *The hydrolysis of disaccharides and absorption of monosaccharides.*

which provide between 30% and 45% of average energy intake (section 7.3.2). The difference between oils and fats is that oils are liquid at room temperature, whereas fats are solid.

- Phospholipids, in which glycerol is esterified to two fatty acids, with a phosphate and a hydrophilic group esterified to carbon-3 (section 4.3.1.2). Phospholipids are major constituents of cell membranes.
- Steroids, including cholesterol and a variety of plant sterols and stanols (section 7.5.1) and extremely small amounts of steroid hormones (section 10.4). Chemically these are completely different from triacylglycerols and phospholipids, and are not a source of metabolic fuel.
- A variety of other compounds, including vitamin A and carotenes (section 11.2), vitamin D (section 11.3), vitamin E (section 11.4) and vitamin K (section 11.5).

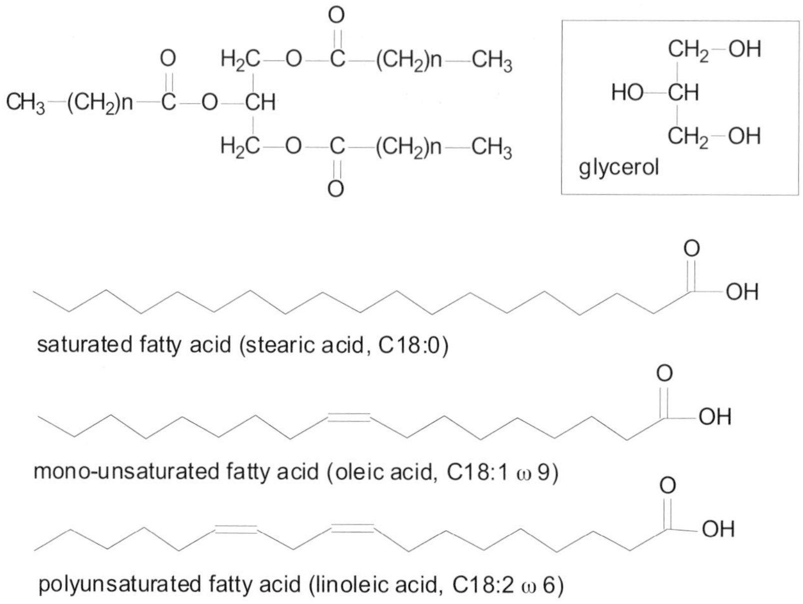

FIGURE 4.10 *The structure of triacylglycerol and types of fatty acids.*

They are absorbed in lipid micelles (section 4.3.2.2), and adequate absorption depends on an adequate intake of fat.

4.3.1.1 Fatty acids

There are a number of different fatty acids, differing in both the length of the carbon chain and whether or not they have one or more double bonds (–CH=CH–) in the chain (see Figure 4.10). Those with no double bonds are saturated fatty acids – the carbon chain is completely saturated with hydrogen. Those with double bonds are unsaturated fatty acids – the carbon chain is not completely saturated with hydrogen. Fatty acids with one double bond are known as monounsaturated, whereas those with two or more double bonds are known as polyunsaturated.

Although it is the fatty acids that are saturated or unsaturated, it is common to discuss saturated and unsaturated fats. Although is not really correct, it is a useful shorthand, reflecting the fact that fats from different sources contain a greater or lesser proportion of saturated and unsaturated fatty acids.

As shown in Table 4.1, there are three different ways of naming the fatty acids:

• Many have trivial names, often derived from the source from which they were originally isolated – thus oleic acid was first isolated from olive oil, stearic acid from beef tallow, palmitic acid from palm oil, linoleic and linolenic acids from linseed oil.

TABLE 4.1 *Fatty acid nomenclature*

	Carbon atoms	Double bonds Number	First	Shorthand
Saturated				
Butyric	4	0	–	C4:0
Caproic	6	0	–	C6:0
Caprylic	8	0	–	C8:0
Capric	10	0	–	C10:0
Lauric	12	0	–	C12:0
Myristic	14	0	–	C14:0
Palmitic	16	0	–	C16:0
Stearic	18	0	–	C18:0
Arachidic	20	0	–	C20:0
Behenic	22	0	–	C22:0
Lignoceric	24	0	–	C24:0
Monounsaturated				
Palmitoleic	16	1	6	C16:1 ω6
Oleic	18	1	9	C18:1 ω9
Cetoleic	22	1	11	C22:1 ω11
Nervonic	24	1	9	C24:1 ω9
Polyunsaturated				
Linoleic	18	2	6	C18:2 ω6
α-Linolenic	18	3	3	C18:3 ω3
γ-Linolenic	18	3	6	C18:3 ω6
Arachidonic	20	4	6	C20:4 ω6
Eicosapentaenoic	20	5	3	C20:5 ω3
Docosatetraenoic	22	4	6	C22:4 ω6
Docosapentaenoic	22	5	3	C22:5 ω3
Docosapentaenoic	22	5	6	C22:5 ω6
Docosahexaenoic	22	6	3	C22:6 ω3

- All have systematic chemical names, based on the number of carbon atoms in the chain and the number and position of double bonds (if any).
- A shorthand notation shows the number of carbon atoms in the molecule, followed by a colon and the number of double bonds. The position of the first double bond from the methyl group of the fatty acid is shown by n- or ω- (the ω-carbon is the furthest from the α-carbon, which is the one to which the carboxyl group is attached; ω (omega) is the last letter of the Greek alphabet).

In the nutritionally important unsaturated fatty acids, the carbon–carbon double bonds are in the *cis*-configuration (see Figure 2.5). The *trans*-isomers of unsaturated fatty acids do occur in foods to some extent, but they do not have the desirable biological actions of the *cis*-isomers, and indeed there is some evidence that *trans*-fatty acids may have adverse effects. As discussed in section 7.3.2.1, it is recommended that the consumption of *trans*-unsaturated fatty acids should not increase above the present average 2% of energy intake.

Polyunsaturated fatty acids have two main functions in the body:

- as major constituents of the phospholipids in cell membranes (section 4.3.1.2);
- as precursors for the synthesis of a group of compounds known as eicosanoids, including prostaglandins, prostacyclins and thromboxanes. These function as local hormones (paracrine agents), being secreted by cells into the extracellular fluid and acting on nearby cells.

The polyunsaturated fatty acids can be interconverted to a limited extent in the body, but there is a requirement for a dietary intake of linoleic acid (C18:2 ω6) and linolenic acid (C18:3 ω3), as these two, which can each be considered to be the precursor of a family of related fatty acids and eicosanoids, cannot be synthesized in the body.

As discussed in section 7.3.2.1, an intake of polyunsaturated fatty acids greater than needed to meet physiological requirements may confer benefits in terms of lowering the plasma concentration of cholesterol and reducing the risk of atherosclerosis and ischaemic heart disease. The requirement is less than 1% of energy intake, but it is recommended that 6% of energy intake should come from polyunsaturated fatty acids.

High intakes of the long-chain ω-3 polyunsaturated fatty acids (as found in fish oils) may additionally provide protection against thrombosis, as they form the 3-series eicosanoids, which inhibit platelet cohesiveness.

4.3.1.2 Phospholipids

Phospholipids are, as their name suggests, lipids that contain a phosphate group. As shown in Figure 4.11, they consist of glycerol esterified to two fatty acids, one of which (esterified to carbon-2 of glycerol) is a polyunsaturated fatty acid. The third hydroxyl group of glycerol is esterified to phosphate. The phosphate, in turn, is esterified to one of a variety of compounds, including the amino acid serine (section 4.4.1), ethanolamine (which is formed from serine), choline (which is formed from ethanolamine), inositol (section 10.3.3) or one of a variety of other compounds.

A phospholipid lacking the group esterified to the phosphate is known as a phosphatidic acid, and the complete phospholipids are called phosphatidylserine, phosphatidylethanolamine, phosphatidylcholine (also called lecithin), phosphatidylinositol, etc.

As shown in Figure 4.12, phospholipids form a lipid bilayer, with the hydrophobic fatty acid chains inside and the hydrophilic groups outside. This is the basic structure of cell membranes; various proteins may be embedded in the membrane at one surface

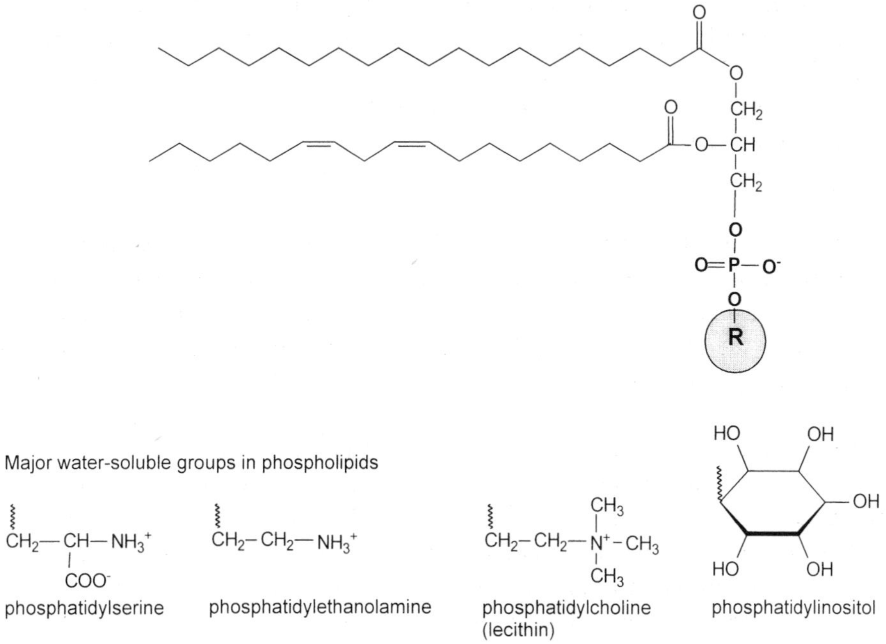

Major water-soluble groups in phospholipids

CH₂—CH—NH₃⁺
|
COO⁻
phosphatidylserine

CH₂–CH₂—NH₃⁺
phosphatidylethanolamine

CH₃
|
CH₂–CH₂—N⁺–CH₃
|
CH₃
phosphatidylcholine
(lecithin)

phosphatidylinositol

FIGURE 4.11 *The structure of phospholipids.*

or the other, or may span the membrane (transmembrane proteins) as either transport proteins (section 3.2.2) or receptors for hormones and neurotransmitters (section 10.3.1). The polyunsaturated fatty acids esterified at carbon-2 of glycerol in phospholipids are essential for membrane fluidity; neither saturated fatty acids nor the *trans*-isomers of polyunsaturated fatty acids will pack to form an adequately fluid membrane. Other lipids, including cholesterol (section 4.4.3.1.3) and vitamin E (section 11.4), are dissolved in the hydrophobic interior of the membrane and are essential to its function.

In addition to its structural role, phosphatidylinositol has a specialized function in membranes, acting as the source of inositol trisphosphate and diacylglycerol, which are produced as intracellular second messengers in response to fast-acting hormones and neurotransmitters (section 10.3.3).

4.3.1.3 Cholesterol and the steroids

As can be seen from Figure 4.13, steroids are chemically completely different from triacylglycerols or phospholipids. The parent compound of all the steroids in the body is cholesterol; different steroids are then formed by replacing one or more of the hydrogens with hydroxyl groups or oxo-groups, and in some cases by shortening the side-chain.

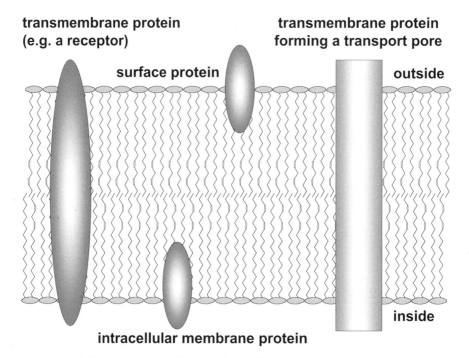

transmembrane protein
(e.g. a receptor)
transmembrane protein
forming a transport pore
surface protein
outside
inside
intracellular membrane protein

FIGURE 4.12 *The arrangement of phospholipids in cell membranes.*

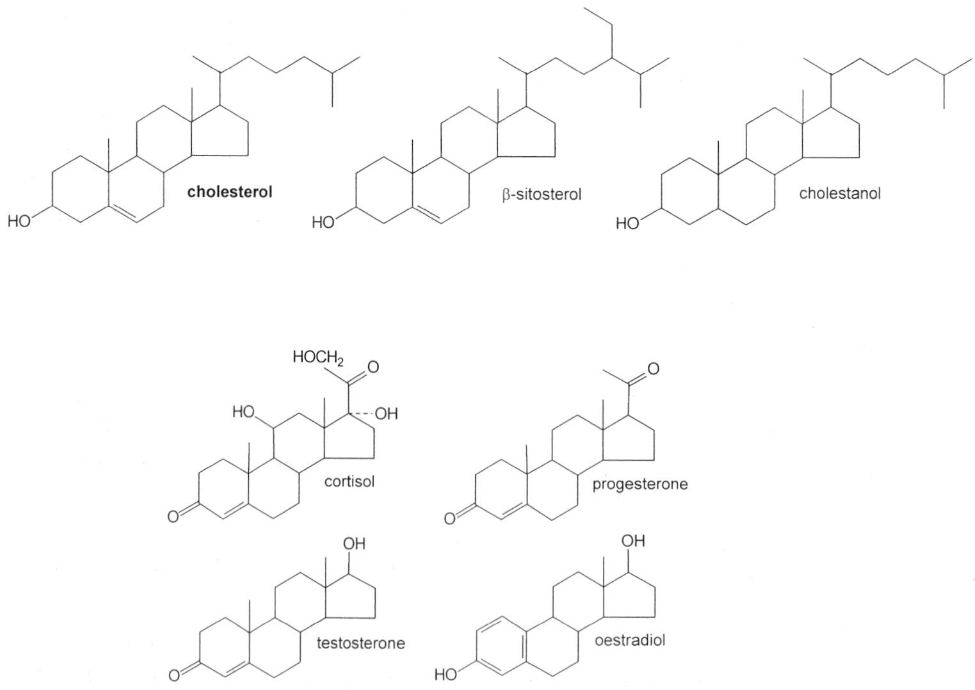

HO
cholesterol
HO
β-sitosterol
HO
cholestanol
HOCH2
O
HO
OH
cortisol
O
O
progesterone
O
OH
testosterone
O
OH
oestradiol
HO

FIGURE 4.13 *Cholesterol and some steroid hormones.*

Apart from cholesterol, which is important in membrane structure and the synthesis of bile salts (section 4.4.3.2.1), the steroids are slow-acting hormones (section 10.4). Vitamin D (section 11.3) is a derivative of cholesterol, and can also be considered to be a steroid hormone.

The cholesterol that is required for membrane synthesis, and the very much smaller amount that is required for the synthesis of steroid hormones, may either be synthesized in the body or provided by the diet; average intakes are of the order of 500 mg (1.3 mmol)/day.

An elevated plasma concentration of cholesterol (in low-density lipoproteins) is a risk factor for atherosclerosis and ischaemic heart disease. As discussed in section 7.3.2.1, the dietary intake of cholesterol is less important as a determinant of plasma cholesterol than is the intake of total and saturated fat, or the intake of compounds that inhibit the reabsorption of cholesterol secreted in bile, or the reabsorption of bile salts themselves (section 4.3.2.1).

4.3.2 DIGESTION AND ABSORPTION OF TRIACYLGLYCEROLS

The digestion of triacylglycerols begins with lipase secreted by the tongue; as discussed in section 1.3.3.1, lingual lipase may be important in permitting the detection of fat in the diet, and hence in determining food choices. It continues in the stomach, where gastric lipase is secreted. As shown in Figure 4.14, hydrolysis of the fatty acids esterified to carbons 1 and 3 of the triacylglycerol results in the liberation of free fatty acids and 2-monoacylglycerol. These have both hydrophobic and hydrophilic regions, and will therefore emulsify the lipid into increasingly small droplets. Triacylglycerol hydrolysis continues in the small intestine, catalysed by pancreatic lipase, which requires a further pancreatic protein, colipase, for activity. Monoacylglycerols are hydrolysed to glycerol and free fatty acids by pancreatic esterase in the intestinal lumen and intracellular lipase within intestinal mucosal cells.

4.3.2.1 Bile salts

The final emulsification of dietary lipids into micelles (droplets that are small enough to be absorbed across the intestinal mucosa) is achieved by the action of the bile salts. The bile salts are synthesized from cholesterol in the liver, and secreted, together with phospholipids and cholesterol, by the gall bladder. As shown in Figure 4.15, some 2 g of cholesterol and 30 g of bile salts are secreted by the gall bladder each day, almost all of which is reabsorbed, so that the total faecal output of steroids and bile salts is 0.2–1 g/day.

The primary bile salts (those synthesized in the liver) are conjugates of chenodeoxycholic acid and cholic acid with taurine or glycine (Figure 4.16). Intestinal bacteria catalyse deconjugation and further metabolism to yield the secondary bile

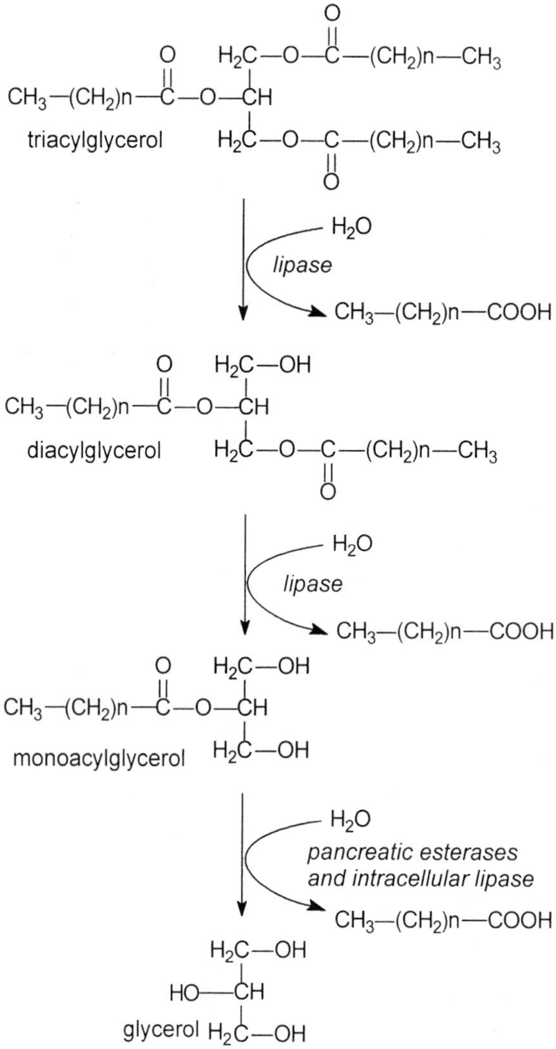

FIGURE 4.14 *Lipase and the hydrolysis of triacylglycerol.*

salts, lithocholic and deoxycholic acids. These are also absorbed from the gut, and are reconjugated in the liver and secreted in the bile.

Both cholesterol and the bile salts can be bound physically by non-starch polysaccharide (section 4.2.1.6) in the gut lumen, so that they cannot be reabsorbed. This is the basis of the cholesterol-lowering effect of moderately high intakes of non-starch polysaccharide (section 7.3.3.2) – if the bile salts are not reabsorbed and reutilized, then there will be further synthesis from cholesterol in the liver, so depleting body cholesterol.

Under normal conditions, the concentration of cholesterol in bile, relative to that of bile salts and phospholipids, is such that cholesterol is at or near its limit of solubility.

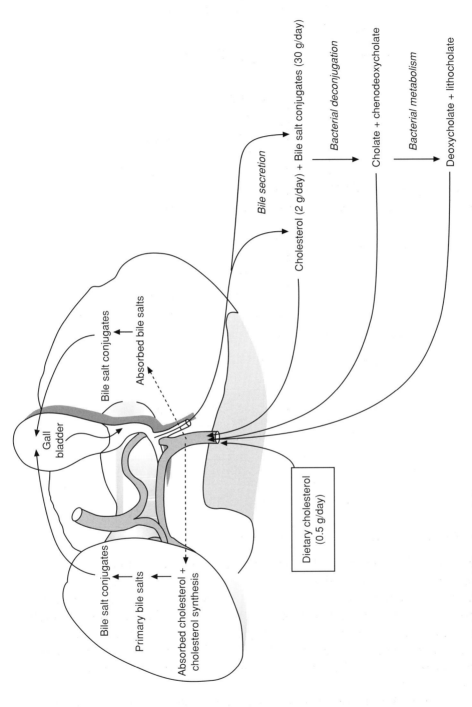

FIGURE 4.15 *Cholesterol and bile salt metabolism.*

Gall bladder

Bile salt conjugates

Absorbed bile salts

Bile salt conjugates

Primary bile salts

Absorbed cholesterol + cholesterol synthesis

Dietary cholesterol (0.5 g/day)

Bile secretion

Cholesterol (2 g/day) + Bile salt conjugates (30 g/day)

Bacterial deconjugation

Cholate + chenodeoxycholate

Bacterial metabolism

Deoxycholate + lithocholate

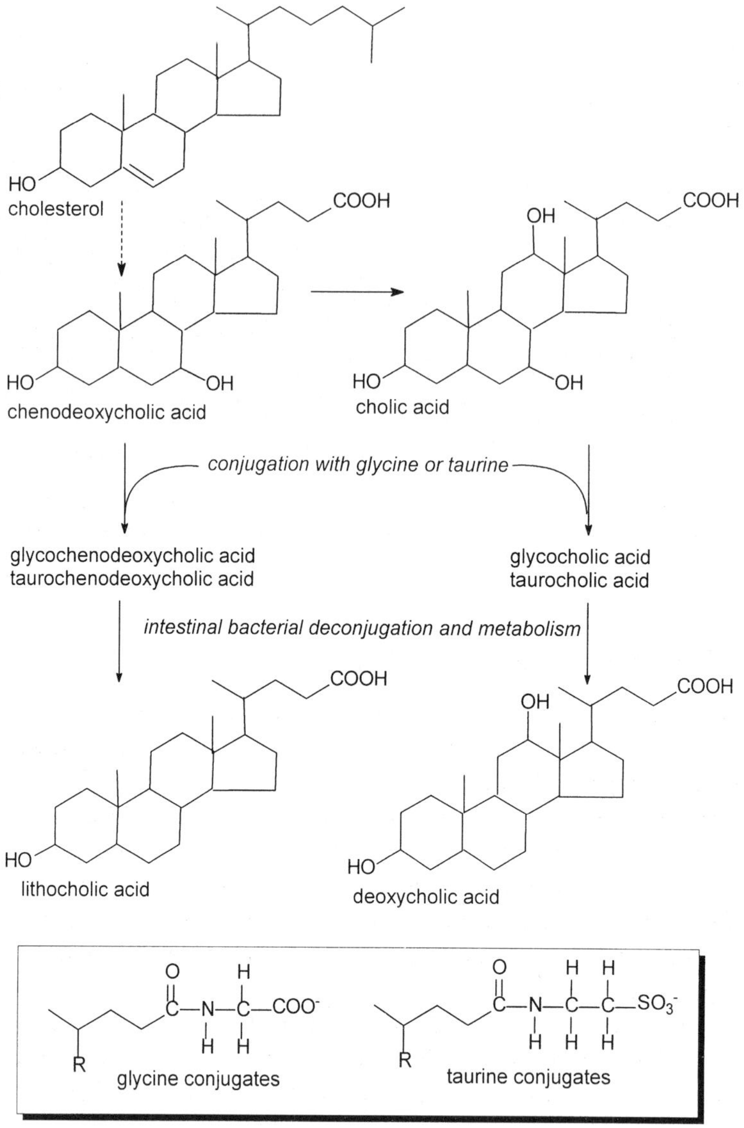

FIGURE 4.16 *The metabolism of bile salts.*

It requires only a relatively small increase in the concentration of cholesterol in bile for it to crystallize out, resulting in the formation of gallstones. Obesity (section 6.2.2) and high-fat diets (especially diets high in saturated fat, which increase the synthesis of cholesterol in the liver) are associated with a considerably increased incidence of gallstones. Figure 4.17 shows the increased risk of developing gallstones with increasing obesity.

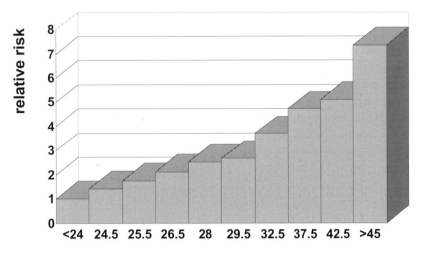

FIGURE 4.17 *The incidence of gallstones with obesity {body mass index = weight (in kg)/height (in m)^2; the desirable range is 20–25}. From data reported by Stampfer MJ et al.,* American Journal of Clinical Nutrition *55: 652–658, 1992.*

4.3.2.2 Lipid absorption and chylomicrons

The finely emulsified lipid micelles, containing free fatty acids with small amounts of intact triacylglycerol, monoacylglycerol, phospholipids, cholesterol and fat-soluble vitamins (see Chapter 11) are absorbed across the intestinal wall into the mucosal cells. Here, fatty acids are re-esterified to form triacylglycerols (see Figure 5.28), and are packaged together with proteins synthesized in the mucosal cells to form chylomicrons. These are secreted into the lacteal in the centre of the villus (see Figure 4.2), and enter the lymphatic system, which drains into the bloodstream at the thoracic duct. See section 5.6.2.1 for a discussion of the metabolism of chylomicrons and other plasma lipoproteins.

In the fed state, in response to the action of insulin (section 10.5) lipoprotein lipase is active at the surface of cells in adipose tissue. It catalyses the hydrolysis of triacylglycerols in chylomicrons, and most of the resultant free fatty acid is taken up by adipose tissue for re-esterification to triacylglycerol for storage. The chylomicron remnants are taken up by the liver, by a process of receptor-mediated endocytosis (section 5.6.2), and most of the residual lipid is secreted, together with triacylglycerol synthesised in the liver, in very low-density lipoproteins (section 5.6.2.2).

4.4 *Digestion and absorption of proteins*

Proteins are large polymers. Unlike starch and glycogen, which are polymers of only a single type of monomer unit (glucose), proteins consist of a variety of amino acids.

There is an almost infinite variety of proteins, composed of different numbers of the different amino acids (between 50 and 1,000 amino acids in a single protein molecule), in different order. There are some 30–50,000 different proteins and polypeptides in the human body. Each protein has a specific sequence of amino acids.

Small proteins have a relative molecular mass of about $50–100 \times 10^3$, whereas some of the large complex proteins have a relative molecular mass of up to 10^6. In addition to proteins, smaller polymers of amino acids, containing up to about 50 amino acids, are important in the regulation of metabolism. Collectively these are known as polypeptides.

4.4.1 THE AMINO ACIDS

Twenty-one amino acids are involved in the synthesis of proteins, together with a number that occur in proteins as a result of chemical modification after the protein has been synthesized. In addition, a number of amino acids occur as metabolic intermediates but are not involved in proteins.

Chemically the amino acids all have the same basic structure – an amino group ($-NH_2$) and a carboxylic acid group ($-COOH$) attached to the same carbon atom (the α-carbon). As shown in Figure 4.18, what differs between the amino acids is the nature of the other group that is attached to the α-carbon. In the simplest amino acid, glycine, there are two hydrogen atoms, while in all other amino acids there is one hydrogen atom and a side-chain, varying in chemical complexity from the simple methyl group ($-CH_3$) of alanine to the aromatic ring structures of phenylalanine, tyrosine and tryptophan. Figure 4.18 does not show the structure of the 21st amino acid, the selenium analogue of cysteine, selenocysteine (section 11.15.2.5).

The amino acids can be classified according to the chemical nature of the side-chain, whether it is hydrophobic (on the left of Figure 4.18) or hydrophilic (on the right of Figure 4.18), and the nature of the group:

- small hydrophobic amino acids: glycine, alanine, proline;
- branched-chain amino acids: leucine, isoleucine, valine;
- aromatic amino acids: phenylalanine, tyrosine, tryptophan;
- sulphur-containing amino acids: cysteine, methionine;
- neutral hydrophilic amino acids: serine and threonine;
- acidic amino acids: glutamic and aspartic acids (the salts of these acids are glutamate and aspartate respectively);
- amides of the acidic amino acids: glutamine and asparagine;
- basic amino acids: lysine, arginine, histidine.

4.4.2 PROTEIN STRUCTURE AND DENATURATION

Proteins are composed of linear chains of amino acids, joined by condensation of the

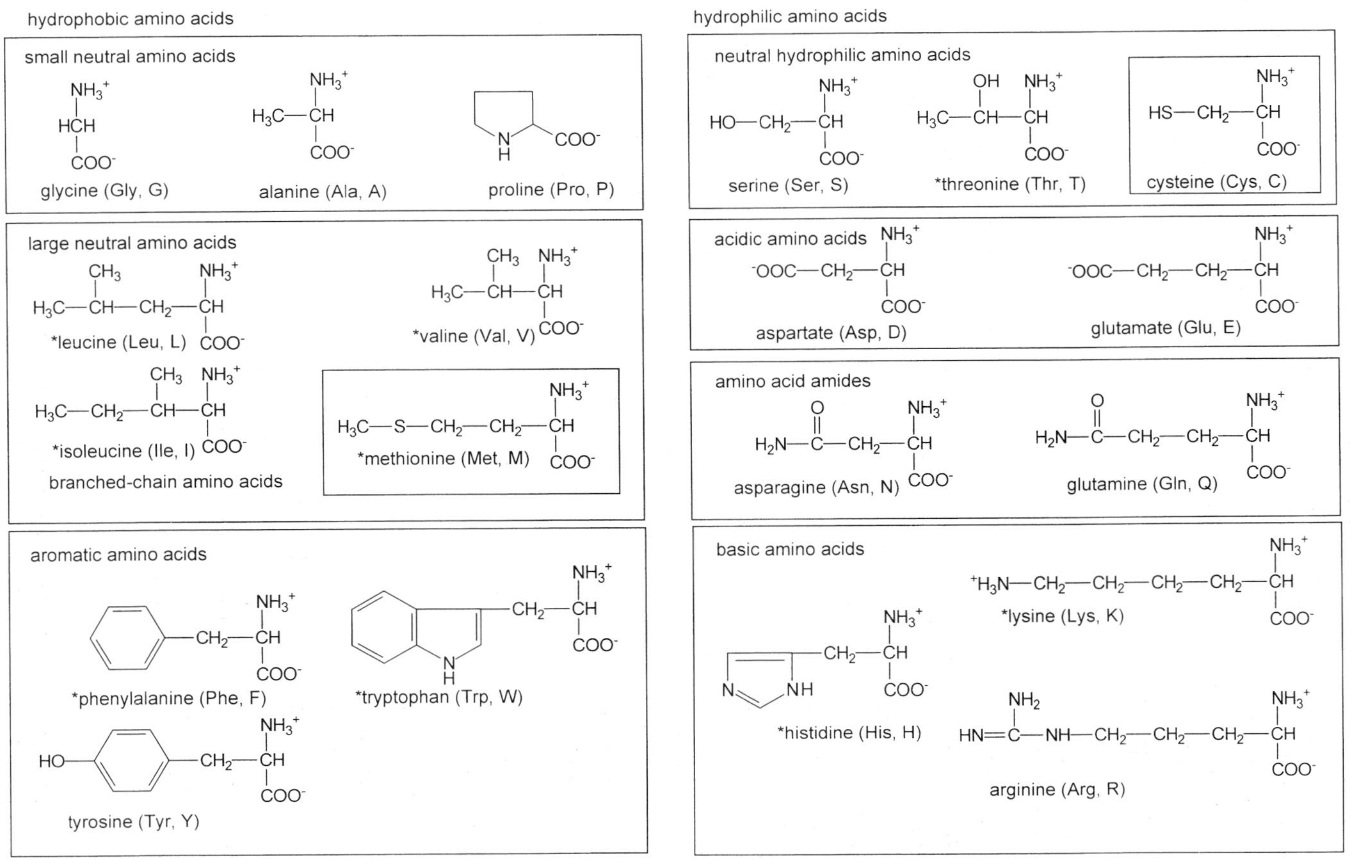

FIGURE 4.18 *The amino acids, showing their three-letter and single-letter codes. *Essential dietary amino acids that cannot be synthesized in the body.*

carboxyl group of one with the amino group of another, to form a peptide bond (Figure 4.19). Chains of amino acids linked in this way are known as polypeptides.

The sequence of amino acids in a protein is its primary structure. It is different for each protein, although proteins that are closely related to each other often have similar primary structures. The primary structure of a protein is determined by the gene containing the information for that protein (section 9.2).

4.4.2.1 Secondary structure of proteins

Polypeptide chains fold up in a variety of ways. Two main types of chemical interaction are responsible for this folding: hydrogen bonds between the oxygen of one peptide bond and the nitrogen of another (Figure 4.20) and interactions between the side-chains of the amino acids. Depending on the nature of the side-chains, different regions of the chain may fold into one of the following patterns:

- α-Helix, in which the peptide backbone of the protein adopts a spiral (helix) form. The hydrogen bonds are formed between peptide bonds which are near each other in the primary sequence.
- β-Pleated sheet, in which regions of the polypeptide chain lie alongside one another, forming a 'corrugated' or pleated surface. The hydrogen bonds are between peptide bonds in different parts of the primary sequence, and the regions of polypeptide chain forming a pleated sheet may run parallel or antiparallel.

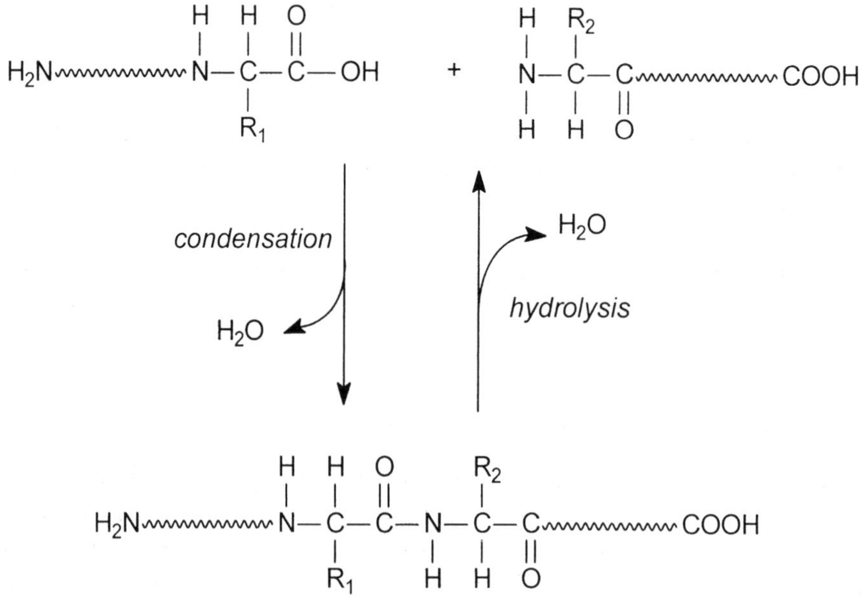

FIGURE 4.19 *Condensation of amino acids to form a peptide bond.*

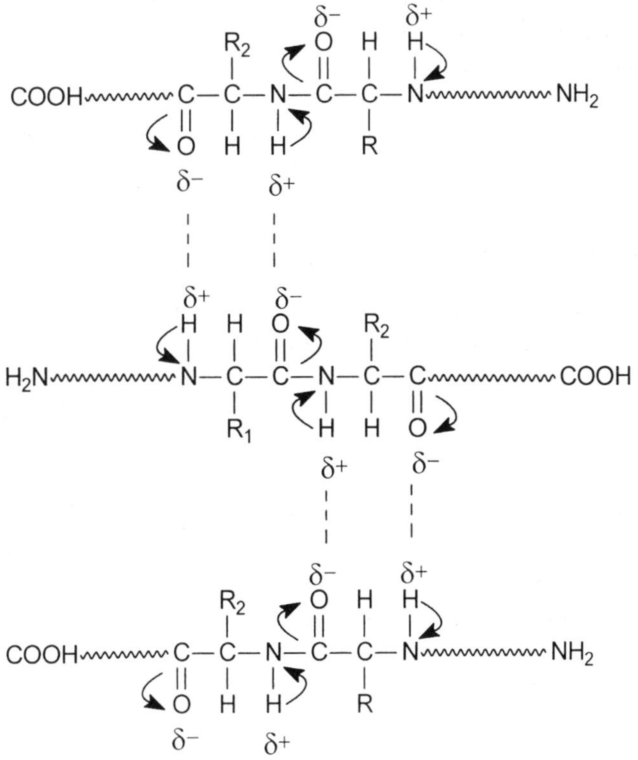

FIGURE 4.20 *Hydrogen bonds between peptide bonds in a peptide chain.*

- Hairpins and loops, in which small regions of the polypeptide chain form very tight bends;
- Random coil, in which there is no recognizable organized structure. Although this appears to be random, for any one protein the shape of a random coil region will always be the same.

A protein may have several regions of α-helix, β-pleated sheet (with the peptide chains running parallel or antiparallel), hairpins and random coil, all in the same molecule.

4.4.2.2 Tertiary and quaternary structures of proteins

Having formed regions of secondary structure, the whole protein molecule then folds up into a compact shape. This is the third (tertiary) level of structure and is largely the result of interactions between the side-chains of the amino acids, both with each other and with the environment. Proteins in an aqueous medium in the cell generally adopt a tertiary structure in which hydrophobic amino acid side-chains are inside the molecule and can interact with each other, whereas hydrophilic side-chains are exposed to interact with water. By contrast, proteins which are embedded in membranes (see Figure 4.12) have a hydrophobic region on the outside, to interact with the membrane lipids.

Two further interactions between amino acid side-chains may be involved in tertiary structure, in this case forming covalent links between regions of the peptide chain (Figure 4.21):

- The ε-amino group on the side-chain of lysine can form a peptide bond with the carboxyl group on the side-chain of aspartate or glutamate. This is nutritionally important, as the side-chain peptide bond is not hydrolysed by digestive enzymes, and the lysine, which is an essential amino acid (section 9.1.3), is not available for absorption.
- The sulphydryl (–SH) groups of two cysteine molecules may be oxidized, to form a disulphide bridge between two parts of the protein chain.

Some proteins consist of more than one polypeptide chain; the way in which the chains interact with each other after they have separately formed their secondary and tertiary structures is the quaternary structure of the protein. Interactions between the subunits of multi-subunit proteins, involving changes in quaternary structure and the conformation of the protein, affecting activity, are important in a number of regulatory enzymes (sections 2.3.3.3 and 10.2.1).

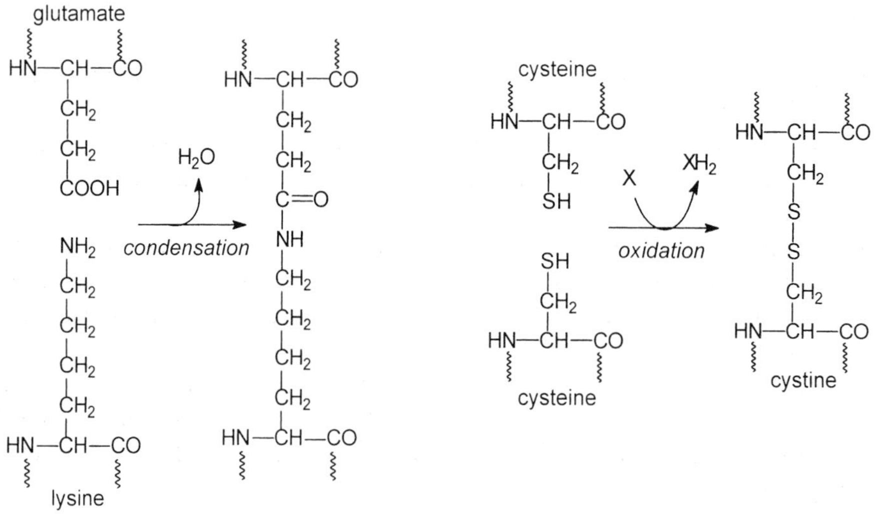

FIGURE 4.21 *Covalent links between peptide chains – on the left a side-chain peptide between the ε-amino group of lysine and the γ-carboxyl group of glutamate; on the right a disulphide bridge formed by oxidation of two cysteine residues.*

4.4.2.3 Denaturation of proteins

Because of their secondary and tertiary structures, most proteins are resistant to digestive enzymes – few bonds are accessible to the proteolytic enzymes that catalyse hydrolysis of peptide bonds. However, apart from covalent links formed by reaction between the side-chains of lysine and aspartate or glutamate, and disulphide bridges, the native structure of proteins is maintained by relatively weak non-covalent forces: ionic interactions, hydrogen bonding and van der Waals forces.

Like all molecules, proteins vibrate, and as the temperature increases so the vibration increases. Eventually, this vibration disrupts the weak non-covalent forces that hold the protein in its organized structure. When this happens, proteins frequently become insoluble. This is the process of denaturation – a loss of the native structure of the protein. In denatured proteins most of the peptide bonds are accessible to digestive enzymes, and consequently denatured (i.e. cooked) proteins are more readily hydrolysed to their constituent amino acids. Gastric acid is also important, as relatively strong acid will also disrupt hydrogen bonds and denature proteins.

4.4.3 PROTEIN DIGESTION

Protein digestion occurs by hydrolysis of the peptide bonds between amino acids. There are two main classes of protein digestive enzymes (proteases), with different specificities for the amino acids forming the peptide bond to be hydrolysed, as shown in Table 4.2:

- *Endopeptidases* cleave proteins by hydrolysing peptide bonds between specific amino acids throughout the molecule.
- *Exopeptidases* remove amino acids one at a time from either the amino or carboxyl end of the molecule, again by the hydrolysis of the peptide bond.

The first enzymes to act on dietary proteins are the endopeptidases: pepsin in the gastric juice and trypsin, chymotrypsin and elastase secreted by the pancreas into the small intestine. (The different specificities of trypsin, chymotrypsin and elastase are discussed in section 2.2.1.)

The result of the combined action of the endopeptidases is that the large protein molecules are broken down into a number of smaller polypeptides with a large number of amino and carboxy terminals for the exopeptidases to act on. There are two classes of exopeptidase:

- Carboxypeptidases, secreted in the pancreatic juice, release amino acids from the free carboxyl terminal of peptides.
- Aminopeptidases, secreted by the intestinal mucosal cells, release amino acids from the amino terminal of peptides.

TABLE 4.2 *Protein digestive enzymes*

	Secreted by	**Specificity**
Endopeptidases		
Pepsin	Gastric mucosa	Adjacent to aromatic amino acid, leucine or methionine
Trypsin	Pancreas	Lysine or arginine esters
Chymotrypsin	Pancreas	Aromatic esters
Elastase	Pancreas	Neutral aliphatic esters
Enteropeptidase	Intestinal mucosa	Trypsinogen $\rightarrow$ trypsin
Exopeptidases		
Carboxypeptidases	Pancreas	Carboxy-terminal amino acids
Aminopeptidases	Intestinal mucosa	Amino-terminal amino acids
Tripeptidases	Mucosal brush border	Tripeptides
Dipeptidases	Mucosal brush border	Dipeptides

4.4.3.1 Activation of zymogens of proteolytic enzymes

The proteases are secreted as inactive precursors (zymogens) – this is essential if they are not to digest themselves and tissue proteins before they are secreted. In each case the active site of the enzyme is masked by a small region of the peptide chain which has to be removed for the enzyme to have activity. This is achieved by hydrolysis of a specific peptide bond in the precursor molecule, releasing the blocking peptide and revealing the active site of the enzyme.

Pepsin is secreted in the gastric juice as pepsinogen, which is activated by the action of gastric acid, and also by the action of already activated pepsin. In the small intestine, trypsinogen, the precursor of trypsin, is activated by the action of a specific enzyme, enteropeptidase (sometimes known by its obsolete name of enterokinase), which is secreted by the duodenal epithelial cells; trypsin can then activate chymotrypsinogen to chymotrypsin, proelastase to elastase, procarboxypeptidase to carboxypeptidase and proaminopeptidase to aminopeptidase.

4.4.3.2 Absorption of the products of protein digestion

The end-product of the action of endopeptidases and exopeptidases is a mixture of free amino acids, di- and tripeptides and oligopeptides, all of which are absorbed:
*   Free amino acids are absorbed across the intestinal mucosa by sodium-dependent active transport, as occurs in the absorption of glucose and galactose (see Figure 4.9). There are a number of different amino acid transport systems with specificity for the chemical nature of the side-chain (large or small neutral, acidic or basic – see Figure 4.18). Similar group-specific amino acid transporters occur in the renal tubules (for reabsorption of amino acids filtered at the glomerulus) and for uptake

of amino acids into tissues. The various amino acids carried by any one transporter compete with each other for absorption and tissue uptake.

- Dipeptides and tripeptides enter the brush border of the intestinal mucosal cells, where they are hydrolysed to free amino acids, which are then transported into the bloodstream.
- Relatively large peptides may be absorbed intact, either by uptake into mucosal epithelial cells (the transcellular route) or by passing between epithelial cells (the paracellular route). Many such peptides are large enough to stimulate antibody formation – this is the basis of allergic reactions to foods.

4.5 *The absorption of minerals*

Most minerals are absorbed by carrier-mediated diffusion into intestinal mucosal cells and accumulated by binding to intracellular proteins. There is then sodium-dependent active transport from the epithelial cells into the bloodstream, where again they are usually bound to transport proteins. Genetic defects of the intracellular binding proteins or the active transport systems at the basal membrane of the mucosal cell can result in functional deficiency despite an apparently adequate intake of the mineral.

The absorption of many minerals is affected by other compounds present in the intestinal lumen. As discussed in section 4.5.1, a number of reducing compounds can enhance the absorption of iron, and a number of chelating compounds enhance the absorption of other minerals. For example, zinc absorption is dependent on the secretion by the pancreas of a zinc-binding ligand (tentatively identified as the tryptophan metabolite picolinic acid). Failure to synthesize and secrete this zinc-binding ligand as a result of a genetic disease leads to the condition of acrodermatitis enteropathica – functional zinc deficiency despite an apparently adequate intake.

Diets based on unleavened wheat bread contain a relatively large amount of phytic acid (inositol hexaphosphate), which can bind calcium, iron and zinc to form insoluble complexes that are not absorbed. Phytases in yeast catalyse dephosphorylation of phytate to products that do not chelate the minerals.

Polyphenols (section 7.5.2.3), and especially tannic acid in tea, can also chelate iron and other minerals, reducing their absorption, and large amounts of free fatty acids in the gut lumen (associated with defects of fat absorption; section 4.3.2) can impair the absorption of calcium and magnesium, forming insoluble soaps.

4.5.1 IRON ABSORPTION

Only about 10% of dietary iron is absorbed, and only as little as 1–5% of that in many plant foods. As discussed in section 11.15.2.3, iron deficiency is a serious problem; some 10–15% of women of child-bearing age have menstrual iron losses greater than can be met from a normal dietary intake. Haem iron in meat is absorbed better than is inorganic iron from plant foods, and by a separate transport system.

Inorganic iron is absorbed only in the Fe^{2+} (reduced) form. This means that a variety of reducing agents present in the intestinal lumen together with dietary iron will enhance its absorption. The most effective such compound is vitamin C (section 11.14.4.1) and, although intakes of 40–60 mg of vitamin C per day are more than adequate to meet requirements, an intake of 25–50 mg per meal is sometimes recommended to enhance iron absorption. Alcohol and fructose also enhance iron absorption.

Like other minerals, iron enters the mucosal cells by carrier-mediated passive diffusion and is accumulated in the cells by binding to a protein, ferritin. Once all the ferritin in the mucosal cell is saturated with iron, no more can be taken up from the gut lumen. Iron can leave the mucosal cell only if there is free transferrin in plasma for it to bind to and, once plasma ferritin is saturated with iron, any that has accumulated in the mucosal cells will be lost back into the intestinal lumen when the cells are shed at the tip of the villus (section 4.1).

The mucosal barrier to the absorption of iron has a protective function. Iron overload is a serious condition, leading to deposition of inappropriately large amounts of iron in tissues, and about 10% of the population are genetically susceptible to iron overload. Once the normal tissue iron-binding proteins are saturated, free iron ions will accumulate in tissues. As discussed in section 7.4.2.4, iron ions in solution are able to generate tissue-damaging oxygen radicals, and this may be a factor in the development of cardiovascular disease and some forms of cancer. Indeed, one of the reasons why women are less at risk of atherosclerosis than men may be that women generally have a lower iron status than men because of menstrual blood losses.

This raises the interesting problem of whether or not it is desirable to recommend high intakes of iron for women of child-bearing age in order to raise their iron reserves to the same level as seen in men. This would prevent the development of iron deficiency but might also put them at risk of iron overload and increased risk of atherosclerosis.

Additional resources

PowerPoint presentation 4 on the CD.
Self-assessment quiz 4 on the CD.

The simulation program Peptide Sequence on the CD lets you sequence a small peptide by a variety of methods, as an example of the way in which we can exploit the specificity of different proteolytic enzymes.

PROBLEM 4.1: *Measurement of urine glucose*

As discussed in section 4.2.1.4, glucose in plasma and urine can be determined in two ways, using an alkaline copper reagent or using glucose oxidase linked to a dyestuff. Both methods were used to determine urine glucose in six people:

A   a person with hitherto undiagnosed diabetes mellitus (section 10.7);

B   a known diabetic patient, with poor glycaemic control, taking supplements of 500 mg of vitamin C per day;

C   a non-diabetic subject taking supplements of 500 mg of vitamin C per day;

D   a person with idiopathic pentosuria (excretion of five-carbon sugars in the urine);

E   a person with idiopathic pentosuria taking supplements of 500 mg of vitamin C per day;

F   a non-diabetic subject taking no supplements.

Which subjects would be expected to give the following results?

- positive using glucose oxidase, positive using alkaline copper reagent;
- positive using glucose oxidase, negative using alkaline copper reagent;
- negative using glucose oxidase, positive using alkaline copper reagent;
- negative using glucose oxidase, negative using alkaline copper reagent.

PROBLEM 4.2: *Ahmed L*

Figure 4.22 shows the results of measuring blood glucose in a group of people after a test dose of 50 g of lactose taken at 08:30 h, before they had eaten breakfast. The two solid lines show the range of results obtained for 10 of the subjects; the dotted line marked with squares shows the results for one subject, Ahmed L.

Can you explain why Ahmed L's results were so different from the others?

About 15 minutes after the test dose of lactose, Ahmed developed severe abdominal pain and had frequent bouts of explosive watery diarrhoea, which persisted for about 2 hours. Can you account for this?

A number of papers in gastroenterological journals have reported fatal explosions during endoscopic removal of colorectal polyps using a heated wire when the gut had been prepared for surgery using an oral dose of the sugar alcohol mannitol (section 4.2.1.2) and it was insufflated with air. How does mannitol prepare the gut for surgery? What caused the explosions?

Very rarely, infants lack lactase, as a result of a genetic defect, and therefore are severely lactose intolerant. They cannot tolerate breast milk or normal infant formula, and have to be fed on special lactose-free formula.

Relatively commonly, people lose intestinal lactase in late adolescence or early

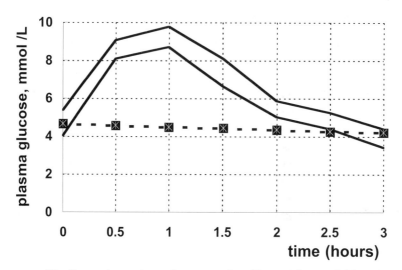

FIGURE 4.22 *The effect on plasma glucose of a 50 g test dose of lactose. The two solid lines show the range of results obtained for 10 of the subjects; the dotted line marked with squares shows the results for one subject, Ahmed L.*

TABLE 4.3 *Lactose intolerance in different population groups*

Population group or country of study	Per cent lactose intolerant
UK white	4.7
Northern Germany*	7.5
Tuareg (nomads of the central Sahara)	12.7
Western Austria*	15.0
Southern Germany*	23.0
Eastern Austria*	25.0
US black	26.2
Turkey	71.2
Sri Lankan	72.5
Italy	75.0
Greece	75.0
South African black	78.0
Japan	89.0
Singapore-born Chinese	92.4
Canadian-born Chinese	97.9
Papua New Guinea	98.0

*The populations of eastern and western Austria are of different origin, as are the populations of northern and southern Germany.

adulthood, and become progressively lactose intolerant. Frequently, they present with a history of abdominal discomfort and diarrhoea. Careful questioning may reveal that this occurs especially after drinking milk, but commonly it is necessary to test their response to a test dose of lactose. As noted above, the classical method was to give a 50 g dose of lactose and measure the glycaemic response – Ahmed L suffered considerable discomfort during this test.

A number of workers have used measurement of hydrogen in exhaled air after a small test dose of lactose as a less unpleasant way of detecting lactose intolerance. Can you explain how measuring breath hydrogen can give information about lactose digestion?

A number of studies have been performed to determine lactose tolerance in adults from different populations; some of the results are shown in Table 4.3. What conclusions can you draw from the results in Table 4.3?

PROBLEM 4.3: *Eddie H*

At the age of 12 Eddie H was referred to the paediatric outpatient clinic at the Middlesex Hospital in early June, suffering from a severe sunburn-like red scaly rash on exposed areas of his skin. His mother said that she thought he was suffering from pellagra (section 11.8.4). His older sister, now aged 20, had been treated for pellagra some 10 years previously.

At the time he had a number of neurological signs that are not characteristic of pellagra. He had an unsteady gait, jerky arm movements and intention tremor. He also showed nystagmus and complained of double vision. His mother stated that several times during childhood he had suffered similar attacks, usually associated with the common winter-time illnesses such as flu, measles and mumps. He had always made a complete recovery after such attacks, which had not been associated with the pellagra-like rash.

A diet history showed that Eddie had a normal, and apparently adequate, intake of tryptophan and niacin. Therefore, dietary deficiency seemed improbable.

Chromatography revealed excretion of a number of amino acids in his urine, with abnormally high concentrations of tryptophan, phenylalanine, tyrosine, leucine, isoleucine and valine. His urine also contained relatively high concentrations of a number of indolic compounds, including indoxyl sulphate (indican), indolyllactate, indolylacetate, indolylacetamide and indolylacetylglutamine, which are not detectable in the urine of normal subjects.

Figure 4.23 shows the effect on Eddie's plasma tryptophan of giving him an oral or intravenous dose of tryptophan of 0.5 mmol/kg body weight, or an equivalent amount of tryptophanyl-glycine by mouth. What conclusions can you draw from this information?

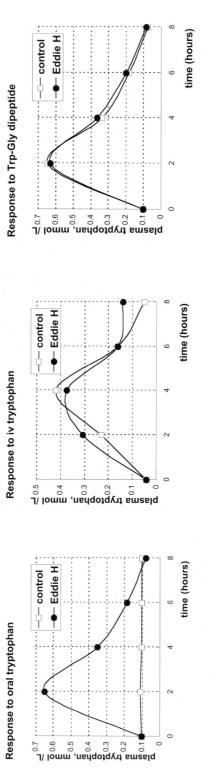

FIGURE 4.23 *The response of plasma tryptophan to 0.5 mmol oral or intravenous tryptophan per kilogram body weight, and to an oral dose of 0.5 mmol/kg body weight tryptophanyl-glycine dipeptide. From data reported by Baron DN et al. (1956) Lancet ii: 421–428.*

5

Energy nutrition – the metabolism of carbohydrates and fats

If the intake of metabolic fuels is equivalent to energy expenditure, there is a state of energy balance. Overall, there will be equal periods of fed-state metabolism (during which nutrient reserves are accumulated as liver and muscle glycogen, adipose tissue triacylglycerols and labile protein stores) and fasting-state metabolism, during which these reserves are utilized. Averaged out, certainly over several days, there will be no change in body weight or body composition.

By contrast, if the intake of metabolic fuels is greater than is required to meet energy expenditure, the body will spend more time in the fed state than the fasting state; there will be more accumulation of nutrient reserves than utilization. The result of this is an increase in body size, and especially an increase in adipose tissue stores. If continued for long enough, this will result in overweight or obesity, with potentially serious health consequences – see Chapter 6.

The opposite state of affairs is when the intake of metabolic fuels is lower than is required to meet energy expenditure. Now the body has to mobilize its nutrient reserves, and overall spends more time in the fasting state than in the fed state. The result of this is undernutrition, starvation and eventually death – see Chapter 8.

Objectives

After reading this chapter you should be able to:

*   define the terms used in energy metabolism, and explain how energy expenditure is measured;
*   describe the sources of metabolic fuels in the fed and fasting states;
*   describe and explain the relationship between energy intake, energy expenditure and body weight;
*   describe the pathway of glycolysis and explain how anaerobic glycolysis under conditions of maximum exertion leads to oxygen debt;
*   describe the pentose phosphate pathway and explain how deficiency of glucose 6-phosphate dehydrogenase results in haemolytic crises;
*   describe the metabolic fates of pyruvate arising from glycolysis;
*   describe the citric acid cycle and explain its role as a central energy-yielding pathway and in the interconversion of metabolites;
*   explain the importance of carnitine in fatty acid uptake into mitochondria, and describe the β-oxidation of fatty acids;
*   describe the formation and utilization of ketone bodies and explain their importance in fasting and starvation;.
*   describe the synthesis of fatty acids and triacylglycerol as a major energy reserve, and explain the importance of plasma lipoproteins;
*   describe the synthesis and utilization of glycogen and the pathways for gluconeogenesis in the fasting state.

5.1 *Estimation of energy expenditure*

Energy expenditure can be determined directly, by measuring heat output from the body. This requires a thermally insulated chamber, in which the temperature can be controlled so as to maintain the subject's comfort and in which it is possible to measure the amount of heat produced – for example by the increase in temperature of water used to cool the chamber. Calorimeters of this sort are relatively small, so that it is only possible for measurements of direct heat production to be made for subjects performing a limited range of tasks, and only for a relatively short time. Most estimates of energy expenditure are based on indirect measurements – either measurement of oxygen consumption and carbon dioxide production (indirect calorimetry; section 5.1.1) or indirect assessment of carbon dioxide production by use of dual isotopically labelled water (section 5.1.2). From the results of a number of studies in which energy expenditure in different activities has been measured, it is possible to calculate total energy expenditure from the time spent in each type of activity (section 5.1.3).

5.1.1 INDIRECT CALORIMETRY AND THE RESPIRATORY QUOTIENT

Energy expenditure can be determined from the rate of consumption of oxygen. This is known as indirect calorimetry, as there is no direct measurement of the heat produced. As shown in Table 5.1, there is an output or expenditure of 20 kJ per litre of oxygen consumed, regardless of whether the fuel being metabolized is carbohydrate, fat or protein. Measurement of oxygen consumption is quite simple using a spirometer. Such instruments are portable, so people can carry on more or less normal activities for several hours at a time, while their energy expenditure is being estimated.

Measurement of oxygen consumption and carbon dioxide production at the same time, again a simple procedure using a spirometer, provides information on the mixture of metabolic fuels being metabolized. In the metabolism of starch, the same amount of carbon dioxide is produced as oxygen is consumed, i.e. the ratio of carbon dioxide produced to oxygen consumed (the respiratory quotient) $= 1.0$. This is because the overall reaction is $C_6H_{12}O_6 + 6O_2 \rightarrow 6CO_2 + 6H_2O$.

Proportionally more oxygen is required for the oxidation of fat. The major process involved is the oxidation of $-CH_2-$ units: $-CH_2 + 1\frac{1}{2} O_2 \rightarrow CO_2 + H_2O$. Allowing for the fact that in triacylglycerols there are also the glycerol and three carboxyl groups to be considered, overall for the oxidation of fat the respiratory quotient $= 0.7$.

The metabolism of proteins gives a ratio of carbon dioxide produced to oxygen consumed that is intermediate between that of carbohydrate and fat – this is because proteins contain relatively more oxygen per carbon than do fats, although less than carbohydrates. For protein metabolism the respiratory quotient $= 0.8$. The amount of protein being oxidized can be determined quite separately, by measurement of the excretion of urea, the end-product of amino acid metabolism (section 9.3.1.4).

Measurement of the respiratory quotient and urinary excretion of urea thus permits calculation of the relative amounts of fat, carbohydrate and protein being metabolized. In the fasting state (section 5.3.2), when a relatively large amount of fat is being used as a fuel, the respiratory quotient is around 0.8–0.85; after a meal, when there is more carbohydrate available to be metabolized (section 5.3.1), the respiratory quotient

TABLE 5.1 *Oxygen consumption and carbon dioxide production in oxidation of metabolic fuels*

	Energy yield (kJ/g)	Oxygen consumed (L/g)	Carbon dioxide produced (L/g)	Respiratory quotient (CO_2/O_2)	Energy/ oxygen consumption (kJ/L oxygen)
Carbohydrate	16	0.829	0.829	1.0	
Protein	17	0.966	0.782	0.809	~ 20
Fat	37	2.016	1.427	0.707	

rises to about 0.9–1.0. If there is a significant amount of lipid being synthesized from carbohydrate (section 5.6.1) then the respiratory quotient may rise above 1.0.

5.1.2 LONG-TERM MEASUREMENT OF ENERGY EXPENDITURE – THE DUAL ISOTOPICALLY LABELLED WATER METHOD

Although indirect calorimetry has considerable advantages over direct calorimetry, it still only permits measurement of energy expenditure over a period of a few hours. A more recent technique permits estimation of total energy expenditure over a period of 1–2 weeks. This method depends on the administration of dual isotopically labelled water, $^2H_2^{18}O$. The rate at which the labelled water is lost from the body is determined by measuring the amounts of these two isotopes in urine or saliva.

The deuterium (^2H) is lost from the body only as water. As shown in Figure 5.1, the labelled oxygen (^{18}O) is lost more rapidly. It can be lost as either water or carbon dioxide, because of the rapid equilibrium between carbon dioxide and bicarbonate: $H_2O + CO_2 \rightleftharpoons H^+ + HCO_3^-$. As all three oxygen atoms in the bicarbonate ion are equivalent, label from $H_2^{18}O$ can be lost in both water and carbon dioxide.

The difference between the rate of loss of the two isotopes from body water (plasma, saliva or urine) thus reflects the total amount of carbon dioxide that has been produced:

$$CO_2 \text{ production} = (0.5 \times \text{total body water})\,(k_O - k_H)$$

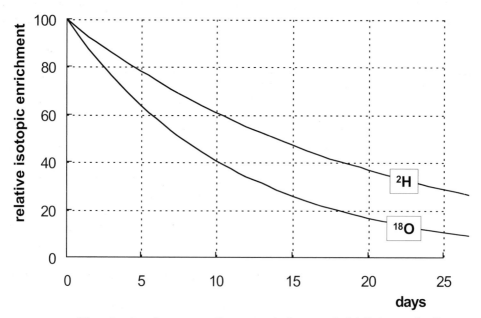

FIGURE 5.1 *The estimation of energy expenditure using dual isotopically labelled water ($^2H_2^{18}O$).*

where k_O = rate constant for loss of label from ^{18}O and k_H = rate constant for loss of label from ^2H.

Estimating the average respiratory quotient over the period from the proportions of fat, carbohydrate and protein in the diet and allowing for any changes in body fat permits calculation of the total amount of oxygen that has been consumed, and hence the total energy expenditure over a period of 2–3 weeks.

5.1.3 CALCULATION OF ENERGY EXPENDITURE

Energy expenditure depends on:

- the requirement for maintenance of normal body structure, function and metabolic integrity – the basal metabolic rate (section 5.1.3.1);
- the energy required for work and physical activity (section 5.1.3.2);
- the energy cost of synthesizing reserves of fat and glycogen and the increase in protein synthesis in the fed state (section 5.1.3.3).

Some common definitions are provided in Table 5.2.

5.1.3.1 Basal metabolic rate (BMR)

Basal metabolic rate is the energy expenditure by the body when at rest, but not asleep, under controlled conditions of thermal neutrality, and about 12 hours after the last meal. It is the energy requirement for the maintenance of metabolic integrity, nerve and muscle tone, circulation and respiration (see Figure 1.2 for the contribution

TABLE 5.2 *Definitions in energy metabolism*

BMR	Basal metabolic rate	Energy expenditure in the post-absorptive state; measured under standardized conditions of thermal neutrality (environmental temperature 26–30 °C) , awake but completely at rest
RMR	Resting metabolic rate	Energy expenditure at rest, not measured under strictly standardized conditions
PAR	Physical activity ratio	Energy cost of physical activity, on a minute by minute basis, expressed as ratio of BMR
IEI	Integrated energy index	Energy cost of an activity over a period of time, including time spent pausing or resting, expressed as the average (integrated) value over the time, as a ratio of BMR
PAL	Physical activity level	Sum of PAR or IEI × time spent in each activity over 24 hours, expressed as ratio of BMR
DIT	Diet-induced thermogenesis	Increased energy expenditure after a meal
TEE	Total energy expenditure	PAL × BMR (+ DIT)

of different organs to BMR). It is important that the subject is awake, as some people show an increased metabolic rate (and hence increased heat output), while others have a reduced metabolic rate and a slight fall in body temperature, when asleep. Where the measurement of metabolic rate has been made under less strictly controlled conditions, the result is more correctly called the resting metabolic rate.

Figure 5.2 shows the variation of BMR with body weight, age and gender:

- Body weight affects BMR because there is a greater amount of metabolically active tissue in a larger body.
- The decrease in BMR with increasing age is due to changes in body composition. With increasing age, even when body weight remains constant, there is loss of muscle tissue and replacement by adipose tissue, which is metabolically very much less active, as 80% of the weight of adipose tissue consists of reserves of triacylglycerol.
- Similarly, the gender difference (women have a significantly lower BMR than do men of the same body weight) is accounted for by differences in body composition. As shown in Figure 5.3, the proportion of body weight that is adipose tissue reserves in lean women is considerably higher than in men. (See also section 6.1.2 for a discussion of methods of estimating the proportions of fat and lean tissue in the body.)

5.1.3.2 Energy costs of physical activity

The most useful way of expressing the energy cost of physical activities is as a multiple of BMR. The physical activity ratio (PAR) for an activity is the ratio of the energy expended while performing the activity to that expended at rest (= BMR). Very gentle, sedentary activities use only about 1.1–1.2 times BMR. By contrast, as shown in Table 5.3, vigorous exertion, such as climbing stairs, cross-country walking uphill, etc. may use 6–8 times BMR.

Using data such as those in Table 5.3 and allowing for the time spent during each type of activity through the day permits calculation of an individual's physical activity level (PAL) – the sum of the PAR of each activity performed multiplied by the time spent in that activity. A desirable level of physical activity, in terms of cardiovascular and respiratory health, is a PAL of 1.7.

Table 5.4 shows the classification of different types of occupational work by PAR. This is the average PAR during the 8-hour working day, and makes no allowance for leisure activities. From these figures it might seem that there would be no problem in achieving the desirable PAL of 1.7. However, in Britain the average PAL is only 1.4, and the desirable level of 1.7 is achieved by only 22% of men and 13% of women.

The energy cost of physical activity is obviously affected by body weight, because more energy is required to move a heavier body. Figure 5.4 shows the effects of body weight on BMR and total energy expenditure at different levels of physical activity.

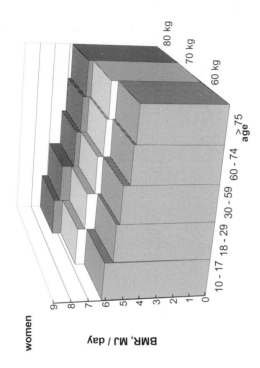

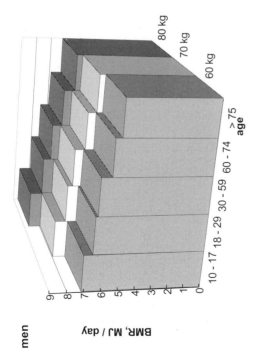

FIGURE 5.2 *The effects of age and gender on basal metabolic rate.*

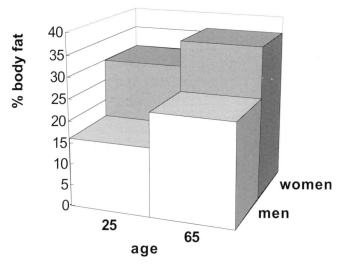

FIGURE 5.3 *Body fat as a percentage of weight with age and gender.*

TABLE 5.3 *Physical activity ratios in different types of activity*

PAR	
1.0–1.4	Lying, standing or sitting at rest, e.g. watching television, reading, writing, eating, playing cards and board games
1.5–1.8	*Sitting*: sewing, knitting, playing piano, driving *Standing*: preparing vegetables, washing dishes, ironing, general office and laboratory work
1.9–2.4	*Standing*: mixed household chores, cooking, playing snooker or bowls
2.5–3.3	*Standing*: dressing, undressing, showering, making beds, vacuum cleaning *Walking*: 3–4 km/h, playing cricket *Occupational*: tailoring, shoemaking, electrical and machine tool industry, painting and decorating
3.4–4.4	*Standing*: mopping floors, gardening, cleaning windows, table tennis, sailing *Walking*: 4–6 km/h, playing golf *Occupational*: motor vehicle repairs, carpentry and joinery, chemical industry, bricklaying
4.5–5.9	*Standing*: polishing furniture, chopping wood, heavy gardening, volley ball *Walking*: 6–7 km/h *Exercise*: dancing, moderate swimming, gentle cycling, slow jogging *Occupational*: labouring, hoeing, road construction, digging and shovelling, felling trees
6.0–7.9	*Walking*: uphill with load or cross-country, climbing stairs *Exercise*: jogging, cycling, energetic swimming, skiing, tennis, football

TABLE 5.4 *Classification of types of occupational work by physical activity ratio; figures show the average PAR throughout an 8-hour working day, excluding leisure activities*

Work intensity	PAR*	
Light	1.7	Professional, clerical and technical workers, administrative and managerial staff, sales representatives, housewives
Moderate	2.2–2.7	Sales staff, domestic service, students, transport workers, joiners, roofing workers
Moderately heavy	2.3–3.0	Machine operators, labourers, agricultural workers, bricklaying, masonry
Heavy	2.8–3.8	Labourers, agricultural workers, bricklaying, masonry where there is little or no mechanization

*Where a range of PAR is shown, the lower figure is for women and the higher for men.

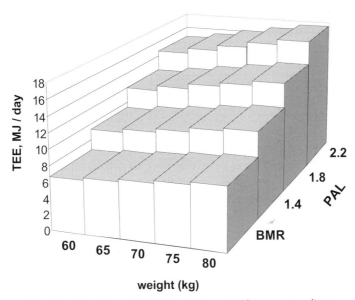

FIGURE 5.4 *The effects of weight and physical activity on total energy expenditure.*

Table 5.5 shows estimated average energy requirements at different ages, assuming average body weight and, for adults, the average PAL of 1.4 × BMR.

5.1.3.3 Diet-induced thermogenesis

There is a considerable increase in metabolic rate in response to a meal. A small part of this is the energy cost of secreting digestive enzymes and the energy cost of active transport of the products of digestion (section 3.2.2). The major part is the energy cost of synthesizing body reserves of glycogen (section 5.5.3) and triacylglycerol (section

TABLE 5.5 *Average requirements for energy, based on average weights, for adults assuming PAL = 1.4*

Age (years)	Males (MJ/day)	Females (MJ/day)
1–3	5.2	4.9
4–6	7.2	6.5
7–10	8.2	7.3
11–14	9.3	7.9
15–18	11.5	8.8
Adults	10.6	8.0

5.6.1), as well as the increased protein synthesis that occurs in the fed state (section 9.2.3.3).

The cost of synthesizing glycogen from glucose is about 5% of the ingested energy, whereas the cost of synthesizing triacylglycerol from glucose is about 20% of the ingested energy. Depending on the relative amounts of fat and carbohydrate in the diet, and the amounts of triacylglycerol and glycogen being synthesized, this diet-induced thermogenesis may account for 10% or more of the total energy yield of a meal.

5.2 *Energy balance and changes in body weight*

When energy intake is greater than energy expenditure (positive energy balance) there is increased storage of excess metabolic fuel, largely as adipose tissue; similarly, if energy intake is inadequate to meet expenditure (negative energy balance), there is utilization of reserves of adipose tissue.

Adipose tissue consists of 80% triacylglycerol (with an energy yield of 37 kJ/g) and 5% protein (energy yield 17 kJ/g) – the remaining 15% is water. Hence, adipose tissue reserves are equivalent to approximately 30 kJ/g or 30 MJ/kg. This means that the theoretical change in body weight is 33 g/MJ energy imbalance per day, or 230 g/MJ energy imbalance per week. On this basis, it is possible to calculate that, even with total starvation, a person with an energy expenditure of 10 MJ/day would lose only 330 g body weight per day or 2.3 kg/week.

These calculations suggest that there should be a constant change of body weight with a constant excessive or deficient energy intake, but this is not observed in practice. As shown in Figure 5.5, with positive energy balance the rate of weight gain is never as great as would be predicted, and gradually slows down, so that after a time the subject regains energy balance, albeit with a higher body weight. Similarly, in negative energy balance weight is not lost at a constant rate; the rate of loss slows down, and (assuming that the energy deficit is not too severe) levels off, and the subject regains energy balance, at a lower body weight.

A number of factors contribute to this adaptation to changing energy balance:

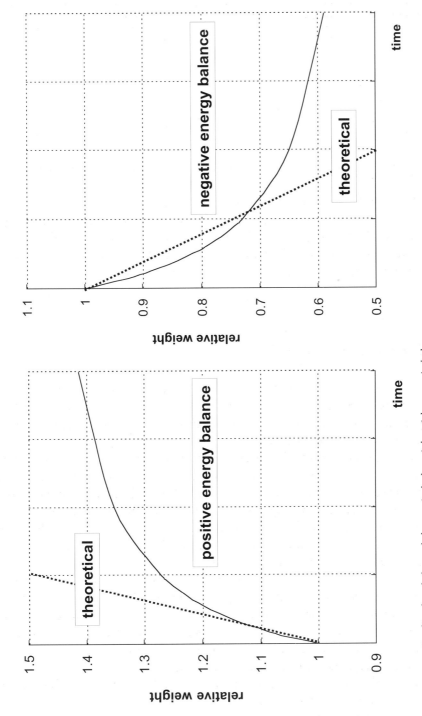

FIGURE 5.5 *Predicted and observed changes in body weight with energy imbalance.*

- As more food is eaten, so there is an increased energy cost of digestion and absorption.
- When food intake is in excess of requirements, a greater proportion is used for synthesis of adipose tissue triacylglycerol reserves, so there is a considerably greater diet-induced thermogenesis. Conversely, in negative energy balance there will be considerably less synthesis of adipose tissue reserves.
- The rate of protein turnover increases with greater food intake (section 9.2.3.3) and decreases with lower food intake.
- Although adipose tissue is less metabolically active than muscle, 5% of its weight is metabolically active, and therefore the BMR changes as body weight changes, increasing as body weight rises and decreasing as body weight falls.
- As shown in Figure 5.4, the energy cost of physical activity is markedly affected by body weight so, even assuming a constant level of physical activity, total energy expenditure will increase with increasing body weight. Furthermore, there is some evidence that people with habitually low energy intakes are more efficient in their movements, and so have a lower cost of activity.

Figure 5.5 shows that in the early stages of negative energy balance the rate of weight loss may be greater than the theoretical rate calculated from the energy yield of adipose tissue. This is because of the loss of relatively large amounts of water associated with liver and muscle glycogen reserves, which are considerably depleted during energy restriction.

5.3 Metabolic fuels in the fed and fasting states

Energy expenditure is relatively constant throughout the day, but food intake normally occurs in two or three meals. There is therefore a need for metabolic regulation to ensure that there is a more or less constant supply of metabolic fuel to tissues, regardless of the variation in intake. See section 10.5 for a more detailed discussion of the hormonal control of metabolism in the fed and fasting states.

5.3.1 THE FED STATE

During the 3–4 hours after a meal, there is an ample supply of metabolic fuel entering the circulation from the gut (Figure 5.6). Glucose from carbohydrate digestion (section 4.2.2) and amino acids from protein digestion (section 4.4.3) are absorbed into the portal circulation, and to a considerable extent the liver controls the amounts that enter the peripheral circulation. By contrast, the products of fat digestion are absorbed into the lymphatic system as chylomicrons (sections 4.3.2.2 and 5.6.2.1), and are available to peripheral tissues before the liver exerts control. Much of the triacylglycerol in chylomicrons goes directly to adipose tissue for storage; when there is a plentiful supply of glucose, it is the main metabolic fuel for most tissues.

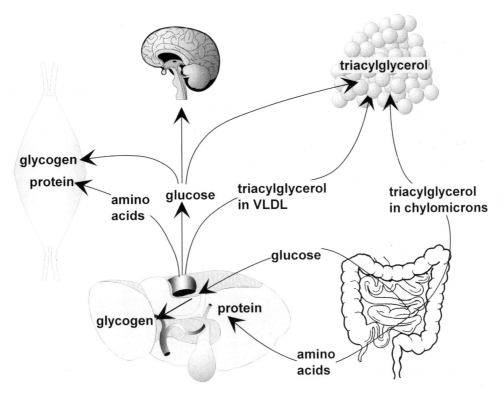

FIGURE 5.6 *An overview of metabolism in the fed state.*

The increased concentration of glucose and amino acids in the portal blood stimulates the β-cells of the pancreas to secrete insulin, and suppresses the secretion of glucagon by the α-cells of the pancreas. Insulin has four main actions:

• Increased uptake of glucose into muscle and adipose tissue. This is effected by recruitment to the cell surface of glucose transporters that are in intracellular vesicles in the fasting state.
• Stimulation of the synthesis of glycogen (section 5.5.3) from glucose in both liver and muscle, by activation of glycogen synthetase (section 10.5).
• Stimulation of fatty acid synthesis in adipose tissue (section 5.6.1) by activation of acetyl CoA carboxylase (section 10.5) and parallel inactivation of hormone-sensitive lipase.
• Stimulation of amino acid uptake into tissues, leading to an increased rate of protein synthesis.

In the liver, glucose uptake is by carrier-mediated diffusion and metabolic trapping as glucose 6-phosphate (section 3.2.2.2), and is independent of insulin. The uptake of glucose into the liver increases very significantly as the concentration of glucose in the portal vein increases, and the liver has a major role in controlling the amount of glucose that reaches peripheral tissues after a meal. There are two isoenzymes that catalyse the formation of glucose 6-phosphate in liver:

- Hexokinase has a K_m of approximately 0.15 mmol/L. This enzyme is saturated, and therefore acting at its V_{max}, under all conditions. It acts mainly to ensure an adequate uptake of glucose into the liver to meet the demands for liver metabolism.
- Glucokinase has a K_m of approximately 20 mmol/L. This enzyme will have very low activity in the fasting state, when the concentration of glucose in the portal blood is between 3 and 4 mmol/L. However, after a meal the portal concentration of glucose may well reach 20 mmol/L or higher, and under these conditions glucokinase has significant activity and there is increased formation of glucose 6-phosphate in the liver. Most of this will be used for synthesis of glycogen (section 5.5.3), although some will also be used for synthesis of fatty acids that will be exported in very low-density lipoprotein (section 5.6.2.2). (See also Problem 2.1 for the role of glucokinase in the pancreatic β-islet cells.)

5.3.2 THE FASTING STATE

In the fasting state (sometimes known as the post-absorptive state, as it begins about 4–5 hours after a meal, when the products of digestion have been absorbed) metabolic fuels enter the circulation from the reserves of glycogen, triacylglycerol and protein laid down in the fed state (Figure 5.7).

As the concentration of glucose and amino acids in the portal blood falls, so the secretion of insulin by the β-cells of the pancreas decreases and the secretion of glucagon by the α-cells increases. Glucagon has two main actions:

- Stimulation of the breakdown of glycogen to glucose 1-phosphate in the liver, resulting in the release of glucose into the circulation. As discussed in section 5.5.3.1, muscle glycogen cannot be used directly as a source of free glucose.
- Stimulation of the synthesis of glucose from amino acids in liver and kidney (the process of gluconeogenesis; section 5.7).

At the same time, the reduced secretion of insulin results in:

- a reduced rate of glucose uptake into muscle;
- a reduced rate of protein synthesis, so that the amino acids arising from protein catabolism (section 9.1.1) are available for gluconeogenesis;
- relief of the inhibition of hormone-sensitive lipase in adipose tissue, leading to release of non-esterified fatty acids.

The metabolic problem in the fasting state is that the brain is largely dependent on glucose as its metabolic fuel, and red blood cells (which lack mitochondria) cannot utilize any metabolic fuel other than glucose. Therefore, those tissues that can utilize

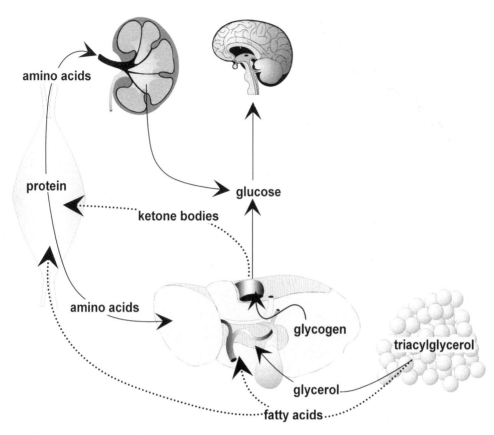

FIGURE 5.7 *An overview of metabolism in the fasting state.*

other fuels do so, in order to spare glucose for the brain and red blood cells. Any metabolites that can be used for gluconeogenesis will be used to supplement the relatively small amount of glucose that is available from glycogen reserves – the total liver and muscle glycogen reserves would only meet requirements for 12–18 hours. The main substrates for gluconeogenesis are amino acids (sections 5.7 and 9.3.2) and the glycerol of triacylglycerol. As discussed in section 5.7, fatty acids can never be substrates for gluconeogenesis.

Tissues other than red blood cells can utilize fatty acids as metabolic fuel, but only to a limited extent, and not enough to meet their energy requirements completely. By contrast, the liver has a greater capacity for the oxidation of fatty acids than is required to meet its own energy requirements. Therefore, in the fasting state, the liver synthesizes ketone bodies (acetoacetate and β-hydroxybutyrate; section 5.5.3), which it exports to other tissues for use as a metabolic fuel.

The result of these metabolic changes in the fasting state is shown in Figure 5.8. The plasma concentration of glucose falls somewhat but is maintained through fasting into starvation as a result of gluconeogenesis. The concentration of free fatty acids in plasma increases in fasting, but does not increase any further in starvation, while the

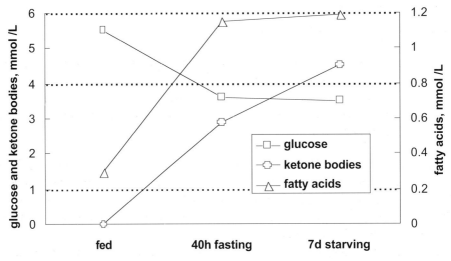

FIGURE 5.8 *Plasma concentrations of metabolic fuels in the fed and fasting states and in starvation.*

concentration of ketone bodies increases continually through fasting into starvation. After about 2–3 weeks of starvation, the plasma concentration of ketone bodies is high enough for them to be a significant fuel for the brain, albeit inadequate to meet all of the brain's energy requirements – this means that in prolonged starvation there is reduction in the amount of tissue protein that needs to be catabolized for gluconeogenesis.

5.4 *Energy-yielding metabolism*

5.4.1 GLYCOLYSIS – THE (ANAEROBIC)
METABOLISM OF GLUCOSE

Overall, the pathway of glycolysis is cleavage of the six-carbon glucose molecule into two three-carbon units. The key steps in the pathway are:

- two phosphorylation reactions to form fructose bisphosphate;
- cleavage of fructose bisphosphate to yield two molecules of triose (three-carbon sugar) phosphate;
- two steps in which phosphate is transferred from a substrate onto ADP, forming ATP (and hence a yield of $4 \times$ ATP per mole of glucose metabolized);
- one step in which NAD^+ is reduced to NADH (equivalent to $3 \times$ ATP per mol of triose phosphate metabolized, or $6 \times$ ATP per mol of glucose metabolized when the NADH is reoxidized in the mitochondrial electron transport chain) (section 3.3.1.2);
- formation of 2 mol of pyruvate per mole of glucose metabolized.

The immediate substrate for glycolysis is glucose 6-phosphate. As shown in Figure 5.9, this may arise from two sources:

- by phosphorylation of glucose, catalysed by hexokinase (and also by glucokinase in the liver in the fed state; section 5.3.1);
- by phosphorolysis of glycogen in liver and muscle to yield glucose 1-phosphate, catalysed by glycogen phosphorylase; glucose 1-phosphate is readily isomerized to glucose 6-phosphate.

The pathway of glycolysis is shown in Figure 5.10. Although the aim of glucose oxidation is to phosphorylate ADP to ATP, the pathway involves two steps in which ATP is used, one to form glucose 6-phosphate when glucose is the substrate and the other to form fructose bisphosphate. In other words, there is a modest cost of ATP to initiate the metabolism of glucose.

As discussed in section 10.2.2, the formation of fructose bisphosphate, catalysed by phosphofructokinase, is an important step for the regulation of glucose metabolism. Once it has been formed, fructose bisphosphate is cleaved into two three-carbon compounds, which are interconvertible. The metabolism of these three-carbon sugars is linked to both the reduction of NAD^+ to NADH and direct (substrate-level) phosphorylation of ADP to ATP (section 3.3). The result is the formation of 2 mol of pyruvate from each mole of glucose.

The oxidation of glucose to pyruvate thus requires the utilization of 2 mol of ATP (giving ADP) per mole of glucose metabolized, but yields $4 \times$ ATP by direct phosphorylation of ADP, and $2 \times$ NADH (formed from NAD^+), which is equivalent

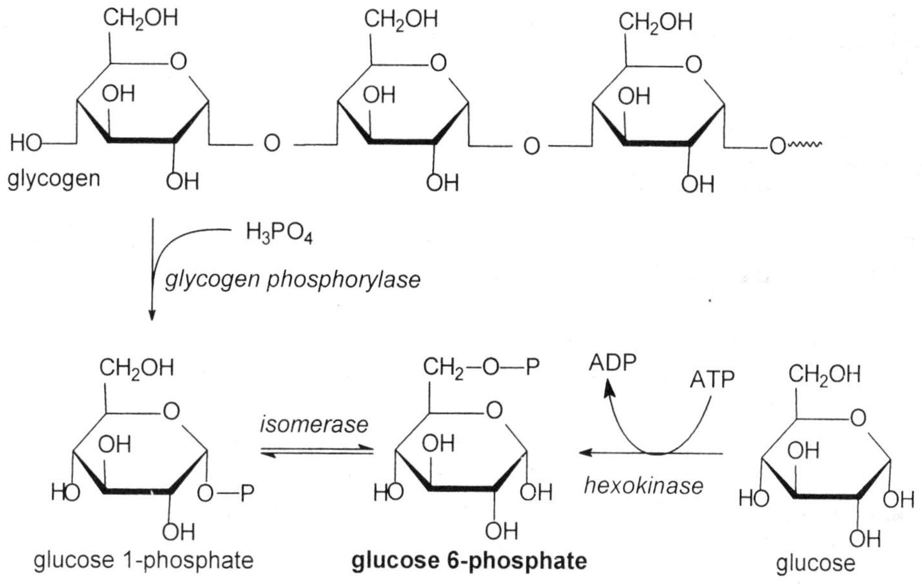

FIGURE 5.9 *Sources of glucose 6-phosphate for glycolysis.*

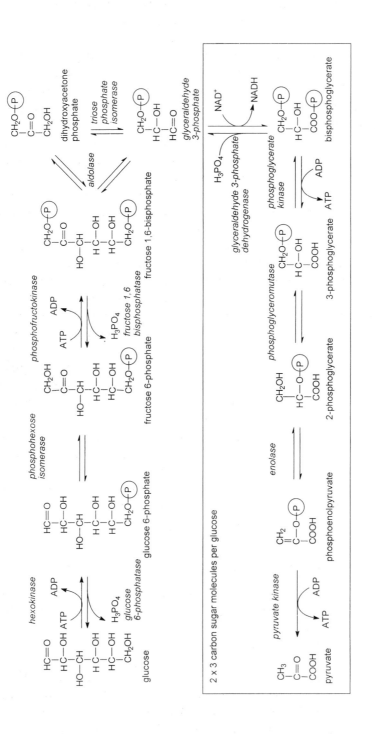

FIGURE 5.10 *Glycolysis.*

to a further 6 × ATP when oxidized in the electron transport chain (section 3.3.2). There is thus a net yield of 8 × ADP + phosphate → ATP from the oxidation of 1 mol of glucose to 2 mol of pyruvate.

As discussed in section 5.7, the reverse of the glycolytic pathway is important as a means of glucose synthesis – the process of gluconeogenesis. Most of the reactions of glycolysis are readily reversible, but at three points (the reactions catalysed by hexokinase, phosphofructokinase and pyruvate kinase) there are separate enzymes involved in glycolysis and gluconeogenesis.

For all of these reactions, the equilibrium is in the direction of glycolysis, because of the utilization of ATP in the reaction and the high ratio of ATP to ADP in the cell. The reactions of phosphofructokinase and hexokinase are reversed in gluconeogenesis by simple hydrolysis of fructose bisphosphate to fructose 6-phosphate plus phosphate (catalysed by fructose bisphosphatase) and of glucose 6-phosphate to glucose plus phosphate (catalysed by glucose 6-phosphatase).

The equilibrium of pyruvate kinase is also strongly in the direction of glycolysis, because the immediate product of the reaction is enolpyruvate, which is chemically unstable. As shown in Figure 5.31, enolpyruvate undergoes a non-enzymic reaction to yield pyruvate. This means that little of the product of the enzymic reaction is available to undergo the reverse reaction in the direction of gluconeogenesis. The conversion of pyruvate to phosphoenolpyruvate in gluconeogenesis is discussed in section 5.7.

The glycolytic pathway also provides a route for the metabolism of fructose, galactose (which undergoes phosphorylation to galactose 1-phosphate and isomerization to glucose 1-phosphate) and glycerol. Some fructose is phosphorylated directly to fructose 6-phosphate by hexokinase, but most is phosphorylated to fructose 1-phosphate by a specific enzyme, fructokinase. Fructose 1-phosphate is then cleaved to yield dihydroxyacetone phosphate and glyceraldehyde; the glyceraldehyde can be phosphorylated to glyceraldehyde 3-phosphate by triose kinase.

Glycerol arising from the hydrolysis of triacylglycerols can be phosphorylated and oxidized to dihydroxyacetone phosphate. In triacylglycerol synthesis (section 5.6.1.2), most glycerol phosphate is formed from dihydroxyacetone phosphate.

5.4.1.1 Transfer of NADH from glycolysis into the mitochondria

The mitochondrial inner membrane is impermeable to NAD, and therefore the NADH produced in the cytosol in glycolysis cannot enter the mitochondria for reoxidation. In order to transfer the reducing equivalents from cytosolic NADH into the mitochondria, two substrate shuttles are used:

- The *malate–aspartate shuttle* (Figure 5.11) involves reduction of oxaloacetate in the cytosol to malate (with the oxidation of cytosolic NADH to NAD^+). Malate enters the mitochondria and is reduced back to oxaloacetate, with the reduction of intramitochondrial NAD^+ to NADH. Oxaloacetate cannot cross the

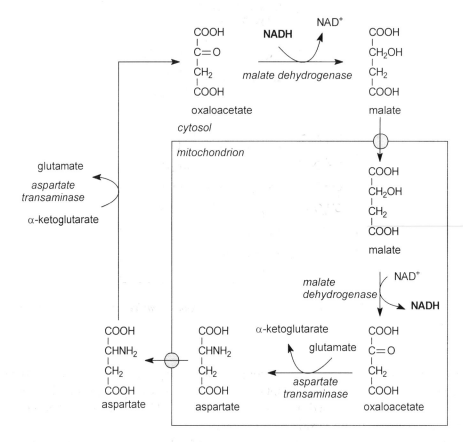

FIGURE 5.11 *The malate–aspartate shuttle for transfer of reducing equivalents from the cytosol into the mitochondrion.*

mitochondrial inner membrane so undergoes transamination to aspartate (section 9.3.1.2), with glutamate acting as amino donor, yielding α-ketoglutarate. α-Ketoglutarate then leaves the mitochondria using an antiporter (section 3.2.2) which transports malate inwards. Aspartate leaves the mitochondria in exchange for glutamate entering; in the cytosol the reverse transamination reaction occurs, forming oxaloacetate (for reduction to malate) from aspartate, and glutamate (for transport back into the mitochondria) from α-ketoglutarate.

• The *glycerophosphate shuttle* (Figure 5.12) involves reduction of dihydroxyacetone phosphate to glycerol 3-phosphate in the cytosol (with oxidation of NADH to NAD^+) and oxidation of glycerol 3-phosphate to dihydroxyacetone phosphate inside the mitochondrion. Dihydroxyacetone phosphate and glycerol 3-phosphate are transported in opposite directions by an antiporter in the mitochondrial membrane.

The cytosolic glycerol 3-phosphate dehydrogenase uses NADH to reduce

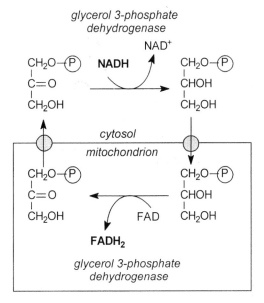

FIGURE 5.12 *The glycerophosphate shuttle for transfer of reducing equivalents from the cytosol into the mitochondrion.*

dihydroxyacetone phosphate to glycerol 3-phosphate, but the mitochondrial enzyme uses FAD to reduce glycerol 3-phosphate to dihydroxyacetone phosphate. This means that when this shuttle is used there is a yield of $\sim 2 \times$ ATP rather than $\sim 3 \times$ ATP as would be expected from reoxidation of NADH.

The malate–aspartate shuttle is sensitive to the $NADH/NAD^+$ ratios in the cytosol and mitochondria, and cannot operate if the mitochondrial $NADH/NAD^+$ ratio is higher than that in the cytosol. However, because it does not use NAD^+ in the mitochondrion, the glycerophosphate shuttle can operate even when the mitochondrial $NADH/NAD^+$ ratio is higher than that in the cytosol.

The glycerophosphate shuttle is important in muscle in which there is a very high rate of glycolysis (especially insect flight muscle); the malate–aspartate shuttle is especially important in heart and liver.

5.4.1.2 The reduction of pyruvate to lactate: anaerobic glycolysis

In red blood cells, which lack mitochondria, reoxidation of NADH formed in glycolysis cannot be by way of the substrate shuttles discussed above (section 5.4.1.1) and the electron transport chain.

Similarly, under conditions of maximum exertion, for example in sprinting, the rate at which oxygen can be taken up into the muscle is not great enough to allow for the reoxidation of all the NADH that is being formed in glycolysis. In order to maintain the oxidation of glucose, and the net yield of $2 \times$ ATP per mol of glucose oxidized (or

3 mol of ATP if the source is muscle glycogen), NADH is oxidized to NAD^+ by the reduction of pyruvate to lactate, catalysed by lactate dehydrogenase (Figure 5.13).

The resultant lactate is exported from the muscle and red blood cells and taken up by the liver, where it is used for the resynthesis of glucose. As shown on the right of Figure 5.13, synthesis of glucose from lactate is an ATP- (and GTP-) requiring process. The oxygen debt after strenuous physical activity is due to an increased rate of energy-yielding metabolism to provide the ATP and GTP that are required for gluconeogenesis from lactate. Although most of the lactate will be used for gluconeogenesis, a proportion will have to undergo oxidation to CO_2 in order to provide the ATP and GTP required for gluconeogenesis (see Problem 5.1).

Lactate may also be taken up by other tissues in which oxygen availability is not a limiting factor, such as the heart. Here it is oxidized to pyruvate, and the resultant NADH is oxidized in the mitochondrial electron transport chain, yielding $3 \times$ ATP. The pyruvate is then a substrate for complete oxidation to carbon dioxide and water, as discussed below (section 5.4.3).

Many tumours have a poor blood supply and hence a low capacity for oxidative

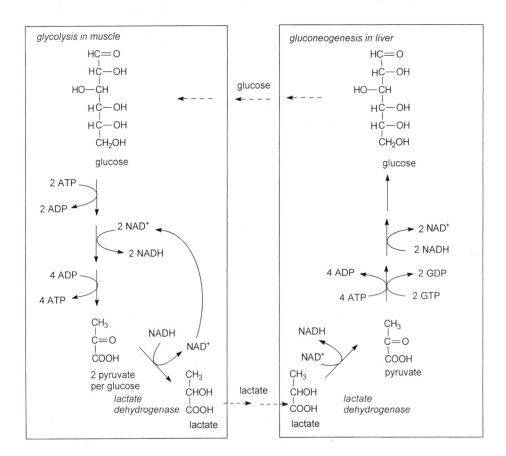

FIGURE 5.13 *The Cori cycle – anaerobic glycolysis in muscle and gluconeogenesis in the liver.*

metabolism, so that much of the energy-yielding metabolism in the tumour is anaerobic. Lactate produced by anaerobic glycolysis in tumours is exported to the liver for gluconeogenesis; as discussed in section 8.4, this increased cycling of glucose between anaerobic glycolysis in the tumour and gluconeogenesis in the liver may account for much of the weight loss (cachexia) that is seen in patients with advanced cancer.

Anaerobic glycolysis also occurs in micro-organisms that are capable of living in the absence of oxygen. Here there are two possible fates for the pyruvate formed from glucose, both of which involve the oxidation of NADH to NAD^+:

- Reduction to lactate, as occurs in human muscle. This is the pathway in lactic acid bacteria, which are responsible for the fermentation of lactose in milk to form yoghurt and cheese, and also for the gastrointestinal discomfort after consumption of lactose in people who lack intestinal lactase (section 4.2.2.2).
- Decarboxylation and reduction to ethanol. This is the pathway of fermentation in yeast, which is exploited to produce alcoholic beverages. Human gastrointestinal bacteria normally produce lactate rather than ethanol, although there have been reports of people with a high intestinal population of yeasts that do produce significant amounts of ethanol after consumption of resistant starch (section 4.2.2.1).

5.4.2 THE PENTOSE PHOSPHATE PATHWAY
– AN ALTERNATIVE TO GLYCOLYSIS

There is an alternative pathway for the conversion of glucose 6-phosphate to fructose 6-phosphate, the pentose phosphate pathway (sometimes known as the hexose monophosphate shunt), shown in Figure 5.14.

Overall, the pentose phosphate pathway produces 2 mol of fructose 6-phosphate, 1 mol of glyceraldehyde 3-phosphate and 3 mol of carbon dioxide from 3 mol of glucose 6-phosphate, linked to the reduction of 6 mol of $NADP^+$ to NADPH. The sequence of reactions is as follows:

- Three mol of glucose are oxidized to yield 3 mol of the five-carbon sugar ribulose 5-phosphate + 3 mol of carbon dioxide.
- Two mol of ribulose 5-phosphate are isomerized to yield 2 mol of xylulose 5-phosphate.
- One mol of ribulose 5-phosphate is isomerized to ribose 5-phosphate.
- One mol of xylulose 5-phosphate reacts with the ribose 5-phosphate, yielding (ultimately) fructose 6-phosphate and erythrose 4-phosphate.
- The other mol of xylulose-5-phosphate reacts with the erythrose 4-phosphate, yielding fructose 6-phosphate and glyceraldehyde 3-phosphate.

This is the pathway for the synthesis of ribose for nucleotide synthesis (section

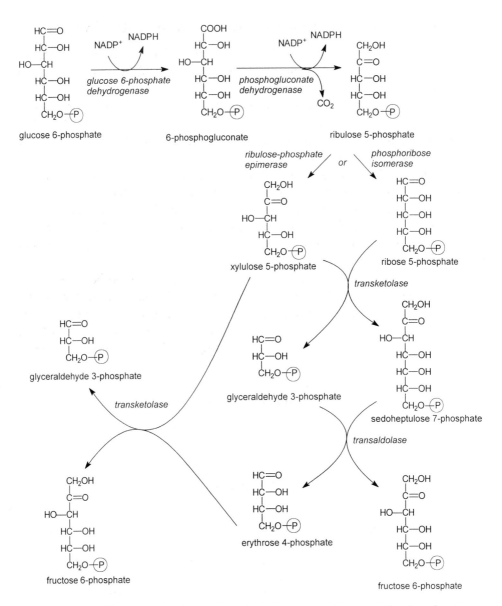

FIGURE 5.14 *The pentose phosphate pathway (also known as the hexose monophosphate shunt).*

9.2.2); more importantly, it is the source of about half the NADPH required for fatty acid synthesis (section 5.6.1); tissues that synthesize large amounts of fatty acids have a high activity of the pentose phosphate pathway. As discussed in section 7.4.2.2, the pentose phosphate pathway is also important in the respiratory burst of macrophages that are activated in response to infection.

5.4.2.1 The pentose phosphate pathway in red blood cells – favism

The pentose phosphate pathway is also important in the red blood cell, where NADPH is required to maintain an adequate pool of reduced glutathione, which is used to remove hydrogen peroxide.

As shown in Figure 5.15, the tripeptide glutathione (γ-glutamyl-cysteinyl-glycine) is the reducing agent for glutathione peroxidase, which reduces H_2O_2 to H_2O and O_2. (Glutathione peroxidase is a selenium-dependent enzyme (section 11.15.2.5), and this explains the antioxidant action of selenium.)

Oxidized glutathione (GSSG) is reduced back to active GSH by glutathione reductase, which uses NADPH as the reducing agent. Glutathione reductase is a flavin-dependent enzyme, and its activity, or its activation after incubation with FAD, can be used as an index of vitamin B_2 status (section 11.7.4.1), in the same way as activation of transketolase by thiamin diphosphate can be used as an index of thiamin status (section 11.6.4.1).

Partial or total lack of glucose 6-phosphate dehydrogenase (and hence impaired activity of the pentose phosphate pathway) is the cause of favism, an acute haemolytic anaemia with fever and haemoglobinuria, precipitated in genetically susceptible people by the consumption of broad beans (fava beans) and a variety of drugs, all of which, like the toxins in fava beans, undergo redox cycling, producing hydrogen peroxide.

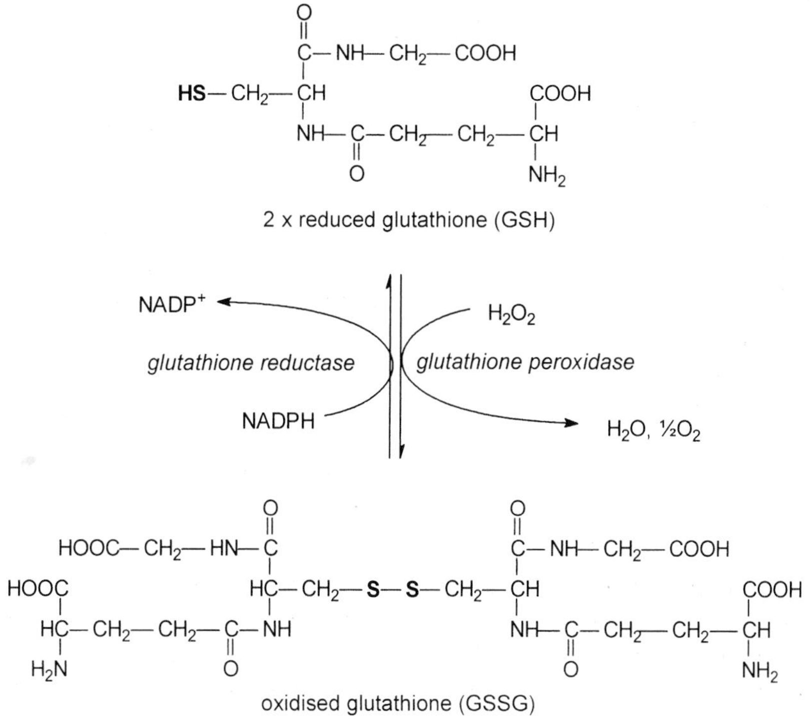

FIGURE 5.15 *The reaction of glutathione peroxidase.*

Infection can also precipitate an attack as a result of the increased production of oxygen radicals as part of the macrophage respiratory burst (section 7.4.2.2).

Because of the low activity of the pentose phosphate pathway in affected people, there is a lack of NADPH in red blood cells, and hence an impaired ability to remove hydrogen peroxide, which causes oxidative damage to the cell membrane lipids, leading to haemolysis. Other tissues are unaffected in favism because there are mitochondrial enzymes that can provide a supply of NADPH; red blood cells have no mitochondria.

Favism is one of the commonest genetic defects; an estimated 200 million people world-wide are affected. It is an X-linked condition, and female carriers are resistant to malaria; this advantage presumably explains why defects in the gene are so widespread. A large number of variant forms of the glucose 6-phosphate dehydrogenase gene are known; some have no effect on the activity of the enzyme, whereas others result in favism. There are two main types of favism:

* A moderately severe form, in which there is between 10% and 50% of the normal activity of glucose 6-phosphate dehydrogenase in red blood cells. The abnormal enzyme is unstable, so that older red blood cells have low activity but younger cells have nearly normal activity. This means that the haemolytic crisis is self-limiting, as only older red blood cells are lysed. This is the form of favism found among people of Afro-Caribbean descent, and crises are rarely precipitated by consumption of fava beans.
* A severe form, in which there is less than 10% of normal activity of glucose 6-phosphate dehydrogenase in red blood cells. In this case the problem is that the enzyme has low catalytic activity or an abnormally high K_m for $NADP^+$. In especially severe cases, haemolytic crises can be occur without the stress of toxin or infection. This is the form of favism found among people of Mediterranean descent.

5.4.3 THE METABOLISM OF PYRUVATE

Pyruvate arising from glycolysis (or from amino acids; section 9.3.2) can be metabolized in three different ways, depending on the metabolic state of the body:

* reduction to lactate (section 5.4.1.2);
* as a substrate for gluconeogenesis (section 5.7);
* complete oxidation to carbon dioxide and water (sections 5.4.3.1 and 5.4.4).

5.4.3.1 The oxidation of pyruvate to acetyl CoA

The first step in the complete oxidation of pyruvate is a complex reaction in which carbon dioxide is lost and the resulting two-carbon compound is oxidized to acetate. The oxidation involves the reduction of NAD^+ to NADH. As 2 mol of pyruvate is formed from each mol of glucose, this step represents the formation of 2 mol of NADH,

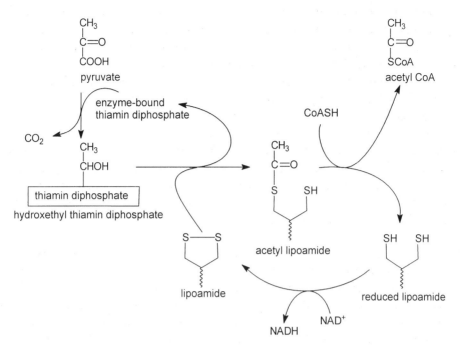

FIGURE 5.16 *The reaction of pyruvate dehydrogenase.*

equivalent to $6 \times ATP$ for each mol of glucose metabolized. The acetate is released from the enzyme esterified to coenzyme A, as acetyl CoA (Figure 5.16). (Coenzyme A is derived from the vitamin pantothenic acid; section 11.13.1.1).

The decarboxylation and oxidation of pyruvate to form acetyl CoA requires the coenzyme thiamin diphosphate, which is formed from vitamin B_1 (section 11.6.2). In thiamin deficiency, this reaction is impaired, and deficient subjects are unable to metabolize glucose normally. Especially after a test dose of glucose or moderate exercise they develop high blood concentrations of pyruvate and lactate. In some cases this may be severe enough to result in life-threatening acidosis.

Thiamin deficiency is not uncommon in alcoholics; apart from a low intake of the vitamin, alcohol inhibits the transport of thiamin from intestinal mucosal cells into the bloodstream. There is little storage of thiamin in the body, and deficiency can develop within a few weeks (see Problem 5.2).

5.4.4 OXIDATION OF ACETYL CoA –
THE CITRIC ACID CYCLE

The acetate of acetyl CoA undergoes a stepwise oxidation to carbon dioxide and water in a cyclic pathway, the citric acid cycle, shown in Figures 5.17 and 5.18. This pathway is sometimes known as the Krebs cycle, after its discoverer, Sir Hans Krebs. For each mole of acetyl CoA oxidized in this pathway, there is a yield of:

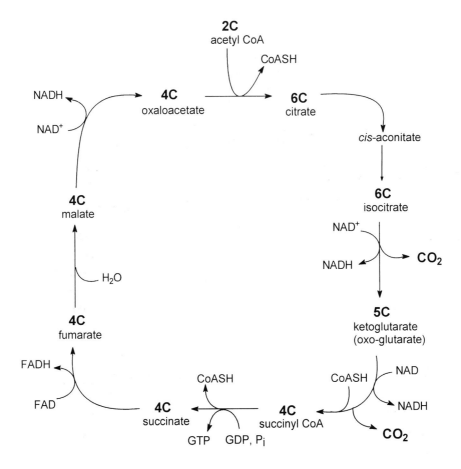

FIGURE 5.17 *An overview of the citric acid cycle (also known as the Krebs cycle or tricarboxylic acid cycle).*

- $3 \times NAD^+$ reduced to NADH, equivalent to $\sim 9 \times ATP$;
- $1 \times$ flavoprotein reduced, leading to reduction of ubiquinone (section 3.3.1.2), equivalent to $\sim 2 \times ADP$;
- $1 \times GDP$ phosphorylated to GTP, equivalent to $1 \times ATP$.

This is a total of $\sim 12 \times ATP$ for each mole of acetyl CoA oxidized; as 2 mol of acetyl CoA are formed from each mol of glucose, this cycle yields $\sim 24 \times ATP$ for each mol of glucose oxidized.

Although it appears complex at first sight, the citric acid cycle is a simple pathway. A four-carbon compound, oxaloacetate, reacts with acetyl CoA to form a six-carbon compound, citric acid. The cycle is then a series of steps in which two carbon atoms are lost as carbon dioxide, followed by a series of oxidation and other reactions,

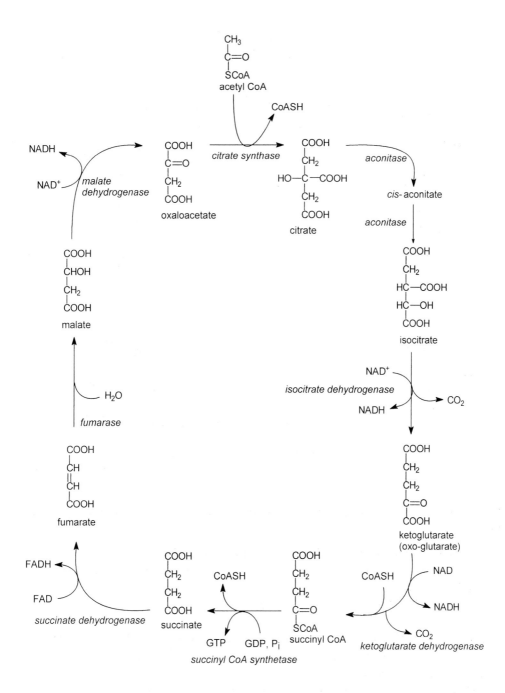

FIGURE 5.18 *The citric acid cycle (also known as the Krebs cycle or tricarboxylic acid cycle).*

eventually reforming oxaloacetate. The CoA of acetyl CoA is released and is available for further formation of acetyl CoA from pyruvate.

The citric acid cycle is also involved in the oxidation of acetyl CoA arising from other sources:

* β-oxidation of fatty acids (section 5.5.2);
* ketone bodies (section 5.5.3);
* alcohol (section 2.6);
* those amino acids that give rise to acetyl CoA or acetoacetate (section 9.3.2).

Although, as discussed below (section 5.7), oxaloacetate is the precursor for gluconeogenesis, fatty acids and other compounds that give rise to acetyl CoA or acetoacetate cannot be used for net synthesis of glucose. As can be seen from Figure 5.18, although two carbons are added to the cycle by acetyl CoA, two carbons are lost as carbon dioxide in each turn of the cycle. Therefore, when acetyl CoA is the substrate, there is no increase in the pool of citric acid cycle intermediates, and therefore oxaloacetate cannot be withdrawn for gluconeogenesis.

α-Ketoglutarate dehydrogenase catalyses a reaction similar to that of pyruvate dehydrogenase – oxidative decarboxylation and formation of an acyl CoA derivative. Like pyruvate dehydrogenase, it is a thiamin diphosphate-dependent enzyme, and the reaction sequence is the same as that shown in Figure 5.16. However, thiamin deficiency does not have a significant effect on the citric acid cycle, because, as shown in Figure 5.19, α-ketoglutarate can undergo transamination to yield glutamate, which is decarboxylated to γ-aminobutyric acid (GABA). In turn, GABA can undergo further metabolism to yield succinate. This pathway (sometimes called the GABA shunt) thus provides an alternative to α-ketoglutarate dehydrogenase in thiamin deficiency, so that oxidation of acetyl CoA and formation of ATP can continue.

The sequence of reactions between succinate and oxaloacetate is chemically the same as that involved in the β-oxidation of fatty acids (section 5.5.2):

* Oxidation to yield a carbon–carbon double bond. Although this reaction is shown in Figure 5.18 as being linked to reduction of FAD, the coenzyme is tightly enzyme bound, and succinate dehydrogenase reacts directly with ubiquinone in the electron transport chain (section 3.3.1.2).
* Addition of water across the carbon–carbon double bond, to yield a hydroxyl group.
* Oxidation of the hydroxyl group, linked to reduction of NAD^+, to yield an oxo-group.

5.4.4.1 The citric acid cycle as pathway for metabolic interconversion

In addition to its role in oxidation of acetyl CoA, the citric acid cycle is an important central metabolic pathway, providing the link between carbohydrate, fat and amino

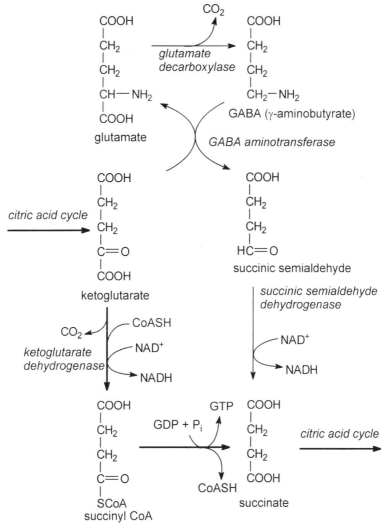

FIGURE 5.19 *The GABA shunt – an alternative to* α*-ketoglutarate dehydrogenase in the citric acid cycle.*

acid metabolism. Many of the intermediates can be used for the synthesis of other compounds:

- α-Ketoglutarate and oxaloacetate can give rise to the amino acids glutamate and aspartate respectively (section 9.3.1.2).
- Oxaloacetate is the precursor for glucose synthesis in the fasting state (section 5.7).
- Citrate is used as the source of acetyl CoA for fatty acid synthesis in the cytosol in the fed state (section 5.6.1).

If oxaloacetate is removed from the cycle for glucose synthesis, it must be replaced, because if there is not enough oxaloacetate available to form citrate the rate of acetyl CoA metabolism, and hence the rate of formation of ATP, will slow down. As shown in Figure 5.20, a variety of amino acids give rise to citric acid cycle intermediates, so replenishing cycle intermediates and permitting the removal of oxaloacetate for gluconeogenesis. In addition, the reaction of pyruvate carboxylase (see Figure 5.20) is a major source of oxaloacetate to maintain citric acid cycle activity.

There is a further control over the removal of oxaloacetate for gluconeogenesis. As shown in Figure 5.18, the decarboxylation and phosphorylation of oxaloacetate to form phosphoenolpyruvate uses GTP as the phosphate donor. In tissues such as liver and kidney, which are active in gluconeogenesis, the major source of GTP in the mitochondria is the reaction of succinyl CoA synthetase. If so much oxaloacetate were withdrawn that the rate of cycle activity fell, there would be inadequate GTP to permit further removal of oxaloacetate. In tissues such as brain and heart, which do not carry out gluconeogenesis, there is a different isoenzyme of succinyl CoA synthetase, which is linked to phosphorylation of ADP rather than GDP.

5.4.4.2 Complete oxidation of four- and five-carbon compounds

Although the citric acid cycle is generally regarded as a pathway for the oxidation of four- and five-carbon compounds arising from amino acids, such as fumarate, oxaloacetate, α-ketoglutarate and succinate (see Figure 5.20), it does not, alone, permit complete oxidation of these compounds. Four-carbon intermediates are not overall consumed in the cycle, as oxaloacetate is reformed. Addition of four- and five-carbon intermediates will increase the rate of cycle activity (subject to control by the requirement for ATP) only until the pool of intermediates is saturated.

Complete oxidation of four- and five-carbon intermediates requires removal of oxaloacetate from the cycle, and conversion to pyruvate, as shown in Figure 5.20. This pyruvate may either undergo decarboxylation to acetyl CoA (see Figure 5.16), which can be oxidized in the cycle, or may be used as a substrate for gluconeogenesis.

Oxidation of four- and five-carbon citric acid cycle intermediates thus involves a greater metabolic activity than oxidation of acetyl CoA. This has been exploited as a means of overcoming the hypothermia that occurs in patients recovering from anaesthesia, by giving an intravenous infusion of the amino acid glutamate. This provides α-ketoglutarate, which will largely be used for gluconeogenesis, and hence causes an increase in metabolic activity and increased heat production.

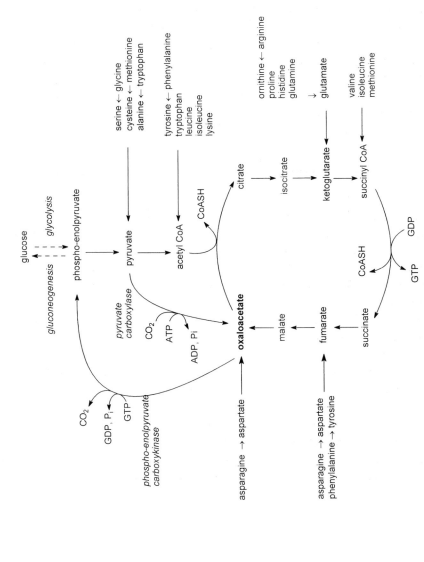

FIGURE 5.20 *The entry of amino acid carbon skeletons into the citric acid cycle for gluconeogenesis.*

5.5 *The metabolism of fats*

As shown in Figure 5.21, fatty acids may be made available to cells in two ways:

- In the fed state, chylomicrons assembled in the small intestine (section 4.3.3.2) and very low-density lipoproteins exported from the liver (section 5.6.2.2) bind to the cell surface, where lipoprotein lipase catalyses hydrolysis of triacylglycerols to glycerol and free fatty acids.
- In the fasting state, hormone-sensitive lipase in adipose tissue is activated in response to falling insulin secretion or the secretion of adrenaline (section 4.3.2.2 and section 10.5.1) and catalyses the hydrolysis of triacylglycerol, releasing free fatty acids into the bloodstream, where they bind to albumin and are transported to tissues.

The glycerol is phosphorylated and converted to dihydroxyacetone phosphate (see Figure 5.10), which may be used either as a metabolic fuel (in the fed state) or for gluconeogenesis (in the fasting state).

The fatty acids are oxidized in the mitochondria by the β-oxidation pathway, in which two carbon atoms at a time are removed from the fatty acid chain as acetyl CoA. This acetyl CoA then enters the citric acid cycle, together with that arising from the metabolism of pyruvate.

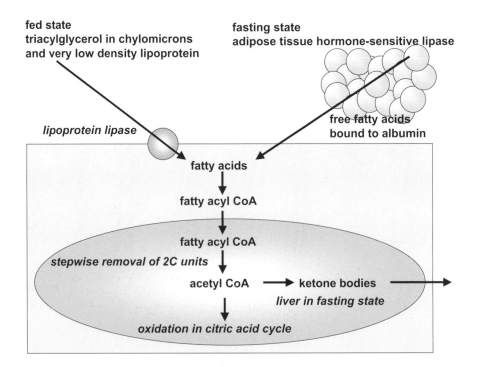

FIGURE 5.21 *An overview of fatty acid metabolism.*

5.5.1 CARNITINE AND THE TRANSPORT
OF FATTY ACIDS INTO THE MITOCHONDRION

As shown in Figure 5.21, fatty acids are esterified with coenzyme A, forming acyl CoA, as they enter the cell. This is necessary to protect the cell membranes against the lytic action of free fatty acids. Fatty acyl CoA cannot cross the mitochondrial membranes to enter the matrix, where the enzymes for β-oxidation are.

On the outer face of the outer mitochondrial membrane, the fatty acid is transferred from CoA onto carnitine, forming acylcarnitine, which enters the inter-membrane space through an acylcarnitine transporter (Figure 5.22). The structures of CoA and carnitine are shown in Figure 5.23.

Acylcarnitine can cross only the inner mitochondrial membrane on a counter-transport system that takes in acylcarnitine in exchange for free carnitine being returned to the inter-membrane space. Once inside the mitochondrial inner membrane, acylcarnitine transfers the acyl group onto CoA ready to undergo β-oxidation. This counter-transport system provides regulation of the uptake of fatty acids into the mitochondrion for oxidation. As long as there is free CoA available in the mitochondrial matrix, fatty acids can be taken up and the carnitine returned to the outer membrane for uptake of more fatty acids. However, if most of the CoA in the mitochondrion is acylated, then there is no need for further fatty uptake immediately and, indeed, it is not possible.

This carnitine shuttle also serves to prevent uptake into the mitochondrion (and hence oxidation) of fatty acids synthesized in the cytosol in the fed state; malonyl

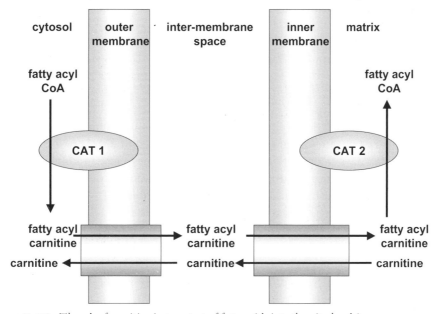

FIGURE 5.22 *The role of carnitine in transport of fatty acids into the mitochondrion.*

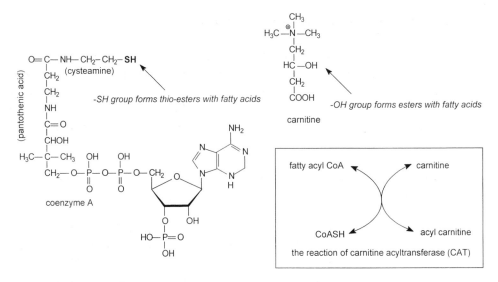

FIGURE 5.23 *The structures of coenzyme A (CoA) and carnitine.*

CoA (the precursor for fatty acid synthesis; section 5.6.1) is a potent inhibitor of carnitine palmitoyl transferase I in the outer mitochondrial membrane.

Tissues that oxidize fatty acids but do not synthesize them, such as muscle, also have acetyl CoA carboxylase and produce malonyl CoA. This seems to be in order to control the activity of carnitine palmitoyl transferase I, and thus control the mitochondrial uptake and β-oxidation of fatty acids. Tissues also have malonyl CoA decarboxylase, which acts to remove malonyl CoA and so reduce the inhibition of carnitine palmitoyl transferase I. The two enzymes are regulated in opposite directions in response to:

- insulin, which stimulates fatty acid synthesis and reduces β-oxidation;
- glucagon, which reduces fatty acid synthesis and increases β-oxidation

As discussed in section 10.6, fatty acids are the major fuel for red muscle fibres, which are the main type involved in moderate exercise. Children who lack one or other of the enzymes required for carnitine synthesis, and are therefore reliant on a dietary intake, have poor exercise tolerance because they have an impaired ability to transport fatty acids into the mitochondria for β-oxidation. Provision of supplements of carnitine to the affected children overcomes the problem. Extrapolation from this rare clinical condition has led to the use of carnitine as a so-called 'ergogenic aid' to improve athletic performance. A number of studies have shown that relatively large supplements of carnitine increase the muscle content of carnitine to only a small extent, and most studies have shown no significant effect on athletic performance or endurance. This is not surprising – carnitine is readily synthesized from lysine and methionine, and there is no evidence that any dietary intake is required.

5.5.2 THE β-OXIDATION OF FATTY ACIDS

Once it has entered the mitochondria, fatty acyl CoA undergoes a spiral series of four reactions, as shown in Figure 5.24, which results in the cleavage of the fatty acid molecule to give acetyl CoA and a new fatty acyl CoA that is two carbons shorter than the initial substrate. This new, shorter, fatty acyl CoA is then a substrate for the same sequence of reactions, which is repeated until the final result is cleavage to yield two molecules of acetyl CoA. This is the pathway of β-oxidation, so called because it is the β-carbon of the fatty acid that undergoes oxidation.

The reactions of β-oxidation are chemically the same as those in the conversion of succinate to oxaloacetate in the citric acid cycle (see Figure 5.18):

- The first step is removal of two hydrogens from the fatty acid, to form a carbon–carbon double bond – an oxidation reaction that yields a reduced flavin, so that for each double bond formed in this way there is a yield of $\sim 2 \times$ ATP.
- The newly formed double bond in the fatty acyl CoA then reacts with water, yielding a hydroxyl group – a hydration reaction.
- The hydroxylated fatty acyl CoA undergoes a second oxidation in which the hydroxyl group is oxidized to an oxo-group, yielding NADH (equivalent to $\sim 3 \times$ ATP).
- The oxo-acyl CoA is then cleaved by reaction with CoA, to form acetyl CoA and the shorter fatty acyl CoA, which undergoes the same sequence of reactions.

There are three separate sets of enzymes catalysing these four reactions, with specificity for long-, medium- and short-chain fatty acyl CoA derivatives. Each set of enzymes is arranged as a membrane-bound array, and the product of one is passed directly to the active site of the next. The result of this is that, although short- and medium-chain fatty acyl CoA derivatives can be detected in the mitochondrial matrix, as they pass from one array of enzymes to the next, none of the intermediates of the reaction spiral can be detected – they remain enzyme bound.

The acetyl CoA formed by β-oxidation then enters the citric acid cycle (see Figure 5.18). Almost all of the metabolically important fatty acids have an even number of carbon atoms, so that the final cycle of β-oxidation is the conversion of a four-carbon fatty acyl CoA (butyryl CoA) to two molecules of acetyl CoA.

5.5.3 KETONE BODIES

Most tissues have a limited capacity for fatty acid oxidation and in the fasting state cannot meet their energy requirements from fatty acid oxidation alone. By contrast, the liver is capable of forming considerably more acetyl CoA from fatty acids than is required for its own metabolism. It takes up fatty acids from the circulation and oxidizes them to acetyl CoA, then synthesizes and exports the four-carbon ketone

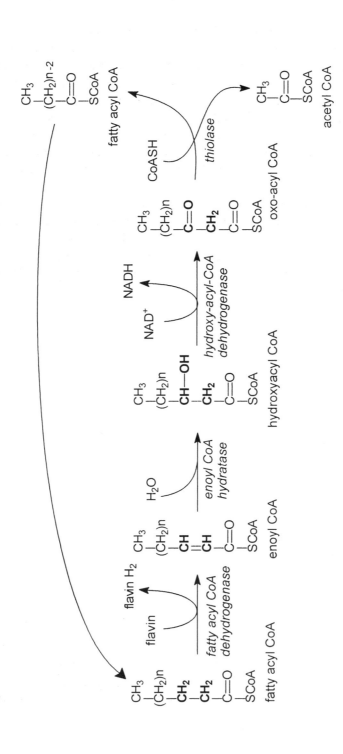

FIGURE 5.24 β-Oxidation of fatty acids.

bodies formed from acetyl CoA to other tissues (especially muscle) for use as a metabolic fuel.

The reactions involved are shown in Figure 5.25. Acetoacetyl CoA is formed by reaction between two molecules of acetyl CoA. This is essentially the reverse of the final reaction of fatty acid β-oxidation (see Figure 5.23). Acetoacetyl CoA then reacts with a further molecule of acetyl CoA to form hydroxymethyl-glutaryl CoA, which then undergoes cleavage to release acetyl CoA and acetoacetate.

Acetoacetate is chemically unstable, and undergoes a non-enzymic reaction to yield acetone, which is only poorly metabolized. Most of it is excreted in the urine and in exhaled air – a waste of valuable metabolic fuel reserves in the fasting state. To avoid this, much of the acetoacetate is reduced to β-hydroxybutyrate before being released from the liver.

The pathway for the utilization of β-hydroxybutyrate and acetoacetate in tissues other than the liver is shown in Figure 5.26. The first step is oxidation of β-hydroxybutyrate to acetoacetate, yielding NADH. The synthesis of β-hydroxybutyrate in the liver can thus be regarded not only as a way of preventing loss of metabolic fuel as acetone, but also effectively as a means of exporting NADH (and therefore effectively ATP) to extrahepatic tissues.

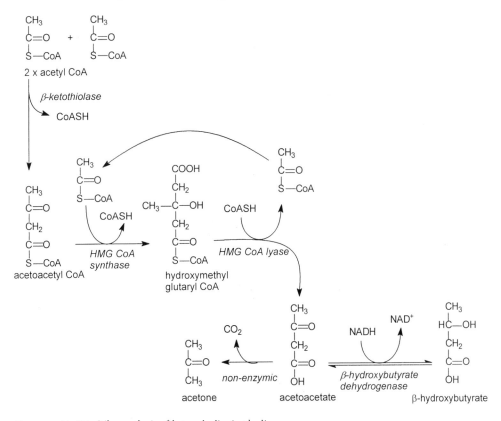

FIGURE 5.25 *The synthesis of ketone bodies in the liver.*

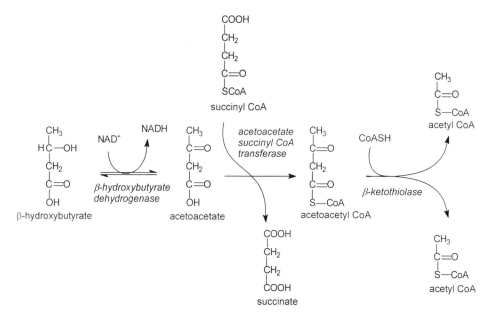

FIGURE 5.26 *The utilization of ketone bodies in extrahepatic tissues.*

The utilization of acetoacetate is controlled by the activity of the citric acid cycle. The reaction of acetoacetate succinyl CoA transferase provides an alternative to the reaction of succinyl CoA synthase (see Figure 5.18), and there will only be an adequate supply of succinyl CoA to permit conversion of acetoacetate to acetoacetyl CoA as long as the rate of citric acid cycle activity is adequate.

Acetoacetate, β-hydroxybutyrate and acetone are collectively known as the ketone bodies, and the occurrence of increased concentrations of these three compounds in the bloodstream is known as ketosis. Actetoacetate and β-hydroxybutyrate are also acids, and will lower blood pH, potentially leading to metabolic acidosis. Although acetone and acetoacetate are chemically ketones, having a –C=O grouping, β-hydroxybutyrate is not chemically a ketone. It is classified with the other two because of its metabolic relationship. See section 10.7 for a discussion of the problems of ketoacidosis in uncontrolled diabetes mellitus.

5.6 *Tissue reserves of metabolic fuels*

In the fed state, as well as providing for immediate energy needs, substrates are converted into storage compounds for use in the fasting state. There are two main stores of metabolic fuels:

- triacylglycerols in adipose tissue;
- glycogen as a carbohydrate reserve in liver and muscle.

In addition, there is an increase in the synthesis of tissue proteins after a meal, as a result of the increased availability of metabolic fuel to provide ATP for protein synthesis (section 9.2.3.3).

In the fasting state, which is the normal state between meals, these reserves are mobilized and used. Glycogen is a source of glucose, while adipose tissue provides both fatty acids and glycerol from triacylglycerol. Some of the relatively labile protein laid down in response to meals is also mobilized in fasting, and the amino acids are used both as a metabolic fuel and, more importantly, a source of citric acid cycle intermediates for gluconeogenesis.

5.6.1 SYNTHESIS OF FATTY ACIDS AND TRIACYLGLYCEROLS

Fatty acids are synthesized by the successive addition of two-carbon units from acetyl CoA, followed by reduction. Like β-oxidation, fatty acid synthesis is a spiral sequence of reactions, with different enzymes catalysing the reaction sequence for synthesis of short, medium- and long-chain fatty acids.

Unlike β-oxidation, which occurs in the mitochondrial matrix, fatty acid synthesis occurs in the cytosol. The enzymes required for fatty acid synthesis form a multienzyme complex, arranged in a series of concentric rings around a central acyl carrier protein (ACP), which carries the growing fatty acid chain from one enzyme to the next. The functional group of the acyl carrier protein is the same as that of CoA, derived from the vitamin pantothenic acid and cysteamine (see Figure 11.26). As the chain grows in length, so the middle then outermost rings of enzymes are used. Short- and medium-chain fatty acids are not released from one set of enzymes to bind to the next, as occurs in β-oxidation.

The only source of acetyl CoA is in the mitochondrial matrix, and, as discussed in section 5.5.1, acetyl CoA cannot cross the inner mitochondrial. For fatty acid synthesis, citrate is formed inside the mitochondria by reaction between acetyl CoA and oxaloacetate (Figure 5.27), and is then transported out of the mitochondria, to undergo cleavage in the cytosol to yield acetyl CoA and oxaloacetate. The acetyl CoA is used for fatty acid synthesis, while the oxaloacetate (indirectly) returns to the mitochondria to maintain citric acid cycle activity.

Fatty acid synthesis can occur only when the rate of formation of citrate is greater than is required for energy-yielding metabolism. Although citrate is a symmetrical molecule, and carbons 1 and 2 are equivalent to carbons 5 and 6, it behaves asymmetrically. The two carbons that are added from acetyl CoA remain in the four carbon intermediates of the citric acid cycle during the first turn. If cells are incubated with [^{14}C]acetate and malonate as an inhibitor of succinate dehydrogenase (see Figure 5.18), no radioactivity is detectable in the carbon dioxide released in the first (partial) turn of the cycle. This is the result of metabolic channelling. Citrate is passed directly from the active site of citrate synthase to that of aconitase. It is only when isocitrate

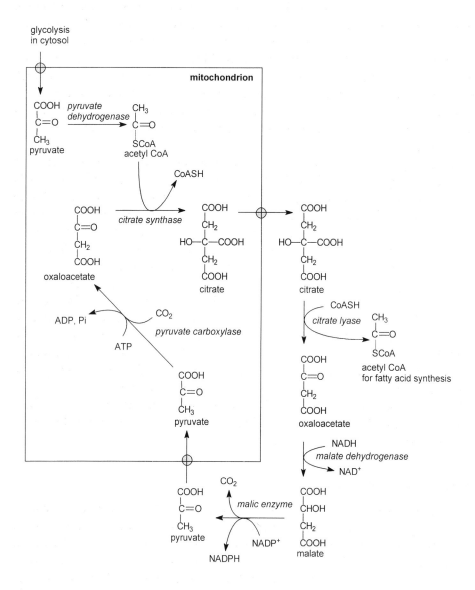

FIGURE 5.27 *The source of acetyl CoA in the cytosol for fatty acid synthesis.*

dehydrogenase is saturated, and hence aconitase is inhibited by its product, that citrate is released from the active site of citrate synthase into free solution, to be available for transport out of the mitochondria.

Oxaloacetate cannot re-enter the mitochondrion directly. As shown in Figure 5.27, it is reduced to malate, which then undergoes oxidative decarboxylation to pyruvate, linked to the reduction of $NADP^+$ to NADPH. This provides about half the NADPH that is required for fatty acid synthesis. The resultant pyruvate enters the mitochondrion and is carboxylated to oxaloacetate in a reaction catalysed by pyruvate carboxylase.

As shown in Figure 5.28, the first reaction in the synthesis of fatty acids is carboxylation of acetyl CoA to malonyl CoA. This is a biotin-dependent reaction (section 11.12.2) and, as discussed above (section 5.5.1), the activity of acetyl CoA carboxylase is regulated in response to insulin and glucagon. Malonyl CoA is not only the substrate for fatty acid synthesis, but also a potent inhibitor of carnitine palmitoyl transferase, so inhibiting the uptake of fatty acids into the mitochondrion for β-oxidation.

The malonyl group is transferred onto an acyl carrier protein, and then reacts with the growing fatty acid chain, bound to the central acyl carrier protein of the fatty acid synthase complex. The carbon dioxide that was added to form malonyl CoA is lost in this reaction. For the first cycle of reactions, the central acyl carrier protein carries an acetyl group, and the product of reaction with malonyl CoA is acetoacetyl-ACP; in subsequent reaction cycles, it is the growing fatty acid chain that occupies the central ACP, and the product of reaction with malonyl CoA is a ketoacyl-ACP.

The ketoacyl-ACP is then reduced to yield a hydroxyl group. In turn, this is dehydrated to yield a carbon–carbon double bond, which is reduced to yield a saturated fatty acid chain. Thus, the sequence of chemical reactions is the reverse of that in β-oxidation (section 5.5.2). For both reduction reactions in fatty acid synthesis, NADPH is the hydrogen donor. One source of this NADPH is the pentose phosphate pathway (section 5.4.2) and the other is the oxidation of malate (arising from oxaloacetate) to pyruvate, catalysed by the malic enzyme (see Figure 5.27).

The end-product of cytosolic fatty acid synthesis is palmitate (C16:0); longer-chain fatty acids (up to C24) and unsaturated fatty acids are synthesized from palmitate in the endoplasmic reticulum and mitochondria.

5.6.1.1 Unsaturated fatty acids

Although fatty acid synthesis involves the formation of an unsaturated intermediate, the next step, reduction to the saturated fatty acid derivative, is an obligatory part of the reaction sequence and cannot be omitted. The product of the fatty acid synthase multienzyme complex is always saturated. Some unsaturated fatty acids can be synthesized from saturated fatty acids, by dehydrogenation to yield a carbon–carbon double bond.

Mammalian tissues have a Δ^9-desaturase, which can introduce a carbon–carbon double bond between carbons 9 and 10 of the fatty acid (counting from the carboxyl group). This will yield oleic acid (C18:1 ω9) from stearic acid (C18:0). Other mammalian desaturases permit insertion of double bonds between Δ^{9-10} and the carboxyl group, but not between Δ^{9-10} and the methyl group.

This means that fatty acids with double bonds between Δ^{9-10} and the methyl group must be provided in the diet. Linoleic acid (C18:2 ω6) is $\Delta^{9-10,\ 12-13}$, and α-linolenic acid (C18:3 ω3) is $\Delta^{9-10,\ 12-13,\ 15-15}$. Both of these are dietary essentials and undergo

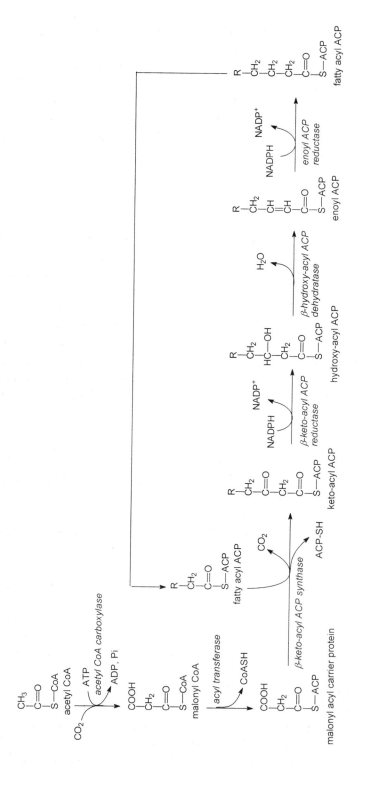

FIGURE 5.28 *The synthesis of fatty acids.*

chain elongation and further desaturation (between Δ^{9-10} and the carboxyl group) to yield the precursors of the eicosanoids.

The same series of enzymes catalyses elongation and desaturation of the $\omega 3$ and $\omega 6$ families of fatty acids, and they compete with each other. Although, as discussed in section 7.3.2.1, it is considered desirable to increase intakes of polyunsaturated fatty acids, there is some concern that an imbalance between intakes of $\omega 6$ polyunsaturated fatty acids (which come mainly from vegetable oils) and the $\omega 3$ series (which come mainly from fish oils) may lead to an undesirable imbalance in the synthesis of the two groups of eicosanoids.

5.6.1.2 Synthesis of triacylglycerols

The storage lipids in adipose tissue are triacylglycerols: glycerol esterified with three molecules of fatty acids. As discussed in section 4.3.1, the three fatty acids in a triacylglycerol molecule are not always the same, and the fatty acid at carbon-2 is usually unsaturated.

Triacylglycerols are synthesized mainly in the liver, adipose tissue and small intestinal mucosa, as well as lactating mammary gland. As shown in Figure 5.29, the substrates for triacylglycerol synthesis are fatty acyl CoA esters (formed by reaction between fatty acids and CoA, linked to the conversion of ATP to AMP plus pyrophosphate), and glycerol phosphate. The main source of glycerol phosphate is by reduction of dihydroxyacetone phosphate (an intermediate in glycolysis; see Figure 5.10); the liver, but not adipose tissue, can also phosphorylate glycerol to glycerol phosphate.

Two molecules of fatty acid are esterified to the free hydroxyl groups of glycerol phosphate, by transfer from fatty acyl CoA, forming monoacylglycerol phosphate and then diacylglycerol phosphate (or phosphatidate). Diacylglycerol phosphate is then hydrolysed to diacylglycerol and phosphate before reaction with the third molecule of fatty acyl CoA to yield triacylglycerol. (The diacylglycerol phosphate can also be used for the synthesis of phospholipids; section 4.3.1.2.)

It is obvious from Figure 5.29 that triacylglycerol synthesis incurs a considerable ATP cost; if the fatty acids are being synthesized from glucose, then overall some 20% of the energy yield of the carbohydrate is expended in synthesizing triacylglycerol reserves. The energy cost is lower if dietary fatty acids are being esterified to form triacylglycerols.

The enzymes for phosphatidate synthesis, acyl CoA synthetase, glycerol 3-phosphate acyltransferase and monoacylglycerol acyltransferase, are on both the outer mitochondrial membrane and the endoplasmic reticulum membrane. Diacylglycerol acyltransferase is only on the endoplasmic reticulum; it may use either diacylglycerol phosphate synthesized on the endoplasmic reticulum or that synthesized on the mitochondrion. Triacylglycerol synthesized on the endoplasmic reticulum membrane may then enter lipid droplets either in the cytosol or, in the liver and intestinal mucosa, the lumen of the endoplasmic reticulum for assembly into lipoproteins – chylomicrons in the intestinal mucosa (section 4.3.2.2) and very low-density lipoprotein in the liver (section 5.6.2).

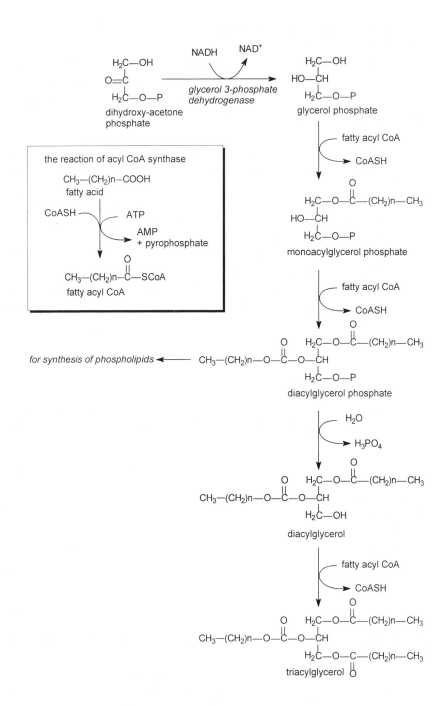

FIGURE 5.29 *The esterification of fatty acids to form triacylglycerol.*

5.6.2 PLASMA LIPOPROTEINS

Triacylglycerol, cholesterol and cholesterol esters, as well as lipid-soluble vitamins, are transported in plasma complexed with proteins. There are four major classes of lipoproteins, classified by their density, which in turn reflects the relative content of lipid and protein, as shown in Table 5.6:

- Chylomicrons, the least dense of the plasma lipoproteins, are formed in the intestinal mucosa and circulate as a source of triacylglycerol in the fed state (section 4.3.2.2).
- Very low-density lipoproteins (VLDL) are assembled in the liver and circulate as a source of cholesterol and triacylglycerol for extrahepatic tissues.
- Low-density lipoproteins (LDL) are formed in the circulation by removal of triacylglycerol from VLDL; intermediate-density lipoproteins (IDL) are an intermediate step in the conversion of VLDL to LDL.
- High-density lipoproteins (HDL). The apoproteins are synthesized in the liver and small intestine and acquire lipids (and especially cholesterol) from tissues for transport back to the liver.

TABLE 5.6 *Major classes of plasma lipoproteins*

	Chylomicrons	VLDL	IDL	LDL	HDL
Density (g/mL)	< 0.95	< 1.006	1.006–1.019	1.020–1.063	1.064–1.210
Diameter (nm)	75–1200	30–80	25–35	18–25	5–12
M_r (10^3 kDa)	400	10–80	5–10	2.3	0.175–0.36
Per cent protein	1.5–2.5	5–10	15–20	20–25	40–55
Per cent phospholipids	7–9	15–20	22	15–20	20–35
Per cent free cholesterol	1–3	5–10	8	7–10	3–4
Per cent triacylglycerol	84–89	50–65	22	7–10	3–5
Per cent cholesteryl esters	3–5	10–15	30	35–40	12
Electrophoretic mobility	At origin	Pre-beta	Between pre-beta and beta	Beta	Alpha
Major apoproteins	A-I, A-II, B-48, C-I, C-II, C-III, E	B-100, C-I, C-II, C-III, E	B-100, C-III, C-I, C-II, C-III, E	B-100	A-I, A-II, B-48, D, E
Turnover in plasma	4–5 minutes	1–3 hours	1–3 hours	45%/day	4 days

5.6.2.1 Chylomicrons

As discussed in section 4.3.2.2, newly absorbed fatty acids are re-esterified to form triacylglycerol in the intestinal mucosal cells, then assembled into chylomicrons, which enter the lacteal of the villus (see Figure 4.2), then the lymphatic system; they enter the bloodstream (the subclavian vein) at the thoracic duct. Chylomicrons begin to appear in the bloodstream about 60 minutes after a fatty meal, and have normally been cleared within 6–8 hours. In the bloodstream they acquire three additional proteins from HDL:

- Apoprotein C-II, which activates lipoprotein lipase at the cell surface, permitting uptake of fatty acids from chylomicron triacylglycerol. The triacylglycerols are hydrolysed extracellularly, and the free fatty acids are then taken into the cell and re-esterified to triacylglycerol. In the fed state the major site of lipoprotein lipase activity is adipose tissue, but other tissues can also hydrolyse chylomicron triacylglycerol as required.
- Apoprotein C-III, which activates lecithin–cholesterol acyltransferase, permitting cells to take up cholesterol from chylomicron cholesteryl esters.
- Apoprotein E, which binds to hepatic receptors for uptake of lipid-depleted chylomicron remnants. Chylomicron remnants are taken into the liver by receptor-mediated endocytosis, followed by hydrolysis of the proteins and the residual lipids.

5.6.2.2 Very low-density lipoproteins (VLDL) and low-density lipoproteins (LDL)

VLDL are assembled in the liver, and contain newly synthesized triacylglycerol, cholesterol and cholesteryl esters and phospholipids as well as lipids from chylomicron remnants. These lipids are taken up by peripheral tissues which have cell-surface lipoprotein lipase, phospholipase and cholesterol esterase.

As the VLDL particles are progressively depleted of lipids, they transfer apoproteins C-I and C-II to HDL, forming intermediate-density lipoprotein particles (IDL). IDL take up cholesteryl esters from HDL, becoming LDL.

LDL are cleared from the circulation by receptor-mediated uptake in the liver. Both the receptor and the LDL are internalized; the LDL is hydrolysed in lysosomes by proteases and lipases, and the receptor is recycled back to the cell surface.

Cholesterol represses synthesis of the LDL receptor, so that when there is an adequate amount of cholesterol in the liver less LDL will be cleared. The hypocholesterolaemic statin drugs both inhibit cholesterol synthesis and also increase clearance of LDL, because there is now less repression of receptor synthesis.

As discussed in section 7.2, elevated LDL cholesterol is one of the major factors in the development of atherosclerosis and ischaemic heart disease. Two factors are involved in elevated LDL cholesterol:

- Increased synthesis and secretion of VLDL – this in turn will be a consequence of a high fat intake, as there is more lipid from chylomicron remnants to be exported from the liver in VLDL.
- Decreased clearance of LDL by receptor-mediated uptake into the liver. This may be due to:
  - Low levels of LDL receptor synthesis (especially when hepatic cholesterol levels are high, but also genetically determined in some of the familial hyperlipidaemias).
  - Poor affinity of some genetic variants of apoprotein E for the LDL receptor. This is the basis of some genetic susceptibility to atherosclerosis.
  - Chemical modification of apoprotein E in the circulation, so reducing its affinity for the hepatic receptors. Commonly, this is secondary to oxidative damage to unsaturated fatty acids in LDL – hence the role of antioxidants in reducing the risk of atherosclerosis (section 7.4.3). High levels of homocysteine (section 11.11.3.3) can also lead to modification of apoprotein E.

LDL that are not cleared by the liver are taken up by the macrophage scavenger receptor; unlike hepatic uptake, this is an unregulated process, and macrophages can take up an almost unlimited amount of lipid from LDL. Lipid-engorged macrophages (foam cells) infiltrate blood vessel endothelium, forming fatty streaks that eventually develop into atherosclerotic plaque.

5.6.2.3 High-density lipoproteins (HDL)

Peripheral tissues take up more cholesterol from VLDL than they require, and export the surplus onto HDL for return to the liver for catabolism. HDL are secreted from the liver as a lipid-poor protein, and take up cholesterol from tissues by the action of lecithin–cholesterol acyltransferase at the lipoprotein surface.

Much of the cholesterol in HDL is transferred to chylomicron remnants and LDL, for receptor-mediated uptake into the liver. However, cholesterol-rich HDL can also bind to a liver receptor that has esterase activity, permitting uptake of cholesterol into the liver. The apoprotein is not internalized, as occurs with chylomicron remnants and LDL, but is released back into the circulation when most of the lipid has been removed.

5.6.3 GLYCOGEN

In the fed state, glycogen is synthesized from glucose in both liver and muscle. The reaction is a stepwise addition of glucose units onto the glycogen that is already present.

As shown in Figure 5.30, glycogen synthesis involves the intermediate formation of UDP-glucose (uridine diphosphate glucose) by reaction between glucose 1-phosphate and UTP (uridine triphosphate). As each glucose unit is added to the growing glycogen

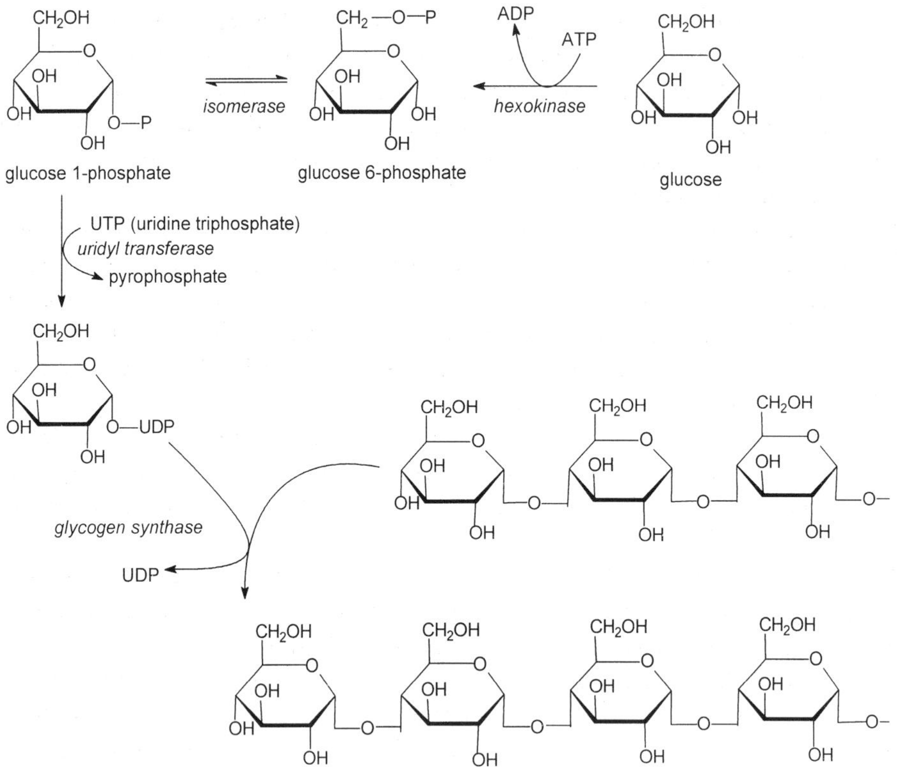

FIGURE 5.30 *The synthesis of glycogen.*

chain, so UDP is released, and must be rephosphorylated to UTP by reaction with ATP. There is thus a significant cost of ATP in the synthesis of glycogen: 2 mol of ATP is converted to ADP plus phosphate for each glucose unit added, and overall the energy cost of glycogen synthesis may account for 5% of the energy yield of the carbohydrate stored.

Glycogen synthetase forms only the $\alpha 1 \rightarrow 4$ links that form the straight chains of glycogen. The branch points are introduced by the transfer of 6–10 glucose units in a chain from carbon-4 to carbon-6 of the glucose unit at the branch point.

The branched structure of glycogen means that it traps a considerable amount of water within the molecule. As discussed in section 5.2, in the early stages of food restriction there is depletion of muscle and liver glycogen, with the release and excretion of this trapped water. This leads to an initial rate of weight loss that is very much greater than can be accounted for by catabolism of adipose tissue, and, of course, it cannot be sustained – once glycogen has been depleted the rapid loss of water (and weight) will cease.

5.6.3.1 Glycogen utilization

In the fasting state, glycogen is broken down by the removal of glucose units one at a time from the many ends of the molecule. As shown in Figure 5.9, the reaction is a phosphorolysis – cleavage of the glycoside link between two glucose molecules by the introduction of phosphate. The product is glucose 1-phosphate, which is then isomerized to glucose 6-phosphate. In the liver glucose 6-phosphatase catalyses the hydrolysis of glucose 6-phosphate to free glucose, which is exported for use especially by the brain and red blood cells.

Muscle cannot release free glucose from the breakdown of glycogen, because it lacks glucose 6-phosphatase. However, muscle glycogen can be an indirect source of blood glucose in the fasting state. Glucose 6-phosphate from muscle glycogen undergoes glycolysis to pyruvate (see Figure 5.10), which is then transaminated to alanine. Alanine is exported from muscle and taken up by the liver for use as a substrate for gluconeogenesis (section 5.7).

Glycogen phosphorylase stops cleaving $\alpha1\rightarrow4$ links four glucose residues from a branch point, and a debranching enzyme catalyses the transfer of a three glucosyl unit from one chain to the free end of another chain. The $\alpha1\rightarrow6$ link is then hydrolysed by a glucosidase, releasing glucose.

The branched structure of glycogen means that there are a great many points at which glycogen phosphorylase can act; in response to stimulation by adrenaline (section 10.3) there can be a very rapid release of glucose 1-phosphate from glycogen.

Endurance athletes require a slow release of glucose 1-phosphate from glycogen over a period of hours, rather than a rapid release. There is some evidence that this is achieved better from glycogen that is less branched, and therefore has fewer points at which glycogen phosphorylase can act. The formation of branch points in glycogen synthesis is slower than the formation of $\alpha1\rightarrow4$ links, and this has been exploited in the process of 'carbohydrate loading' in preparation for endurance athletic events. The athlete exercises to exhaustion, when muscle glycogen is more or less completely depleted, then consumes a high-carbohydrate meal, which stimulates rapid synthesis of glycogen with fewer branch points than normal. There is little evidence to show whether or not this improves endurance performance; such improvement as has been reported may be the result of knowing that one has made an effort to improve performance rather than any real metabolic effect.

5.7 *Gluconeogenesis – the synthesis of glucose from non-carbohydrate precursors*

Because the brain is largely dependent on glucose as its metabolic fuel (and red blood cells are entirely so) there is a need to maintain the blood concentration of glucose between about 3 and 5 mmol/L in the fasting state. If the plasma concentration of glucose falls below about 2 mmol/L there is a loss of consciousness – hypoglycaemic coma.

To a considerable extent the plasma concentration of glucose is maintained in short-term fasting by the use of glycogen, and by releasing free fatty acids from adipose tissues and ketone bodies from the liver, which are preferentially used by muscle, so sparing such glucose as is available for use by the brain and red blood cells.

However, the total body content of glycogen would be exhausted within 12–18 hours of fasting if there were no other source of glucose. This is the process of gluconeogenesis – the synthesis of glucose from non-carbohydrate precursors: amino acids from the breakdown of protein and the glycerol of triacylglycerols. It is important to note that, although acetyl CoA, and hence fatty acids, can be synthesized from pyruvate (and therefore from carbohydrates), the decarboxylation of pyruvate to acetyl CoA cannot be reversed. Pyruvate cannot be formed from acetyl CoA. As two molecules of carbon dioxide are formed for each two-carbon acetate unit metabolized in the citric acid cycle (see Figure 5.18), there can be no net formation of oxaloacetate from acetate. *It is not possible to synthesize glucose from acetyl CoA, and fatty acids and ketone bodies cannot serve as a precursor for glucose synthesis under any circumstances.*

The pathway of gluconeogenesis is essentially the reverse of the pathway of glycolysis, shown in Figure 5.10. However, at three steps there are separate enzymes involved in the breakdown of glucose (glycolysis) and gluconeogenesis. As discussed in section 5.4.1, the reactions of pyruvate kinase, phosphofructokinase and hexokinase cannot readily be reversed (i.e. they have equilibria which are strongly in the direction of the formation of pyruvate, fructose bisphosphate and glucose 6-phosphate respectively).

There are therefore separate enzymes, under distinct metabolic control, for the reverse of each of these reactions in gluconeogenesis:

- Pyruvate is converted to phosphoenolpyruvate for glucose synthesis by a two-step reaction, with the intermediate formation of oxaloacetate. As shown in Figure 5.31, pyruvate is carboxylated to oxaloacetate in an ATP-dependent reaction in which the vitamin biotin (section 11.12) is the coenzyme. This reaction can also be used to replenish oxaloacetate in the citric acid cycle when intermediates have been withdrawn for use in other pathways, and is involved in the return of oxaloacetate from the cytosol to the mitochondrion in fatty acid synthesis – see Figure 5.26. Oxaloacetate then undergoes a phosphorylation reaction, in which it also loses carbon dioxide, to form phosphoenolpyruvate. The phosphate donor for this reaction is GTP; as discussed in section 5.4.4, this provides regulation over the use of oxaloacetate for gluconeogenesis if citric acid cycle activity would be impaired.
- Fructose bisphosphate is hydrolysed to fructose 6-phosphate by a simple hydrolysis reaction catalysed by the enzyme fructose bisphosphatase.
- Glucose 6-phosphate is hydrolysed to free glucose and phosphate by the action of glucose 6-phosphatase.

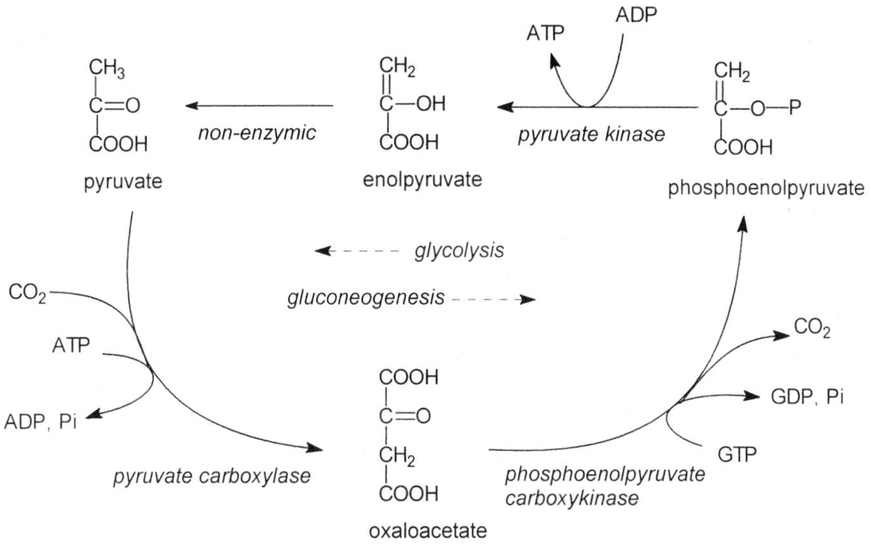

FIGURE 5.31 *Reversal of the reaction of pyruvate kinase for gluconeogenesis – pyruvate carboxylase and phosphoenolpyruvate carboxykinase.*

The other reactions of glycolysis are readily reversible, and the overall direction of metabolism, either glycolysis or gluconeogenesis, depends mainly on the relative activities of phosphofructokinase and fructose bisphosphatase, as discussed in section 10.2.2.

As discussed in section 5.4.4.2 and section 9.3.2, many of the products of amino acid metabolism can also be used for gluconeogenesis, as they are sources of pyruvate or one of the intermediates in the citric acid cycle, and hence give rise to oxaloacetate. The requirement for gluconeogenesis from amino acids in order to maintain a supply of glucose explains why there is often a considerable loss of muscle in prolonged fasting or starvation, even if there are apparently adequate reserves of adipose tissue to meet energy needs.

Additional resources

PowerPoint presentation 5 on the CD.
Self-assessment quiz 5 on the CD.

PROBLEM 5.1: *Winston B*

Winston is a 75-kg man who takes part in a 100 m sprint. His plasma lactate was 0.5 mmol/L before the race and 11.5 mmol/L immediately after the race. Thirty minutes later, when his breathing had returned to normal, it was 1.0 mmol/L.

Assuming that extracellular fluid is 20% of body weight, what is the total amount of lactate that he metabolizes during this 30 minutes?

Most of this lactate will be metabolized in the liver, undergoing gluconeogenesis, followed by release of glucose into the bloodstream and uptake into muscle for synthesis of glycogen to replace that used during the race.

What is the total cost in mol ATP and/or GTP per mol of lactate converted to glycogen?

How much ATP would be required to convert all of the lactate that is metabolized into muscle glycogen?

How much lactate must undergo total oxidation to CO_2 and water (via lactate dehydrogenase, pyruvate dehydrogenase and the citric acid cycle) to provide this ATP?

The oxidation of lactate, like that of glucose, consumes 0.746 L of oxygen per gram. The molecular mass of lactate is 90.1. What is his additional oxygen requirement (in litres of oxygen) over the 30 minutes after the end of the race?

Assuming that his total energy expenditure is 14 MJ/day, and that regardless of the fuel being oxidized the energy yield is 20 kJ per litre of oxygen consumed, what is the percentage increase in his oxygen consumption during this 30 minutes?

PROBLEM 5.2: *Peter C*

Peter is a 50-year-old man, 174 cm tall and weighing 105 kg. He is an engineer, and works on secondment in one of the strict Islamic states in the Gulf, where alcohol is prohibited. At the beginning of August he returned to England for his annual leave. According to his family, he behaved as he usually did when on home leave, consuming a great deal of alcohol and refusing meals. He was known to be drinking 2 L of whisky, two or three bottles of wine and a dozen or more cans of lager each day; his only solid food consisted of sweets and biscuits.

On 1 September he was admitted to the Accident and Emergency Department of UCL (University College London) Hospital, semiconscious, and with a rapid respiration rate (40/min). His blood pressure was 90/60 and his pulse rate was 136/min. His temperature was normal (37.1 °C). Emergency blood gas analysis revealed severe acidosis (pH 7.02) and base excess (−23) with a Po_2 of 91 mmHg and Pco_2 of 10 mmHg. He was transferred to intensive care and given intravenous bicarbonate.

His pulse rate remained high, and his blood pressure low, so emergency cardiac catheterization was performed; this revealed a cardiac output of 23 L/min (normal 4–6). A chest radiograph showed significant cardiac enlargement.

TABLE 5.7 *Clinical chemistry results for a plasma sample from Peter C taken in the fasting state*

Concentration (mmol/L)	Peter C	Reference range
Glucose	10.6	3.5–5.0
Sodium	142.0	131–151
Potassium	3.9	3.4–5.2
Chloride	91.0	100–110
Bicarbonate	5.0	21–29
Lactate	18.9	0.9–2.7
Pyruvate	2.5	0.1–0.2

Table 5.7 shows the clinical chemistry results from a plasma sample taken shortly after Peter was admitted.

What is the likely biochemical basis of Peter's problem, which led to his emergency hospitalization?

What additional test(s) might you request to confirm your assumption?

What emergency treatment would you suggest?

This information is from the case notes of a patient in the ITU at UCL Hospital/ The Middlesex Hospital – I am grateful to Dr Hugh Montgomery for drawing my attention to this case, and for permission to repeat data from the patient's notes.

PROBLEM 5.3: *The citric acid cycle*

The key experiments that led to elucidation of the citric acid cycle (tricarboxylic acid cycle) were described by Krebs and Johnson in 1937. They measured the consumption of oxygen by a preparation of minced pigeon breast muscle when incubated with various additions. The results in Table 5.8 show the volume of oxygen consumed during the incubation by 460 mg wet weight of tissue (the complete oxidation of 1 mmol of citrate to CO_2 and H_2O consumes 100 µL of O_2).

Previous studies had shown a similar effect of adding fumarate, oxaloacetate or succinate. What conclusions can you draw from these results?

Isolated hepatocytes were incubated for 40 minutes in a phosphate–bicarbonate–CO_2 buffer system, with [U-^{14}C]palmitate (i.e. palmitate labelled with ^{14}C in all 16 carbon atoms), at a specific radioactivity of 10^3 dpm (radioactive disintegrations per minute) per micromole, with and without the addition of 60 mmol/L malonate and/ or oxaloacetate.

One set of incubations was set up to act as a control, in which the perchloric acid was added at the beginning of the experiment.

After collection of the CO_2 for measurement of the radioactivity incorporated, the denatured incubation mixture was extracted with a chloroform–methanol mixture to separate unmetabolized palmitate (in the organic phase) from water-soluble metabolites

TABLE 5.8 *Oxygen consumption by pigeon breast muscle with and without added citrate*

Incubation time (min)	Oxygen consumed (μL)		
	No citrate	Plus citrate	Difference
30	645	682	+37
60	1055	1520	+465
90	1132	1938	+806

Source: From data reported by Krebs HA and Johnson WA, *Enzymologia* 4: 148–156, 1937.

TABLE 5.9 *Recovery of radioactivity from {U-^{14}C}palmitate in isolated hepatocytes*

	Radioactivity (10^3 dpm/min/g cells) found in		
	CO_2	Organic phase	Aqueous phase
Control (unincubated)	0	10.0	0
No addition	2.3	7.5	0.2
Plus malonate	0	9.8	0.2
Plus oxaloacetate	4.8	5.0	0.2
Plus malonate + oxaloacetate	0	5.0	5.0

TABLE 5.10 *Metabolism of palmitate, lactate and glutamate in isolated hepatocytes*

Substrate	Change (μmol/min/g cells)			
	Lactate	Palmitate	Glutamate	Glucose
Lactate	−4.11	+0.21	0	+0.60
Palmitate	0	−0.35	0	0
Palmitate + lactate	−2.4	−0.59	0	+1.20
Glutamate	0	0	−3.42	+0.81

TABLE 5.11 *Recovery of radioactivity from {^{14}C-2}lactate and {U-^{14}C}palmitate in isolated hepatocytes*

Substrate	Radioactivity (10^3 dpm/min/g cells) found in	
	CO_2	Glucose
[^{14}C-2]Lactate	3.71	1.20
[U-^{14}C]Palmitate	3.71	0
[U-^{14}C]Palmitate + glutamate	7.75	0.51

(which remained in the aqueous layer). The radioactivity in both phases was determined, and the results are shown in Table 5.9.

Can you account for these observations?

What is the water-soluble compound that accumulates in the presence of malonate?

Isolated hepatocytes were incubated with lactate, glutamate and/or palmitate as substrates. At the end of the experiment lactate, palmitate, glutamate, glucose (after acid hydrolysis of glycogen) and total ketone bodies (acetoacetate plus β-hydroxybutyrate) were determined. The results have been expressed as change during the incubation, compared with similar incubations which were stopped with perchloric acid at the beginning of the experiment, and are shown in Table 5.10.

What conclusions can you draw from these results?

Isolated hepatocytes were incubated with lactate labelled with ^{14}C in carbon-2 ($[^{14}C\text{-}2]$lactate) or palmitate labelled with ^{14}C in all carbon atoms ($[U\text{-}^{14}C]$palmitate); in each case the specific radioactivity of the labelled substrate in the incubation medium was 10^3 dpm/μmol. In a further series of incubations with $[U\text{-}^{14}C]$palmitate, non-radioactive glutamate was also added. The results are shown in Table 5.11.

What conclusions can you draw from these results?

Overweight and obesity

As discussed in section 5.2, if the intake of metabolic fuels (in other words the total intake of food) is greater than is required to meet energy expenditure, the result is storage of the excess, largely as triacylglycerols in adipose tissue. This chapter is concerned with the problems associated with excessive accumulation of body fat: overweight and obesity.

Objectives

After reading this chapter you should be able to:

- explain what is meant by desirable body weight, calculate body mass index and determine whether it is within the desirable range or not;
- describe the methods that are available to determine body fat content;
- describe the health hazards associated with overweight and obesity;
- explain the cause and treatment of obesity.

6.1 Desirable body weight

Figure 6.1 shows the relationship between body weight and premature death. It is based on a study of 750,000 people, who were classified according to their percentage of the average weight of the study group, then followed for 15 years. There is a steady

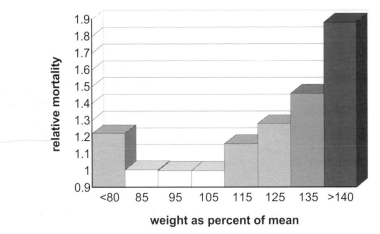

FIGURE 6.1 *Excess mortality with obesity. From data reported by Garfinkel L (1986) Cancer 58: 1826–1829.*

increase in mortality with increasing body weight above average, so that people who were 50–60% over average weight were twice as likely to die prematurely as those of average weight.

People who were significantly below average weight at the beginning of the study were also more at risk of premature death. However, this may be because those people who were significantly underweight were already seriously ill (section 8.4), rather than implying that a moderate degree of underweight is undesirable or poses any health hazards.

Figure 6.1 also shows that people whose weight was about 90% of the average were less likely to die prematurely than those of average weight. Such data make it possible to define a range of body weight, somewhat below average weight, which is associated with optimum life expectancy. The ranges of desirable weight for height, based on insurance company data of life expectancy, are shown in Figure 6.2.

6.1.1 BODY MASS INDEX

As an alternative to using tables of weight and height, it is possible to calculate a simple numerical index from height and weight, and to use this to establish acceptable ranges. The most commonly used such index is the body mass index (BMI), sometimes also called Quetelet's index, after Quetelet, who first demonstrated its usefulness in nutritional studies.

Body mass index is calculated from the weight (in kilograms) divided by the square of the height (in metres) – i.e. $BMI = weight (kg)/height^2 (m)$. The desirable range, associated with optimum life expectancy, is between 20 and 25. As discussed in section 8.2, values of BMI below 20 are associated with undernutrition. Table 6.1 shows the classification of overweight and obesity by BMI. For older people, there is some evidence

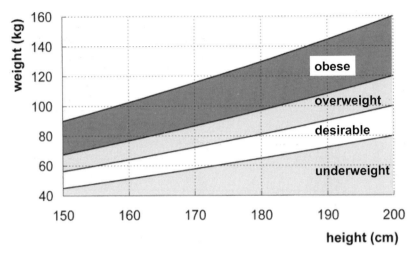

FIGURE 6.2 *Weight for height as an index of overweight and obesity.*

that a higher body weight is associated with better health and survival; Table 6.2 shows the desirable ranges of BMI at different ages.

6.1.2 MEASUREMENT OF BODY FAT

Although BMI is widely used to assess overweight and obesity, what is important for health and life expectancy is the body content of fat, and it is important to be able to determine the proportion of body weight that is fat. This is termed adiposity; a number of techniques are available for assessing adiposity, although most of them are research techniques and are not appropriate for routine screening of the general public.

6.1.2.1 Determination of body density

The density of body fat is 0.9 g/mL, whereas that of the fat-free body mass is 1.10 g/mL. This means that, if the density of the body can be calculated, then the proportion of fat and lean tissue can be calculated.

   Density is determined by weighing in air, and again totally submerged in water (the density of water = 1.0 g/mL), or by determining the volume of the body by its displacement of water when submerged. Neither procedure is particularly pleasant for the experimental subject, and considerable precision is necessary in the measurements; at 10% of body weight as fat, which is extremely low, density = 1.08 g/mL, while at 50% fat, which is very high, density = 1.00 g/mL.

   Although direct determination of body density is the standard against which all the other techniques listed below must be calibrated, it is clearly a research technique and not appropriate for general use.

TABLE 6.1 *Classification of overweight and obesity by body mass index*

	BMI	Excess weight (kg)	Per cent of desirable weight
Desirable	20–25	–	100
Acceptable but not desirable	25–27	< 5	100–110
Overweight	25–30	5–15	110–120
Obese	30–40	15–25	120–160
Severely obese	> 40	> 25	> 160

$BMI = $ weight (kg)/height^2 (m).

TABLE 6.2 *Desirable ranges of body mass index with age*

Age (years)	Desirable BMI
19–24	19–24
25–34	20–25
35–44	21–26
45–54	22–27
55–64	23–28
> 65	24–29

6.1.2.2 Determination of total body water or potassium

The water content of fat (i.e. pure triacylglycerol, not adipose tissue) is zero, while the fat-free mass of the body is 73% water. The total amount of water in the body can be determined by giving a dose of water labelled with ^{2}H or ^{18}O, and then measuring the dilution of the label in urine or saliva.

An alternative approach is to measure the total body content of potassium; again, fat contains no potassium, which occurs only in the fat-free mass of the body. There is a gender difference here: in males the fat-free mass contains 60 mmol potassium/kg, and in females 66 mmol/kg. The radioactive isotope of potassium, ^{40}K, occurs naturally. It is a weak γ-emitter, and therefore total body potassium can be determined by measuring the γ-radiation of the appropriate wavelength emitted by the body. This requires total enclosure in a shielded whole-body counter for about 15 minutes to achieve adequate precision, and because of this, and the cost of the equipment required, this is again purely a research technique.

6.1.2.3 Imaging techniques

Fat, bone and lean tissues absorb X-rays and ultrasound to different extents, and therefore either a radiograph or ultrasound image will permit determination of the amounts of different tissues in the body, by measuring the areas (or volumes if scanning imaging techniques are used) occupied by each type of tissue. Such imaging techniques permit determination not only of the total amount of fat in the body, but also of its distribution. As discussed in section 6.2.3, the distribution of body fat is an important factor in the adverse effects of excess adiposity.

6.1.2.4 Measurement of whole-body electrical conductivity

Fat is an electrical insulator, whereas lean tissue, being a solution of electrolytes, will conduct an electric current. If electrodes are attached to the hand and foot, and an extremely small alternating electric current (typically 80 μA at 50 MHz) is passed between them, measurement of the fall in voltage permits calculation of the conductivity of the body. The percentage of fat and lean tissue can be calculated from equations based on a series of studies in which this technique has been calibrated against direct determination of density (section 6.1.2.1).

Measurements of either total body electrical conductivity (TOBEC) or bioelectrical impedance (BIE) are used mainly in research, but as the equipment becomes more widely available these methods will become the methods of preference for routine estimation of body fat.

6.1.2.5 Measurement of skinfold thickness

The most widely used technique for estimating body fat reserves is measurement of the thickness of subcutaneous adipose tissue, using standardized calipers that exert a moderate pressure (10 g/mm^2 over an area of 20–40 mm^2) and hence cause some temporary discomfort. For greatest precision, the mean of the skinfold thickness at four sites should be calculated:

1 over the triceps, at the mid-point of the upper arm;
2 over the biceps, at the front of the upper arm, directly above the cubital fossa, at the same level as the triceps site;
3 subscapular, just below and laterally to the angle of the shoulder blade, with the shoulder and arm relaxed;
4 suprailiac, on the mid-axillary line immediately superior to the iliac crest.

The approximate desirable ranges of mean skinfold thickness are: men 3–10 mm; women 10–22 mm.

6.2 *The problems of overweight and obesity*

Historically, a moderate degree of overweight was considered desirable. In a society in which food was scarce, fatness demonstrated greater than average wealth and prosperity.

This attitude persists in many developing countries today; food is scarce, and few people have enough to eat, let alone too much.

There is a good biological (evolutionary) argument in favour of a modest degree of overweight. A person who has reserves of fat is more likely to be able to survive a period of food deprivation or famine than a person with smaller fat reserves. So, at least in times past, fatter people may have been at an advantage. This is no longer so in developed countries, where there are no longer seasonal shortages of food. Widespread hunger is not been a problem in Western Europe or North America, although, as discussed in Chapter 8, lack of food is still a major problem in many countries.

Figure 6.3 shows that in 1998 (the most recent year for which data are available) more than half of all people in Britain were classified as overweight (i.e. BMI > 25); 17% of men and 21% of women were classified as obese (i.e. BMI > 30). Perhaps more seriously, the proportion of people who were classified as obese increased almost threefold in the period 1980 to 1998, and there is no evidence of any reversal of this trend. There has been a similar increase in the prevalence of obesity in most developed countries over the same period.

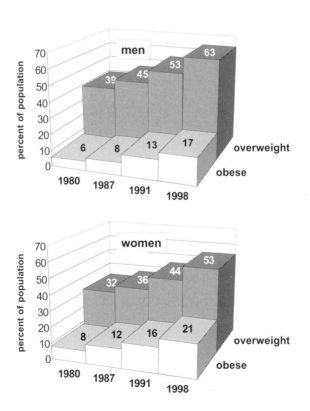

FIGURE 6.3 *The increasing prevalence of overweight and obesity in UK, 1980–98, from UK Department of Health data.*

6.2.1 SOCIAL PROBLEMS OF OBESITY

As food supplies have become more assured, so perceptions have changed. Fatness is no longer regarded as a sign of wealth and prosperity. No longer are the overweight in society envied. Rather, they are likely to be mocked, reviled and made deeply unhappy by the unthinking comments and prejudices of their lean companions.

Because society at large considers obesity undesirable, and fashion emphasizes slimness, many overweight and obese people have problems of a poor self-image and low self-esteem. Obese people are certainly not helped by the all too common prejudice against them, the difficulty of buying clothes that will fit and the fact that they are often regarded as a legitimate butt of crude and cruel humour. This may lead to a sense of isolation and withdrawal from society, and may frequently result in increased food consumption, for comfort, thus resulting in yet more weight gain, a further loss of self-esteem, further withdrawal and more eating for compensation.

The psychological and social problems of the obese spill over to people of normal weight as well. There is continual advertising pressure for 'slimness', and newspapers and magazines are full of propaganda for slimness and 'diets' for weight reduction. This may be one of the factors in the development of major eating disorders such as anorexia nervosa and bulimia (section 8.3.1.1).

6.2.2 THE HEALTH RISKS OF OBESITY

As shown in Figure 6.1, people who are overweight are significantly more likely to die prematurely, and at 50% over desirable weight there is a twofold risk of premature death. Figure 6.4 shows the main causes of premature death that are associated with overweight and obesity, expressed as the ratio of that condition as a cause of death in obese people to the expected rate in lean people.

Obesity, and especially abdominal obesity (section 6.2.3), is strongly associated with insulin resistance and the development of non-insulin-dependent diabetes mellitus (section 10.7). This is largely the result of increased circulating concentrations of non-esterified fatty acids (released from plasma lipoproteins by lipoprotein lipase; section 5.5.6.2). Non-esterified fatty acids decrease muscle uptake and utilization of glucose and may also antagonize insulin action. Weight loss results in a considerable improvement in glycaemic control in patients with early non-insulin-dependent diabetes.

In addition to the diseases caused by, or associated with, obesity, obese people are considerably more at risk of death during surgery and post-operative complications. There are three main reasons for this:

- Surgery is longer and more difficult when the surgeon has to cut through large amounts of subcutaneous and intra-abdominal adipose tissue.
- Induction of anaesthesia is more difficult when veins are not readily visible through subcutaneous adipose tissue, and maintenance of anaesthesia is complicated by

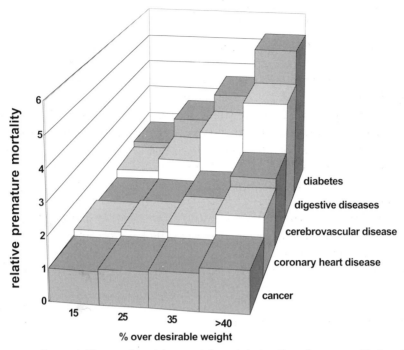

Figure 6.4 *Cause-specific mortality with overweight and obesity. From data reported by Lew EA and Garfinkel L (1979)* Journal of Chronic Diseases *12: 563–576.*

the solubility of anaesthetic agents in fat, so that there is a large buffer pool in the body, and adjustment of the dose is difficult.

- Most importantly, anaesthesia depresses lung function (as does being in a supine position) in all subjects. Obese people suffer from impaired lung function under normal conditions, largely as a result of adipose tissue in the upper body segment; total lung capacity may be only 60% of that in lean people, and the mechanical workload on the respiratory muscles may be twice that of lean people. Therefore, they are especially at risk during surgery.

Because of their impaired lung function, obese people are more at risk of respiratory distress, pneumonia and bronchitis than are lean people. In addition, excess body weight is associated with increased morbidity from such conditions as:

- arthritis of the hips and knees, associated with the increased stress on weight-bearing joints;
- varicose veins and haemorrhoids, associated with increased intra-abdominal pressure, which possibly are due more to a low intake of dietary fibre (section 4.2.1.6 and section 7.3.3.2) and hence straining on defecation than a direct result of obesity.

6.2.3 THE DISTRIBUTION OF EXCESS ADIPOSE TISSUE

The adverse effects of obesity are due not only to the excessive amount of body fat, but also to its distribution in the body. In most studies of coronary heart disease patients there is a threefold excess of men compared with women, a difference that persists even when the raw data are corrected for such known risk factors as blood pressure, cholesterol in low-density lipoproteins, body mass index, smoking and physical activity. However, as shown in Figure 6.5, if the data are corrected for the ratio of the diameter of the waist to hip, there is now only a 1.4-fold excess of men over women.

The waist–hip ratio provides a convenient way of defining two patterns of adipose tissue distribution:

- predominantly in the upper body segment (thorax and abdomen) – the classical male pattern of obesity, sometimes called apple-shaped obesity;
- predominantly in the lower body segment (hips) – the classical female pattern of obesity, sometimes called pear-shaped obesity.

It is the male pattern of upper body segment obesity that is associated with the major health risks, and in a number of studies assessment of the pattern of fat distribution by measurement of either the waist–hip ratio or the subscapular skinfold thickness (section 6.1.2.5) shows a greater correlation with the incidence of hypertension, diabetes and coronary heart disease than does BMI alone.

Abdominal adipose tissue produces less leptin (section 1.3.2) than does subcutaneous adipose tissue, so that abdominal fat will have less effect on long-term regulation of food intake and energy expenditure (section 1.3.2).

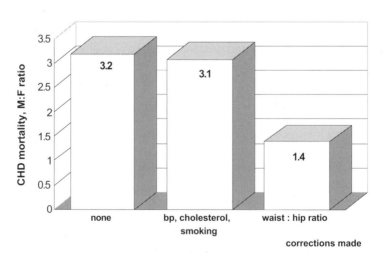

FIGURE 6.5 *Body fat distribution and the gender difference in coronary heart disease mortality.*

6.3 *The causes and treatment of obesity*

The cause of obesity is an intake of metabolic fuels greater than is required for energy expenditure, so that excess is stored, largely as fat in adipose tissue reserves. The simple answer to the problem of obesity is therefore to reverse the balance: reduce food intake and increase physical activity and hence energy expenditure.

6.3.1 ENERGY EXPENDITURE

Part of the problem is the relatively low level of physical activity of many people in Western countries. The dramatic increase in overweight and obesity between 1980 and 1998 shown in Figure 6.3 occurred at a time when average food consumption was static or decreasing. As discussed in section 5.1.3.2, the average physical activity level in Britain is only 1.4; physical activity accounts for only 40% more energy expenditure than basal metabolic rate. At the same time, food is always readily available, with an ever-increasing array of attractive snack foods, which are easy to eat, and many of which are high in fat and sugar.

Sometimes, the problem can be attributed to a low rate of energy expenditure despite a reasonable level of physical activity. There is a range of individual variation as much as 30% above and below the average BMR (section 5.1.3.1). This means that some people will have a very low BMR, and hence a very low requirement for food. Despite eating very little compared with those around them, they may gain weight. Equally, there are people who have a relatively high BMR and are able to eat a relatively large amount of food without gaining weight.

Lean people can increase their energy expenditure to match their food intake; leptin (section 1.3.2) increases the activity of mitochondrial uncoupling proteins (section 5.1.3.1). The result of this is an increased rate of metabolism of metabolic fuels and increased heat output from the body, especially after meals and while asleep.

Other people seem to be much more energy efficient, and their body temperature may drop slightly while they are asleep. This means that they are using less metabolic fuel to maintain body temperature, and so are able to store more as adipose tissue. Such people tend to be overweight. (This response, lowering body temperature and metabolic rate to conserve food, is seen in a more extreme form in animals that hibernate. During their long winter sleep these animals have a very low rate of metabolism, and hence a low rate of utilization of the fuel they have stored in adipose tissue reserves.)

6.3.2 CONTROL OF APPETITE

Most people manage to balance their food intake with energy expenditure remarkably precisely. Indeed, even people who are overweight or obese are in energy balance and their weight is more or less constant. As discussed in section 1.3.2, leptin is central to the control of both food intake and energy expenditure, and there are a number of mechanisms involved in short-term control of food intake, with regulation of both hunger and satiety.

Very rarely, people are overweight or obese as a result of a physical defect of the appetite control centres in the brain – for example, some tumours can cause damage to the satiety centre, so that the patient feels hunger, but not the sensation of satiety, and has no physiological cue to stop eating.

More commonly, obesity can be attributed to a psychological failure of appetite control. At its simplest, this can be blamed on the variety of attractive foods available. People can easily be tempted to eat more than they need, and it may take quite an effort of will-power to refuse a choice morsel. Even when hunger has been satisfied, the appearance of a different dish can stimulate the appetite. Experimental animals, which normally do not become obese, can be persuaded to overeat and become obese by providing them with a 'cafeteria' array of attractive foods.

A number of studies comparing severely obese people with lean people have shown that obese people do not respond to the normal cues for hunger and satiety. Rather, in many cases, it is the sight of food that prompts them to eat, regardless of whether they are 'hungry' or not. If no food is visible, they will not feel hungry; conversely, if food is still visible they will not feel satiety. There have been no similar studies involving more moderately overweight people, so it is not known whether the apparent failure of appetite regulation is a general problem or whether it affects only severely obese people with body mass index > 40.

6.3.3 HOW OBESE PEOPLE CAN BE HELPED TO LOSE WEIGHT

In considering the treatment of obesity, two different aspects of the problem must be considered:

* The initial problem, which is to help the overweight or obese person to reduce his or her weight to within the desirable range, where life expectancy is maximum.
* The long-term problem of helping the now lean person to maintain desirable body weight. This is largely a matter of education, increasing physical activity and changing eating habits. The same guidelines for a prudent diet (discussed in section 7.3) apply to the slimmed-down, formerly obese, person as to anyone else.

The aim of any weight reduction regime is to reduce the intake of food to below the level needed for energy expenditure, so that body reserves of fat will have to be used. As discussed in section 5.2, the theoretical maximum possible rate of weight loss is 230 g per megajoule energy imbalance per week; for a person with an energy expenditure of 10 MJ/day, total starvation would result in a loss of 2.3 kg/week. In practice, the rate of weight loss is lower than this theoretical figure because of the changes in metabolic rate and energy expenditure that occur with changes in both body weight and food intake.

Very often, the first one or two weeks of a weight-reducing regime are associated with a very much greater loss of weight than this. Obviously, this cannot be due to loss of fat. It is due to loss of the water associated with glycogen (section 4.2.1.5). Although it is not sustained, the initial rapid rate of weight loss can be extremely encouraging for the obese person. The problem is to ensure that he or she realizes that it will not, and indeed cannot, be sustained. It also provides excellent advertising copy for less than totally scrupulous vendors of slimming diets, who make truthful claims about the weight loss in the first week or two and omit any information about the later weeks and months needed to achieve goal weight.

6.3.3.1 Starvation

More or less total starvation has been used in a hospital setting to treat seriously obese patients, especially those who are to undergo elective surgery. Vitamins and minerals have to be supplied (see Chapter 11), as well as fluid, but apart from this an obese person can lose weight at about the predicted rate of 2.3 kg/week if starved completely. There are two major problems with total starvation as a means of rapid weight loss:

- The problem of enforcement. It is very difficult to deprive someone of food and to prevent them finding more or less devious means of acquiring it – by begging or stealing from other patients, visitors and hospital volunteers, or even by walking down to the hospital shop or out-patients cafeteria.
- As much as half the weight lost in total starvation may be protein from muscle and other tissues, in order to provide a source of amino acids for gluconeogenesis to maintain blood glucose (section 5.5.7) This is not desirable; the stress of surgery causes a considerable loss of protein (section 9.1.2.2), and it would be highly undesirable to start this loss before surgery.

6.3.3.2 Very low-energy diets

Many of the problems associated with total starvation can be avoided by feeding a very low energy intake, commonly 1–1.5 MJ/day, in specially formulated meal replacements that provide adequate intakes of vitamins and minerals. Such regimes have shown excellent results in the treatment of severe obesity. There is very much less loss of tissue protein than in total starvation, and with this small intake people feel less hungry than those who are starved completely.

If very low-energy diets are used together with a programme of exercise, the rate of weight loss can be close to the theoretical maximum of 2–2.5 kg/week. Such diets should probably be regarded as a treatment of last resort, for people with a serious problem of obesity which does not respond to more conventional diet therapy.

6.3.3.3 Conventional diets

For most people, the problem is not one of severe obesity, but a more modest excess body weight. Even for people who have a serious problem of obesity, it is likely that less drastic measures than those discussed above will be beneficial. The aim is to reduce energy intake to below expenditure, and so ensure the utilization of adipose tissue reserves. To anyone who has not tried to lose weight, the answer would appear to be simply to eat less. Obviously it is not so simple. As shown in Figure 6.3, there is a considerable, and increasing, problem of obesity in Western countries – and a vast array of diets, slimming regimes, special foods and appetite suppressants is available.

The ideal approach to the problem of obesity and weight reduction would be to provide people with the information they need to choose an appropriate diet for themselves. This is not easy. It is not simply a matter of reducing energy intake, but of ensuring at the same time that intakes of protein, vitamins and minerals are adequate. The preparation of balanced diets, especially when the total energy intake is to be reduced, is a highly skilled job, and is one of the main functions of the professional dietitian. Furthermore, there is the problem of long-term compliance with dietary restrictions – the diet must not only be low in energy and high in nutrients, it must also be attractive and pleasant to eat in appropriate amounts.

A simple way of helping people to select an appropriate diet for weight reduction is to offer three lists of foods:

- Energy-rich foods, which should be avoided. These are generally foods rich in fat and sugar but providing little in the way of vitamins and minerals. Such foods include oils and fats, fried foods, fatty cuts of meat, cakes, biscuits, etc. and alcoholic beverages. They should be eaten extremely sparingly, if at all.
- Foods which are relatively high in energy yield but also good sources of protein, vitamins and minerals. They should be eaten in moderate amounts.
- Foods which are generally rich sources of vitamins and minerals, high in starch and non-starch polysaccharide and low in fat and sugars (i.e. nutrient dense). These can be eaten (within reason) as much as is wanted.

An alternative method is to provide people with a series of meal plans and menus, designed to be nutrient dense and energy low, and providing sufficient variety from day to day to ensure compliance.

To make this less rigid and prescriptive, it is easy to provide a list of foods with 'exchange points', permitting one food to be substituted for another. At its simplest, such a list would give portions of foods with approximately the same energy yield.

A more elaborate exchange list calculates 'points' for foods based on their energy yield, nutrient density and total or saturated fat content. The consumer is given a target number of 'points' to be consumed each day, depending on gender, physical activity and the amount of weight to be lost, and can make up a diet to meet this target. An advantage of this is that foods that might be considered forbidden in a simple energy-counting diet can be permitted – but a single portion may constitute a whole day's points.

An interesting variant of the exchange points system also allocates (negative) points to physical activity, so promoting physical activity as well as sound eating habits.

6.3.3.4 Low-carbohydrate (ketogenic) diets

At one time, there was a vogue for low-carbohydrate diets for weight reduction. These were soundly based on the fact that fat and protein are more slowly digested and absorbed than carbohydrates and therefore have greater satiety value. At the same time, a severe restriction of carbohydrate intake would limit the intake of other foods as well – one argument was that without bread there was nothing on which to spread butter.

There is certainly a benefit in reducing the intake of carbohydrates with a high glycaemic index (section 4.2.2), as these lead to a larger insulin response, and hence result in more triacylglycerol synthesis in response to insulin than an equivalent amount of carbohydrate with a low glycaemic index.

Nowadays a low-carbohydrate diet would not be recommended for weight reduction, as the aim for general health promotion is to reduce the proportion of energy from fat and increase that from starches (section 7.3). Furthermore, storage of dietary fat in adipose tissue is metabolically more efficient than synthesis of triacylglycerol from carbohydrate (see sections 5.6.1 and 5.6.3), so that dietary fat will contribute more to adipose tissue reserves than will an equivalent amount of dietary carbohydrate. Nevertheless, to those raised in the belief that carbohydrates are fattening (as is any food in excess) it is a strange concept that weight reduction is helped by increased starch consumption.

6.3.3.5 High-fibre diets

One of the persistent problems raised by many people who are restricting their food intake to lose excess weight is that they continually feel hungry. Quite apart from true physiological hunger, the lack of bulk in the gastrointestinal tract may well be a factor here. This problem can be alleviated by increasing the intake of dietary fibre or non-starch polysaccharide (section 4.2.1.6) – increased amounts of whole-grain cereal products, fruits and vegetables. Such regimes are certainly successful, and again represent essentially a more extreme version of the general advice for a prudent diet.

It is generally desirable that the dietary sources of non-starch polysaccharides should be ordinary foods, rather than 'supplements'. However, as an aid to weight reduction, a number of preparations of dietary fibre are available. Some of these are more or less ordinary foods, but containing added fibre, which gives texture to the food, and increases the feeling of fullness and satiety. Some of the special slimmers' soups, biscuits, etc. are of this type. They are formulated to provide about one-third of a day's requirement of protein, vitamins and minerals, but with a low energy yield. They are supposed to be taken in place of one meal each day, and to aid satiety they contain carboxymethylcellulose or another non-digested polysaccharide.

An alternative approach is to take tablets or a suspension of non-starch polysaccharide before a meal. This again creates a feeling of fullness, and so reduces the amount of food that is eaten.

6.3.3.6 'Diets' that probably won't work

Weight reduction depends on reducing the intake of metabolic fuels but ensuring that the intake of nutrients is adequate to meet requirements. Equally important is the problem of ensuring that the weight that has been lost is not replaced – in other words, eating patterns must be changed after weight has been lost, to allow for maintenance of a body weight with a well-balanced diet.

There is a bewildering array of different diet regimes on offer to help the overweight and obese to lose weight. Some of these are based on sound nutritional principles and provide about half the person's energy requirement, together with adequate amounts of protein, vitamins and minerals. They permit a sustained weight loss of about 1–1.5 kg/week.

Other 'diets' are neither scientifically formulated nor based on sound nutritional principles, and indeed frequently depend on pseudo-scientific mumbo-jumbo to attempt to give them some validity. They frequently make exaggerated claims for the amount of weight that can be lost, and rarely provide a balanced diet. Publication of testimonials from 'satisfied clients' cannot be considered to be evidence of efficacy, and publication in a book that is a best-seller, or in a magazine with wide circulation, cannot correct the underlying flaws in many of these 'diets'.

Some of the more outlandish diet regimes depend on such nonsensical principles as eating protein and carbohydrates at different meals (so-called food combining) – ignoring the fact that such 'carbohydrate' foods as bread and potatoes provide a significant amount of protein as well (see Figure 9.3). Others depend on a very limited range of foods. The most extreme have allowed the client to eat bananas, grapefruit or peanuts (or some other food) in unlimited amounts, but little else. Other diet regimes ascribe almost magical properties to certain fruits (e.g. mangoes and pineapples), again with a very limited range of other foods allowed.

The idea is that if someone is permitted to eat as much they wish of only a very limited range of foods, even desirable and much liked foods, they will end up eating very little, because even a favourite food soon palls if it is all that is permitted. In practice, these 'diets' do neither good nor harm. People get so bored that they give up before there can be any significant effect on body weight, or any adverse effects of a very unbalanced diet. This is all to the good – if people did stick to such diets for any length of time they might well encounter problems of protein, vitamin and mineral deficiency.

6.3.3.7 Slimming patches

Basal metabolic rate is controlled to a considerable extent by the thyroid hormone tri-iodothyronine, and iodine deficiency (section 11.15.3.3) results in impaired synthesis of thyroid hormone, a low metabolic rate and hence ready weight gain. Pathological overactivity of the thyroid gland results in increased synthesis and secretion of thyroid hormone, and an increased basal metabolic rate, with weight loss.

The synthesis of thyroid hormone is regulated, and in the absence of thyroid disease provision of additional iodine does not increase hormone secretion except in people who were iodine deficient. Nevertheless, there are people who market various iodine-rich preparations to aid weight loss. Foremost among these are the so-called slimming patches, which contain seaweed extract as a source of iodine which is supposed to be absorbed from a small patch applied to the skin. There is no evidence that such patches have any beneficial effect at all.

6.3.3.8 Sugar substitutes

As discussed in section 7.3.3.1, the average consumption of sugar is higher than is considered desirable. There is a school of thought that blames the ready availability of sugar for much of the problem of overweight and obesity in Western countries. Simply omitting the sugar in tea and coffee would make a significant contribution to reduction of energy intake. A teaspoon of sugar is 5 g of carbohydrate, and thus provides 80 kJ. Two spoons of sugar in each of six cups of tea or coffee a day would thus account for some 960 kJ – almost 10% of the average person's energy expenditure. Quite apart from this obvious sugar, there is a great deal of sugar in beverages – for example, a standard 330 mL can of lemonade provides 20 g of sugar (= 320 kJ).

Because many people like their tea and coffee sweetened, and to replace the sugar in lemonades etc., there is a range of sugar substitutes. These are synthetic chemicals that are very much sweeter than sugar but are not metabolized as metabolic fuels. Even those that can be metabolized (for example aspartame, which is an amino acid derivative) are taken in such small amounts that they make no significant contribution to intake. All of these compounds have been extensively tested for safety, but as a result of concerns about possible hazards some are not permitted in some countries although they are widely used elsewhere.

6.3.3.9 Pharmacological treatment of obesity

A number of compounds act either to suppress the activity of the hunger centre in the hypothalamus or to stimulate the satiety centre. Sometimes this is an undesirable side-effect of drugs used to treat disease and can contribute to the undernutrition seen in chronically ill people (section 8.4). As an aid to weight reduction, especially in people who find it difficult to control their food intake, drugs that suppress appetite can be useful. Three compounds are in relatively widespread use as appetite suppressants: fenfluramine (and more recently the D-isomer, dexfenfluramine), diethylpropion and mazindol. The combination of phentermine and fenfluramine was withdrawn in the 1990s, after a number of reports associating it with cardiac damage, and there is some evidence of psychiatric disturbance and possible problems of addiction with these drugs. They should be used for only a limited time, and only under strict medical supervision. The action of appetite suppressants decreases after a few weeks, as tolerance or resistance to their action develops.

A number of compounds have been marketed as 'carbohydrate blockers', which are supposed to act by inhibiting amylase (section 4.2.2.1), and so reducing the digestion of starch. There is no evidence that they are effective, and none has been licensed for pharmaceutical use.

Inhibitors of pancreatic lipase (section 4.3.2) do reduce lipid digestion and absorption, and some have been licensed for pharmaceutical use. The problem with their use is that undigested fat in the gastrointestinal tract can cause discomfort and, if enough is present, foul-smelling fatty diarrhoea (steatorrhoea).

6.3.3.10 Surgical treatment of obesity

Severe obesity may be treated by surgical removal of much of the excess adipose tissue – a procedure known as liposuction. Two further surgical treatments have also been used:

- Intestinal by-pass surgery, in which the jejunum is connected to the distal end of the ileum, so by-passing much of the small intestine in which the digestion and absorption of food occurs (section 4.1). The resultant malabsorption means that the subject can, and indeed must, eat a relatively large amount of food but will only absorb a small proportion. There are severe side-effects of intestinal by-pass surgery, including persistent foul-smelling diarrhoea and flatulence and failure to absorb medication, as well as problems of mineral and vitamin deficiency. This procedure has been more or less abandoned in most centres.
- Gastroplasty, in which the physical capacity of the stomach is reduced to half or less. This limits the amount of food that can be consumed at any one meal. While the results of such surgery appear promising, long-term follow-up suggests that a significant number of patients experience serious side-effects, and many regret undergoing the procedure.

6.3.3.11 Help and support

Especially for the severely obese person, weight loss is a lengthy and difficult experience. Friends and family can be supportive, but frequently specialist help and advice are needed. To a great extent, this is the role of the dietitian and other health care professionals. In addition, there are a number of organizations, normally of formerly obese people, who can offer a mixture of professional nutritional and dietetic advice together with practical help and counselling. The main advantage of such groups is that they provide a social setting, rather than the formal setting of the dietitian's office in an out-patient clinic, and all the members have experienced similar problems.

Many people find the sharing of the problems and experiences of weight reduction extremely helpful.

Additional resources

PowerPoint presentation 6 on the CD.
Self-assessment exercise 6 on the CD.

The simulation program Energy Balance on the CD permits you to vary physical activity by keeping an activity diary, and see the effects of varying physical activity and energy intake on body weight.

PROBLEM 6.1: *Janice W*

Janice is a 40-year-old woman who is 162 cm tall and weighs 85 kg.
    What is her BMI? Is this within the desirable range?
    How much weight could she lose per megajoule energy deficit?
    For the purpose of these calculations, you may assume that all of the weight loss will be adipose tissue: 15% water, 5% protein (with an energy yield of 17 kJ/g) and 80% triacylglycerol (with an energy yield of 37 kJ/g). You should ignore the (probably considerable) loss of muscle tissue to provide amino acids for gluconeogenesis.
    Her total energy expenditure is 10 MJ/day. Assuming that she maintains her habitual level of physical activity, how much weight could she expect to lose per week:

1 if she reduced her food intake by 10%;
2 if she halved her food intake;
3 if she replaced all meals with a specially formulated very low-energy diet providing 2 MJ/day
4 if she starved completely?

For a woman age 40, and weighing 85 kg, BMR will be about 6.6 MJ/day. What is her PAL?
    Rather than reducing her food intake, she decides that she would prefer to increase her physical activity. What would be the effect on her body weight per week of walking moderately briskly for 1 hour per day (PAR = 3.0)
    After her exercise, she is thirsty, and drinks a pint of lager. The energy yield of lager is 130 kJ/100 mL. What is the effect of this drink on her overall energy balance and weight loss?

7

Diet and the diseases of affluence

Human beings have evolved in a hostile environment in which food has always been scarce. It is only in the last half-century, and only in Western Europe, North America and Australasia, that there is a surplus of food. As discussed in Chapter 8, food is still short in much of Africa, Asia and Latin America.

This chapter is concerned with the role of diet and nutrition in the so-called *diseases of affluence*: the health problems of developed countries, associated with a superabundant availability of food.

Objectives

After reading this chapter you should be able to:

- explain the types of evidence that link diet with the diseases of affluence;
- describe and explain the guidelines for a prudent diet and explain the recommendations concerning dietary fat and carbohydrate;
- explain what is meant by a free radical, how oxygen radicals cause tissue damage and the main sources of oxygen radicals;
- describe the main antioxidant nutrients and explain how they are believed to protect against cancer and heart disease;
- describe the various protective non-nutrient compounds that are found in a variety of foods and explain their protective actions.

7.1 *The diseases of affluence*

Despite the problems to be discussed in this chapter, which are major causes of premature death, people in developed countries have a significantly greater life expectancy than those in developing countries.

The major causes of death in developed countries today are heart disease, high blood pressure, strokes and cancer. These are not just diseases of old age, although it is true to say that the longer people live, the more likely they are to develop cancer. Heart disease is a major cause of premature death, striking a significant number of people aged under 40. This is not solely a Western phenomenon. As countries develop, so people in the prosperous cities begin to show a Western pattern of premature death from these same diseases.

Diet is, of course, only one of the differences between life in the developed countries of Western Europe, North America and Australasia and that in developing countries; there are a great many other differences in environment and living conditions. In addition, genetic variation will affect susceptibility to nutritional and environmental factors, and there is evidence that nutritional status *in utero* and infancy affects responses to diet in adult life.

It can be assumed that human beings and their diet have evolved together. Certainly, we have changed our crops and farm animals by selective breeding over the last 10,000 years, and it is reasonable to assume that we have evolved by natural selection to be suited to our diet. The problem is that evolution is a slow process, and there have been major changes in food availability in developed countries over the last century. As recently as the 1930s (very recent in evolutionary terms) it was estimated that up to one-third of households in Britain could not afford an adequate diet. Malnutrition was a serious problem, and the provision of 200 mL of milk daily to schoolchildren had a significant effect on their health and growth.

Foods that were historically scarce luxuries are now commonplace and available in surplus. Sugar was an expensive luxury until the middle of the nineteenth century; traditionally, fat was also scarce, and every effort was made to save and use all the fat (dripping) from a roast joint of meat.

There are thus two separate, but related, questions to be considered:

*   Is diet a factor in the aetiology of diseases of affluence that are major causes of premature death in developed countries?
*   Might changes in average Western diets reduce the risk of developing cancer and cardiovascular disease?

7.2 *Types of evidence linking diet and diseases of affluence*

The main evidence linking diet with the diseases of affluence is epidemiological; animal studies are used to test hypotheses derived from epidemiology, and to test the effects of specific nutritional changes. When there is a substantial body of evidence then there can be direct intervention studies, in which the diets of large numbers of people are changed (e.g. by providing supplements of nutrients for which there is epidemiological evidence of a protective effect), and they are followed for 5–10 or more years, to see whether the intervention has any effect on disease incidence or mortality.

7.2.1 SECULAR CHANGES IN DIET AND DISEASE INCIDENCE

The first type of evidence comes from studying changes in disease incidence and diet (but also other factors) over time. Table 7.1 shows the changes in diet in rural south-west Wales between 1870 and 1970. This was a century during which there was a marked decrease in hunger-related diseases and a marked increase in premature death from coronary heart disease – to the extent that in 1970 this region had one of the highest rates of coronary heart disease in Europe.

The major changes over this period were an increase in the proportion of energy derived from fat and an increase in the proportion of dietary fat that was saturated (section 4.3.1.1). At the same time there was a considerable increase in cholesterol consumption as a result of increased consumption of animal (saturated) fats and a significant decrease in the proportion of energy derived from starch, although sugar consumption increased considerably. Intake of cereal fibre also decreased. This suggests that increased intakes of fat (and especially saturated fat), cholesterol and sugar and reduced intakes of starch and cereal fibre may be factors in the development of coronary heart disease.

7.2.2 INTERNATIONAL CORRELATIONS BETWEEN DIET AND DISEASE INCIDENCE

World-wide there are very considerable differences in mortality from cancer and heart

TABLE 7.1 *Secular changes in diet with changes in disease incidence – changes in diet in rural Wales between 1870 and 1970*

	1870	1970	
Protein	11	11	% of energy
Fat	25	42	% of energy
Sugar	4	17	% of energy
Starch	60	30	% of energy
Unsaturated fat	19	9	% of total fat
Cholesterol	130	517	mg/day
Dietary fibre	65	21	g/day

disease. Incidence of breast cancer ranges from 34/million in the Gambia to 1002/ million in Hawaii and the incidence of prostate cancer from 12/million in the Gambia to 912/million among black Americans. Coronary heart disease accounts for 4.8% of deaths in Japan, but 31.7% of deaths in Northern Ireland.

Assuming that there are adequate and comparable data available for food consumption in different countries, it is possible to plot graphs such as that in Figure 7.1, which shows a highly significant positive association between fat consumption and breast cancer. It is important to note that this statistical correlation does not imply cause and effect; indeed, further analysis of the factors involved in breast cancer suggest that it is not dietary fat intake, but rather adiposity, or total body fat content, that is the important factor. Obviously, dietary fat intake is a significant factor in the development of obesity and high body fat reserves.

Figure 7.2 shows a highly significant negative correlation between mortality from coronary heart disease and the serum concentration of vitamin E, suggesting that vitamin E may be protective against the development of atherosclerosis and coronary heart disease.

7.2.3 STUDIES OF MIGRANTS

People who migrate from one country to another provide an excellent opportunity to study the effects of dietary and environmental factors on disease; their first-degree relatives who have not migrated provide a genetically matched control group for comparison.

Both breast and prostate cancer are rare in China and Japan compared with the

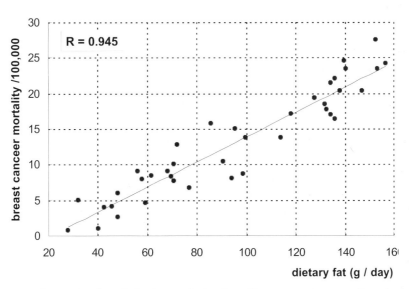

FIGURE 7.1 *International correlation between fat intake and breast cancer in women. From data reported by Caroll KK (1975)* Cancer Research 35: 3374–3383.

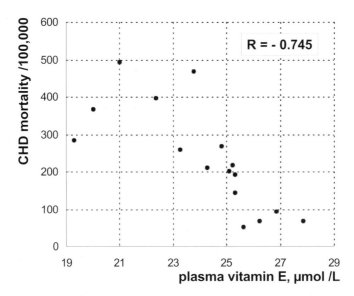

FIGURE 7.2 *The relationship between plasma vitamin E levels and coronary heart disease. From data reported by Gey KF et al. (1991)* American Journal of Clinical Nutrition *53 (supplement 1): 326–334s.*

incidence of both in USA. Figure 7.3 shows that people who have migrated from China and Japan to Hawaii or San Francisco have a considerably higher incidence of both cancers than their relatives who did not migrate and retained their traditional diet and lifestyle.

Similar studies of adult immigrants in the mid-twentieth century from Poland (where gastric cancer was common and colorectal cancer rare) to Australia (where gastric cancer is rare and colorectal cancer relatively common) found a significant increase in colorectal cancer among the immigrants, whereas the incidence of gastric cancer remained at the relatively high Polish level (although second-generation Polish-Australians have the low Australian incidence of gastric cancer (Figure 7.4). This suggests that dietary or environmental factors involved in the development of colorectal cancer may act relatively late in life, whereas factors that predispose to gastric cancer act earlier in life.

7.2.4 CASE–CONTROL STUDIES

A more precise technique for studying relationships between diet and disease is to compare people suffering from the disease with disease-free subjects who are matched as closely as possible for gender, ethnicity, age, lifestyle and as many other factors as possible. Figure 7.5 shows the results of a series of such case–control studies, which show that the serum concentration of β-carotene (section 7.4.3.4) is significantly lower in people with a variety of cancers than in disease-free control subjects. Such data have been widely interpreted as suggesting that β-carotene has a protective effect

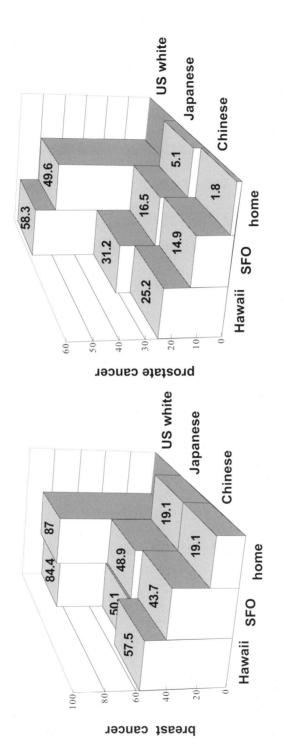

FIGURE 7.3 *Cancer of the breast and prostate in Chinese and Japanese immigrants to the USA compared with incidence of the diseases in first-degree relatives in China and Japan and the local population in the USA (SFO, San Francisco). From data reported by Haenzel W and Kurihawa M (1965) Journal of the* National Cancer Institute *40: 43–68, and Yu H et al. (1991)* International Journal of Epidemiology *20: 76–81.*

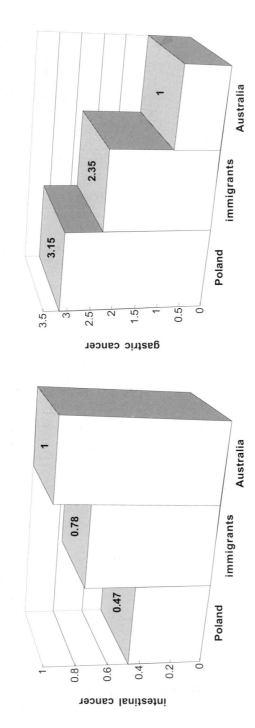

FIGURE 7.4 *Gastric and colorectal cancer in Polish immigrants to Australia compared with rates in Poland and among the local population in Australia. From data reported by Staszewski J et al. (1971)British Journal of Cancer 25: 599–610, and McMichael AJ et al. (1980) International Journal of Cancer 25: 431–437.*

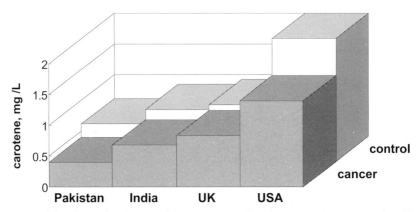

FIGURE 7.5 *The relationship between plasma carotene and various cancers – case–control studies. From data reported by Peto R et al. (1981)* Nature *290: 201–208.*

against a variety of cancers; equally, it could be interpreted as suggesting that a variety of cancers affect carotene metabolism.

7.2.5 PROSPECTIVE STUDIES

Once dietary factors that seem to pose a hazard or offer a protective effect have been identified by the types of study discussed above, the next step is to undertake a prospective study. In these studies, a group of people are grouped according to their status with respect to the nutrient in question then followed for 5–10 or more years to see whether there is any significant difference in disease incidence between people with high or low intakes of the nutrient in question. Figure 7.6 shows the results of such a prospective study in which people were grouped according to their plasma

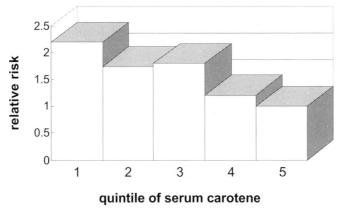

FIGURE 7.6 *The relationship between plasma carotene and lung cancer – a prospective study. From data reported by Peto R et al. (1981)* Nature *290: 201–208.*

concentration of β-carotene; those with the lowest initial concentration of serum carotene were 2.2 times more likely to die from lung cancer during the study period than those with the highest concentration. As with the case–control studies (Figure 7.5) this suggests a protective effect of β-carotene, but in this case the subjects were presumably free from cancer at the beginning of the study, so there is not the confounding problem that the disease may have affected carotene metabolism rather than carotene affecting the chance of developing cancer.

7.2.6 INTERVENTION STUDIES

The next step is to test the hypothesis derived, from epidemiological and prospective studies, that a change in diet, or provision of a nutritional supplement, will reduce the risk of developing a disease. Figure 7.7 shows the results of such an intervention trial in Finland in the 1980s to test the protective effect of β-carotene against lung cancer. Altogether some 10,000 people were involved – half received supplements of β-carotene and half did not, and they were followed for 5–10 years. The results were disappointing – not only did the supplements not reduce the incidence of lung cancer in the test group, but there was an increased incidence of lung, prostate and bladder cancer among those receiving β-carotene. A similar intervention trial of β-carotene in USA was terminated early because of the increased incidence of cancer among those receiving the supplements.

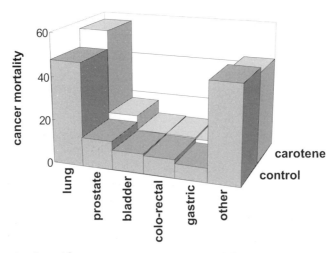

FIGURE 7.7 *The effects of β-carotene supplementation on death from lung and other cancers. From data reported by the Alpha-Tocopherol Beta-Carotene Cancer Prevention Study Group (1994)* New England Journal of Medicine *330: 1029–1035.*

7.3 *Guidelines for a prudent diet*

Despite the disappointing results of the intervention trials with β-carotene discussed in section 7.2.6, epidemiological studies of the type discussed in section 7.2 do provide useful information on dietary factors that may be important in the development of the diseases of affluence. Diet is not the sole cause, as these diseases are all due to interactions of multiple factors, including heredity, a variety of environmental factors, smoking and exercise (or the lack of it). Nonetheless, diet is a factor that is readily amenable to change. Individuals can take decisions about diet, smoking and exercise, whereas they can do little about the stresses of city life, environmental pollution or the other problems of industrial society, and nothing, of course, to change their genetic make-up, which determines the extent to which they are at risk from various environmental and nutritional factors.

The epidemiological evidence linking dietary factors with the diseases of affluence shows that in countries or regions with, for example, a high intake of saturated fat there is a higher incidence of cardiovascular disease and some forms of cancer than in regions with a lower intake of fat. It does not show that people who have been living on a high-fat diet will necessarily benefit from a relatively abrupt change to a low-fat diet. Indeed, the results of a number of intervention studies, in which large numbers of people have been persuaded to change their diets, have been disappointing. Overall, premature death from cardiovascular disease is reduced, but the total death rate remains unchanged, with an increase in suicide, accidents and violent death.

Nevertheless, the epidemiological data are irrefutable, and there is general agreement among nutritionists and medical scientists about changes in the average Western diet that would be expected to reduce the prevalence of the diseases of affluence. Changing diets in the way suggested below is not a guarantee of immortality, and indeed some of the evidence is conflicting. As new data are gathered, old data reinterpreted and the results of long-term studies become available, it is inevitable that opinions as to what constitutes a prudent or desirable diet will change.

7.3.1 ENERGY INTAKE

Obesity involves both an increased risk of premature death from a variety of causes and increased morbidity from conditions such as diabetes, varicose veins and arthritis (section 6.2.2). On the other hand, people who are significantly underweight are also at increased risk of illness as a result of undernutrition (see Chapter 8). For people whose body weight is within the desirable range, energy intake should be adequate to maintain a reasonably constant body weight, with an adequate amount of exercise. Energy expenditure in physical activity and appropriate levels of energy intake are discussed in section 6.1.

Figure 7.8 shows the average percentage of energy intake from each of fat,

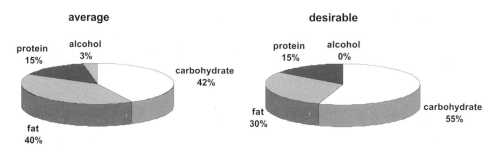

FIGURE 7.8 *Average and desirable percentage of energy intake from different metabolic fuels.*

carbohydrate, protein and alcohol in the diets of adults in Britain in the 1990s, compared with the guidelines for a prudent diet.

7.3.2 FAT INTAKE

Dietary fat includes not only the obvious fat in the diet (the visible fat on meat, cooking oil, butter or margarine spread on bread), but also the hidden fat in foods. This latter may be either the fat naturally present in foods (e.g. the fat between the muscle fibres in meat, the oils in nuts, cereals and vegetables) or fat used in cooking and manufacture of foods. There are two problems associated with a high intake of fat:

- The energy yield of fat (37 kJ/g) is more than twice that of protein (16 kJ/g) or carbohydrate (17 kJ/g). This means that foods which are high in fat are also concentrated energy sources. It is easier to have an excessive energy intake on a high-fat diet, and hence a high-fat diet can be a factor in the development of obesity (see Chapter 6).
- There is good epidemiological evidence that fat intake is correlated with premature death from a variety of conditions, including especially atherosclerosis and ischaemic heart disease and cancer of the colon, prostate, breast and uterus.

From the results of epidemiological studies, it seems that diets providing about 30% of energy from fat are associated with the lowest risk of ischaemic heart disease. There is no evidence that a fat intake below about 30% of energy intake confers any additional benefit, although a very low-fat diet is specifically recommended as part of treatment for some people with pathological hyperlipidaemia.

As an aid to reducing fat intake, a number of low-fat versions of foods that are traditionally high in fat are available. Some of these are meat products which make use of leaner (and more expensive) cuts of meat for the preparation of sausages, hamburgers and pies. Low-fat minced meat (containing about 5–10% fat by weight, instead of the more usual 20%) is widely available in supermarkets, although it is, of course, more expensive, and low-fat cheeses and patés are also available, as are salad dressings made with little or no oil. There are also a number of low-fat spreads to replace butter or margarine. Skimmed and semiskimmed milk are now widely available, providing very much less fat than full-cream milk, although full-cream milk is an important source of vitamins A and D, especially for children.

A more recent advance has been the development of compounds that will replace fat more or less completely while retaining the texture and flavour of traditional fatty foods. Two such compounds are Simplesse, which is a modified protein used in low-fat spreads but is not suitable for cooking, and Olestra (also known as Olean), which is a fatty acid ester of sucrose (and hence chemically related to fats; section 4.3.1) but is not absorbed. It is stable to cooking and can be used to prepare fat-free potato crisps etc.

7.3.2.1 The type of fat in the diet

Figure 7.9 shows the relationship between the concentration of cholesterol (section 4.3.1.3) in plasma, and specifically cholesterol in plasma low-density lipoproteins (LDL; section 5.6.2.2), and premature death from ischaemic heart disease. The main dietary factor affecting the concentration of cholesterol in plasma is the intake of fat.

Both the total intake of fat and, more importantly, the relative amounts of saturated and unsaturated fats affect the concentration of cholesterol in LDL. Figure 7.10 shows the results of a number of studies of the effects of different types of dietary fat on serum LDL cholesterol:

- It increases by a factor related to 2 × the intake of saturated fat.

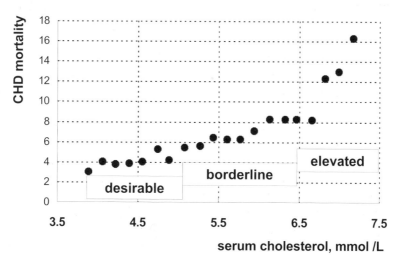

FIGURE 7.9 *The relationship between serum cholesterol and coronary heart disease mortality. From data reported by the Multiple Risk Factor Intervention Trial Research Group (1982)* Journal of the American Medical Association *248: 1465–1475.*

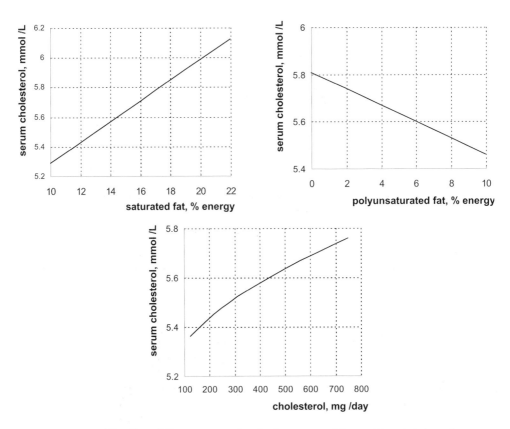

FIGURE 7.10 *The effects of dietary saturated and polyunsaturated fatty acids and cholesterol on serum cholesterol. From data reported by Keys A et al. (1965)* Metabolism *14: 747–787.*

- It decreases by a factor related to 1 × the intake of unsaturated fat.
- It increases by a factor related to the square root of cholesterol intake (see section 7.5.1 for a discussion of the effects of dietary cholesterol on synthesis of cholesterol in the body).

Diets that are relatively rich in polyunsaturated fatty acids result in decreased synthesis of fatty acids in the liver (section 5.6.1); this means that there is less export of lipids from the liver in VLDL (section 5.6.2.2), which are the precursors of LDL in the circulation. Polyunsaturated fatty acids (or their derivatives) act via nuclear receptors (section 10.4) to reduce the transcription of the genes coding for acetyl CoA carboxylase and other key enzymes of fatty acid synthesis (section 5.6.1).

In addition, the polyunsaturated fatty acids in fish oil (the ω3 series of long-chain polyunsaturated fatty acids; section 4.3.1.1) have a further protective effect, reducing the stickiness of blood platelets, and hence reducing the risk of blood clot formation. Figure 7.11 shows the beneficial effect of consuming a modest amount of oily fish on the incidence of coronary heart disease – even one fish meal a week reduces the risk to

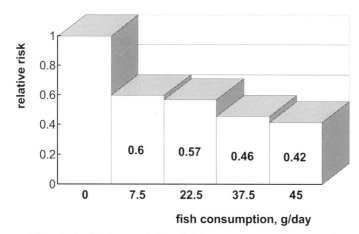

FIGURE 7.11 *The relationship between habitual fish consumption and coronary heart disease. From data reported by Kromhout D et al. (1985)* New England Journal of Medicine *312: 1205–1209.*

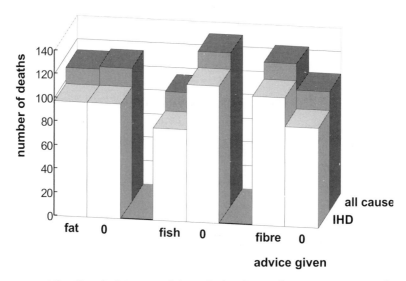

FIGURE 7.12 *The effect of advice to eat fish (and other dietary changes) on recurrence of myocardial infarction in middle-aged men who have suffered one infarction. From data reported by Burr ML et al. (1989)* Lancet *ii: 757–761.*

60% of that in people who eat no fish. Figure 7.12 shows the beneficial effect of following advice to eat fish regularly in a group of men who had already suffered one myocardial infarction.

Figure 7.13 shows the average and desirable proportions of energy coming from saturated, monounsaturated and polyunsaturated fatty acids in the dietary fat. As a general rule, animal foods (meat, eggs and milk products) are rich sources of saturated fats, whereas oily fish and vegetables are rich sources of unsaturated fats.

The recommendation is to reduce intake of saturated fats considerably more than

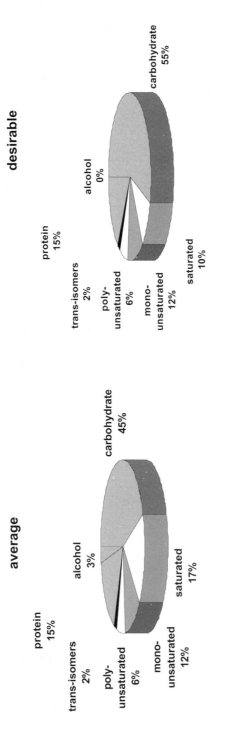

FIGURE 7.13 *Average and desirable percentage of energy intake from different types of fat.*

just in proportion to the reduction in total fat intake. Total fat intake should be 30% of energy intake, with no more than 10% from saturated fats (compared with the present average of 17% of energy from saturated fat). Current average intakes of 6% of energy from polyunsaturated and 12% from monounsaturated fats match what is considered to be desirable, on the basis of epidemiological studies. About 2% of energy intake is accounted for by the *trans*-isomers of unsaturated fatty acids (section 4.3.1.1), and it is considered that this should not increase.

7.3.3 CARBOHYDRATE INTAKE

If the total energy intake is to remain constant, as it should for people who are not overweight, and the proportion derived from fat is to be reduced from 40% to 30% of total, then the proportion of energy derived from another metabolic fuel must be increased. It is not considered desirable to increase the proportion derived from protein from the current 15% of energy intake, so the proportion derived from carbohydrates should increase, from the current 45% of energy to 55%.

7.3.3.1 Sugars in the diet

Average intakes of sugars (and especially sucrose) are generally considered to be higher than is desirable. The adverse effects of an excessive intake of sugars include:

- *Dental decay.* Although many sugars in free solution (extrinsic sugars; section 4.2.1) will promote the growth of oral bacteria that produce acids and cause dental decay, sucrose is especially undesirable, as it specifically promotes the growth of plaque-forming bacteria that coat the teeth.
- *Obesity.* Sugars added to foods increase the energy yield of the food and increase the pleasure of eating (section 1.3.3.1), so that it is relatively easy to consume an excessive amount.
- *Diabetes mellitus.* Sugars and other carbohydrates with a high glycaemic index (section 4.2.2) lead to a higher post-prandial insulin response, which results in increased lipogenesis and secretion of VLDL from the liver (section 5.6.2.2). This has been associated with the development of insulin resistance and non-insulin-dependent (type II) diabetes (section 10.7). There is, however, a strong genetic predisposition to type II diabetes, and it is difficult to determine the relative importance of heredity and sucrose consumption.
- *Atherosclerosis and coronary heart disease.* There is some evidence that a high consumption of sucrose is a factor in the development of atherosclerosis and coronary heart disease, although the evidence is less convincing than that for the effects of a high (saturated) fat intake.

Because of this, it is considered desirable that sucrose should provide no more than

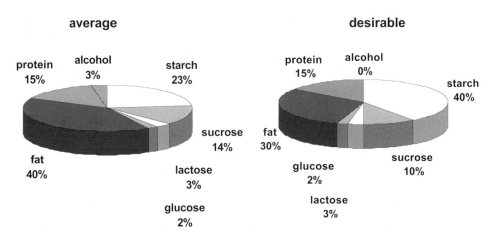

FIGURE 7.14 *Average and desirable percentage of energy intake from different types of carbohydrate.*

10% of energy (compared with the current average of 14%). Intakes of other sugars (mainly glucose and fructose in fruits, and lactose from milk) are considered to be appropriate. Therefore, as shown in Figure 7.14, the increased proportion of energy from carbohydrates should be from increased consumption of starches.

7.3.3.2 Undigested carbohydrates (dietary fibre)

The residue of plant cell walls is not digested by human enzyme, but provides bulk in the diet (and hence in the intestines). It is measured by weighing the fraction of foods that remains after treatment with a variety of digestive enzymes. This is what is known as dietary fibre. It is a misleading term, as not all the components of dietary fibre are fibrous; some are soluble and form viscous gels.

A more precise analytical method permits measurement of the specific polysaccharides other than starch (section 4.2.1.6) that are the main constituents of dietary fibre; the results of such analysis are quoted as non-starch polysaccharides (nsp).

The two methods of analysis give different results. Measurement of non-starch polysaccharides in the diet gives average intakes in Britain of between 11 and 13 g/day, compared with an intake of dietary fibre of about 20 g/day as measured by the less specific method. Non-starch polysaccharides are found only foods of vegetable origin, and vegetarians have a higher intake than omnivores.

Non-starch polysaccharides have little nutritional value in their own right, as they are compounds that are not digested or absorbed to any significant extent. Nevertheless, they are a valuable component of the diet, and some of the products of fermentation by colonic bacteria can be absorbed and utilized as metabolic fuel. Together with non-starch polysaccharides, we have to consider that proportion of starch that is (relatively) resistant to digestion in the small intestine (section 4.2.2.1), because it too is a substrate for bacterial fermentation.

The main products of bacterial fermentation of non-starch polysaccharides and resistant starch are short-chain fatty acids such as propionate and butyrate. In addition to being absorbed, and hence used as metabolic fuels, they have an antiproliferative effect on tumour cells in culture, and there is some evidence that they provide protection against the development of colorectal cancer.

Diets low in non-starch polysaccharides are associated with the excretion of a small bulk of faeces, and frequently with constipation and straining while defecating. This has been linked with the development of haemorrhoids, varicose veins and diverticular disease of the colon. These diseases are commoner in Western countries, where people generally have a relatively low intake of non-starch polysaccharide, than in parts of the world where the intake is higher.

Some types of non-starch polysaccharides bind a number of potentially undesirable compounds in the intestinal lumen, and so reduce their absorption. Again this may be protective against colorectal cancer. A number of compounds that are believed to be involved in causing or promoting cancer of the colon occur in the contents of the intestinal tract, both because they are present in foods and as a result of bacterial metabolism in the colon. They are adsorbed by non-starch polysaccharides, and so cannot interact with the cells of the gut wall but are eliminated in the faeces.

Although epidemiological studies show that diets high in non-starch polysaccharides are associated with a low risk of colon cancer, such diets also provide relatively large amounts of fruit and vegetables, and are therefore rich in vitamins C and E and carotene, which may have protective effects against the development of cancers (section 7.4.3). Furthermore, because they provide more fruit and vegetables, and less meat, such diets are also relatively low in saturated fats, and there is evidence that a high intake of saturated fats is a separate risk factor for colon cancer.

As discussed in section 4.3.2.1, the bile salts required for the absorption of dietary fat are synthesized in the liver from cholesterol. Normally about 90–95% of the 30 g of bile salts secreted daily is reabsorbed and reutilized. Non-starch polysaccharides adsorb bile salts, so that they are excreted in the faeces. This means that there has to be increased synthesis *de novo* from cholesterol to replace the lost bile salts, so reducing the total body content of cholesterol.

A total intake of about 18 g of non-starch polysaccharides per day is recommended (equivalent to about 30 g/day of dietary fibre). In general, this should come from fibre-rich foods – whole-grain cereals and wholemeal cereal products, fruits and vegetables – rather than supplements. This is because as well as the nsp, these fibre-rich foods are valuable sources of a variety of nutrients. There is no evidence that intakes of fibre over about 30 g/day confer any benefit, other than in the treatment of established bowel disease. Above this level of intake it is likely that people would reach satiety (or at least feel full, or even bloated) without eating enough food to satisfy energy needs. This may be a problem for children fed on a diet that is very high in fibre – they may be physically full but still physiologically hungry.

7.3.4 SALT

There is a physiological requirement for the mineral sodium, and salt (chemically sodium chloride) is the major dietary source of sodium. One of the basic senses of taste is for saltiness – a pleasant sensation (section 1.3.3.1). However, average intakes of salt in Western countries are considerably higher than the physiological requirement for sodium. Most people are able to cope with this excessive intake adequately by excreting the excess. However, people with a genetic predisposition to develop high blood pressure are sensitive to the amount of sodium in their diet. One of the ways of treating dangerously high blood pressure (hypertension) is by a severe restriction of salt intake. It is estimated that about 10% of the population are salt sensitive, and epidemiologically there is a relationship between sodium intake and the increase in blood pressure that occurs with increasing age.

The problem in terms of public health and dietary advice to the population at large (as opposed to specific advice to people known to be at risk of, or suffering from, hypertension) is one of extrapolating from clinical studies in people who have severe hypertension, and who benefit from a severe restriction in salt intake, to the rest of the healthy population. It is not clear whether a modest reduction in salt intake will benefit those salt-sensitive individuals who might go on to develop severe hypertension. Nevertheless, it is prudent to recommend reducing the average intake of salt by about one-quarter, to a level that meets requirements for sodium without providing so great an excess over requirements as is seen in average diets at present.

7.3.5 ALCOHOL

A high intake of alcoholic drinks can be a factor in causing obesity, both as a result of the energy yield of the alcohol itself and also because of the relatively high carbohydrate content of many alcoholic beverages. People who satisfy much of their energy requirement from alcohol frequently show vitamin deficiencies, because they are meeting their energy needs from drink, and therefore are not eating enough food to provide adequate amounts of vitamins and minerals. Deficiency of vitamin B_1 is especially a problem among heavy drinkers (section 11.6.3).

In moderate amounts, alcohol has an appetite-stimulating effect, and may also help the social aspect of meals. Furthermore, there is good epidemiological evidence that modest consumption of alcohol is protective against atherosclerosis and coronary heart disease. However, alcohol has harmful effects in excess, not only in the short term, when drunkenness may have undesirable consequences, but also in the longer term.

Figure 7.15 shows the relationship between alcohol consumption and mortality from various causes – it is a classical 'J-shaped' curve, with a protective effect of modest consumption compared with abstinence but a sharp increase in mortality with excessive consumption.

Opinions differ as to whether the protective effect of modest alcohol consumption

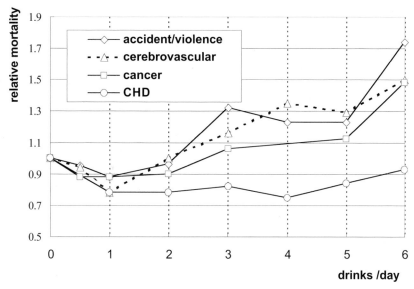

FIGURE 7.15 *The effects of habitual alcohol consumption on mortality from various causes. From data reported by Boffetta P and Garfinkel L,* Epidemiology *1: 342–348, 1990.*

is a protective effect of the alcohol itself or due to some other constituent of the alcoholic beverages. Figure 7.16 shows that there are differences between the effects of wine, beer and spirits, regardless of the amount of alcohol consumed. Some studies have shown the same protective of red wine and dealcoholized wine, suggesting that alcohol is not the protective factor; the various polyphenols in red wine may well have an antioxidant action (section 7.4.3.6).

One problem in interpreting the data on alcohol consumption is that those who consume no alcohol will include not only those who for religious or other reasons choose to abstain from alcohol, but also those whose health has already been damaged by excessive consumption.

Habitual excess consumption of alcohol is associated with long-term health problems, including loss of mental capacity, liver damage and cancer of the oesophagus. Continued abuse can lead to physical and psychological addiction. The infants of mothers who drink more than a very small amount of alcohol during pregnancy are at risk of congenital abnormalities, and heavy alcohol consumption during pregnancy can result in the fetal alcohol syndrome – low birth weight and lasting impairment of intelligence, as well as congenital deformities.

The guidelines on alcohol intake, the prudent upper limits of habitual consumption, are summarized in Table 7.2, and the alcohol content of beverages in Table 7.3.

7.4 *Free radicals and antioxidant nutrients*

A compound that loses or gains a single electron, and thus has an unpaired electron in

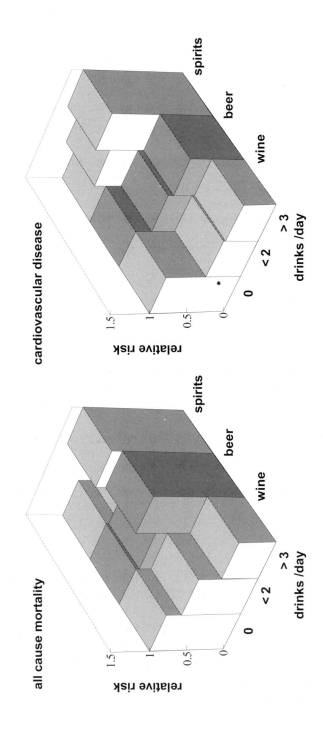

FIGURE 7.16 *The effects of different alcoholic beverages on mortality. From data reported by Grøbbæk M et al. (1995) British Medical Journal 310: 1165–1169.*

TABLE 7.2 *Prudent upper limits of alcohol consumption*

Royal College of Physicians		
Men	21 units	(= 168 g alcohol)/week
Women	14 units	(= 112 g alcohol)/week
Department of Health (1995)		
Men	4 units	(= 32 g alcohol)/day
Women	3 units	(= 24 g alcohol)/day

TABLE 7.3 *Amounts of beverages providing 1 unit of alcohol*

8 g absolute alcohol
$^1/_2$ pint of beer (300 mL)
1 glass of wine (100 mL)
Single measure of spirits (25 mL)

its outermost shell, is extremely unstable and very highly reactive. Such compounds are known as free radicals.

Free radicals usually exist for only extremely short periods of time, of the order of nanoseconds (10^{-9} seconds) or less, before they react with another molecule, either gaining or losing a single electron in order to achieve a stable configuration. However, this reaction, in turn, generates another molecule with an unpaired electron. Each time a radical reacts with a molecule to lose its unpaired electron and achieves stability, it in turn generates another radical that is again short-lived and highly reactive. This is a chain reaction.

To show that a compound is a free radical, its chemical formula is shown with a dot (•) to represent the unpaired electron – for example, the hydroxyl radical is •OH.

If two radicals react together, each contributes its unpaired electron to the formation of a new, stable bond. This means that the chain reaction, in which reaction of radicals with other molecules generates new radicals, is stopped. This is quenching of the chain reaction, or quenching of the radicals. As radicals are generally so short-lived, it is rare for two radicals to come together to quench each other in this way.

Some radicals are relatively stable. This applies especially to those which are formed from molecules with aromatic rings or conjugated double-bond systems. A single unpaired electron can be distributed or delocalized through such a system of double bonds, and the resultant radical is less reactive and longer-lived than most radicals. Compounds that are capable of forming relatively stable radicals are important in quenching radical chain reactions. Their radicals frequently have a long enough life to permit two such stable radicals to come together, react with each other and so terminate the chain. Vitamin E (sections 7.4.3.3 and 11.4)) and carotene (section 7.4.3.4) are especially important in quenching radical reactions in biological systems.

7.4.1 TISSUE DAMAGE BY OXYGEN RADICALS

Radicals may interact with any compounds present in the cell, and the result may be initiation of cancer, heritable mutations, atherosclerosis and coronary heart disease or autoimmune disease. The most important, and potentially damaging, such interactions are:

1 With DNA in the nucleus, causing chemical changes in the nucleic acid bases (section 9.2.1) or breaks in the DNA strand. This damage may result in heritable mutations if the damage is to ovaries or testes, or the induction of cancer in other tissues. Although much damage to DNA is detected and repaired by the DNA repair system in cells, some will escape detection.
2 With individual amino acids in proteins. This results in a chemical modification of the protein, which may therefore be recognized as foreign by the immune system, leading to the production of antibodies against the modified protein that will also react with the normal, unmodified body protein. This may be an important factor in the development of autoimmune disease.
3 Some modified amino acids (e.g. dihydroxyphenylalanine) are capable of undergoing non-enzymic redox cycling, resulting in the production of more oxygen radicals.
4 With unsaturated fatty acids in cell membranes. This leads to the formation of dialdehydes, which react with DNA, causing chemical modification, and hence may result in either heritable mutations or initiation of cancer. Dialdehydes can also react with amino acids in proteins, leading to modified proteins that stimulate the production of autoantibodies.
5 With unsaturated fatty acids or amino acids in LDL (section 5.6.2.2). Oxidized LDL are not recognized and taken up by the LDL receptors in the liver but are recognized and taken up by scavenger receptors in macrophages. Macrophage uptake of LDL is unregulated, and the cells become engorged with lipid. These lipid-rich macrophages (called foam cells, because of their microscopic appearance) then infiltrate the epithelium of blood vessel walls, leading to the development of fatty streaks, and eventually atherosclerosis.

7.4.2 SOURCES OF OXYGEN RADICALS

Oxygen radicals arise in the body in four main ways.

7.4.2.1 Reoxidation of reduced flavins

Oxygen radicals may be generated by normal oxidative metabolism, and especially reactions involving the reoxidation of reduced flavin coenzymes (sections 3.3.1.2 and 11.7.2.1). During the reoxidation of flavins a number of radicals are generated as transient intermediates. If the whole sequence of reactions continues then there is no problem. However, by their very nature, radicals are unpredictable, and there will always be some escape of radicals from the reaction sequence. Overall, some 3–5% of the 30 mol of oxygen consumed by an adult each day is converted to oxygen radicals rather than undergoing complete reduction to water in the mitochondrial electron transport chain (section 3.3.1.2). There is, thus, a total daily formation of some 1.5 mol of reactive oxygen species that are potentially able to cause damage to tissues.

7.4.2.2 The macrophage respiratory burst

The cytotoxic action of macrophages is due to production of radicals, including halogen, nitric oxide and oxygen radicals. This means that infection can lead to a considerable increase in the total radical burden in the body. As discussed in section 8.5.1, this may be an important factor in the protein–energy deficiency disease kwashiorkor.

Stimulation of macrophages leads to a considerable increase in the consumption of glucose (the respiratory burst), which is metabolized by the pentose phosphate pathway (section 5.4.2), leading to increased production of NADPH. The respiratory burst oxidase (NADPH oxidase) is a flavoprotein that transfers electrons from NADPH onto cytochrome b_{558}, which then reduces oxygen to superoxide. The reaction is:

$$NADPH + 2\, O_2 \rightarrow NADP^+ + 2{}^{\bullet}O_2^- + 2H^+$$

The respiratory burst oxidase is a transmembrane multienzyme complex that is activated in response to:

* complement fragment C_{5a} which arises from the antibody–antigen reaction;
* peptides containing N-formyl-Met-Leu-Phe, which may be bacterial or arise from the mitochondria of damaged tissue;
* cytokines and other signalling molecules released in response to infection, including platelet-activating factor, leukotrienes and interleukins.

7.4.2.3 Formation of nitric oxide

Production of nitric oxide ($NO^{\bullet}$), by hydroxylation of arginine, is a part of normal cell signalling. In addition to being a radical, and hence potentially damaging in its own right, nitric oxide can react with superoxide to form peroxynitrite, which in turn decays to yield the more damaging hydroxyl radical. Nitric oxide was first discovered as the endothelium-derived relaxation factor, and this loss of nitric oxide by reaction with superoxide may be an important factor in the development of hypertension.

7.4.2.4 Non-enzymic formation of radicals

A variety of transition metal ions react with oxygen or hydrogen peroxide in solution:

$$M^{n+} + H_2O_2 \rightarrow M^{(n+1)+} + {}^{\bullet}OH + OH^-$$

Physiologically important metal ions include iron, copper, cobalt and nickel. Normally, metal ions are not present in free solution to any significant extent, but are bound to transport proteins (in plasma) or storage proteins and enzymes (in cells). Thus, iron is bound to transferrin (in plasma) and haemosiderin and ferritin in tissues, copper is bound to caeruloplasmin in plasma, and metallothionein in plasma binds a wide variety of metal ions. The adverse effects of iron overload (section 4.5.1) are the result of free iron, not bound to storage proteins, acting as a source of oxygen radicals.

Ionizing radiation such as X-rays, the radiation from radioactive isotopes and ultraviolet from sunlight cause lysis of water to yield hydroxyl and other radicals.

7.4.3 ANTIOXIDANT NUTRIENTS AND NON-NUTRIENTS – PROTECTION AGAINST RADICAL DAMAGE

Apart from avoidance of exposure to ionizing radiation, there is little that can be done to prevent the formation of radicals, as they are the result of normal metabolic processes and responses to infection. There are, however, a number of mechanisms to minimize the damage done by radical action. As the important radicals are oxygen radicals, and the damage done is oxidative damage, the protective compounds are known collectively as antioxidants.

Antioxidants such as vitamin E (sections 7.4.3.3 and 11.4), carotene (section 7.4.3.4) and ubiquinone (section 3.3.1.2) owe their antioxidant action to the fact that they can form stable radicals, in which an unpaired electron can be delocalized in the molecule. Such stable radicals persist long enough to undergo reaction to yield non-radical products. However, because they are stable, they are also capable of penetrating further into cells or lipoproteins, and hence causing damage to DNA in the nucleus or lipids in the core of the lipoprotein. Therefore, as well as being protective antioxidants, these compounds are also capable of acting as potentially damaging pro-oxidants, especially at high concentrations. This may explain the disappointing results of trials of β-carotene against lung cancer (section 7.2.6).

7.4.3.1 Superoxide dismutase, peroxidases and catalase

Superoxide is a substrate for the enzyme superoxide dismutase, which catalyses the reaction:

$$ {}^{\bullet}O_2^- + H_2O \rightarrow O_2 + H_2O_2 $$

In turn, hydrogen peroxide is removed by catalase and a variety of peroxidases:

$$ 2\,H_2O_2 \rightarrow 2\,H_2O + O_2 $$

As a further protection, many of the reactions in the cell that generate superoxide or hydrogen peroxide occur in the peroxisomes – intracellular organelles that also contain superoxide dismutase, catalase and peroxidases.

7.4.3.2 Glutathione peroxidase

Lipid peroxides formed by radical action on unsaturated fatty acids in membranes and LDL can be reduced to unreactive alcohols by the enzyme glutathione peroxidase, with the oxidation of the tripeptide glutathione (γ-glutamyl-cysteinyl-glycine, GSH) to the disulphide-linked GSSG. In turn, oxidized glutathione is reduced back to the active peptide by glutathione reductase, as shown in Figure 5.15.

Glutathione reductase has selenium at the catalytic site, as a selenocysteine residue (section 11.15.2.5); this explains the role of selenium as an antioxidant nutrient. Glutathione reductase is a flavoprotein, and is especially sensitive to riboflavin (vitamin B$_2$) depletion; as discussed in section 11.7.4.1, measurement of glutathione reductase is used as a means of assessing riboflavin status.

7.4.3.3 Vitamin E

Vitamin E (section 11.4) forms a stable radical that can persist long enough to undergo reaction to yield non-radical products. As shown in Figure 7.17, tocopherol reacts with lipid peroxides to form stable fatty acids and the tocopheroxyl radical. In turn,

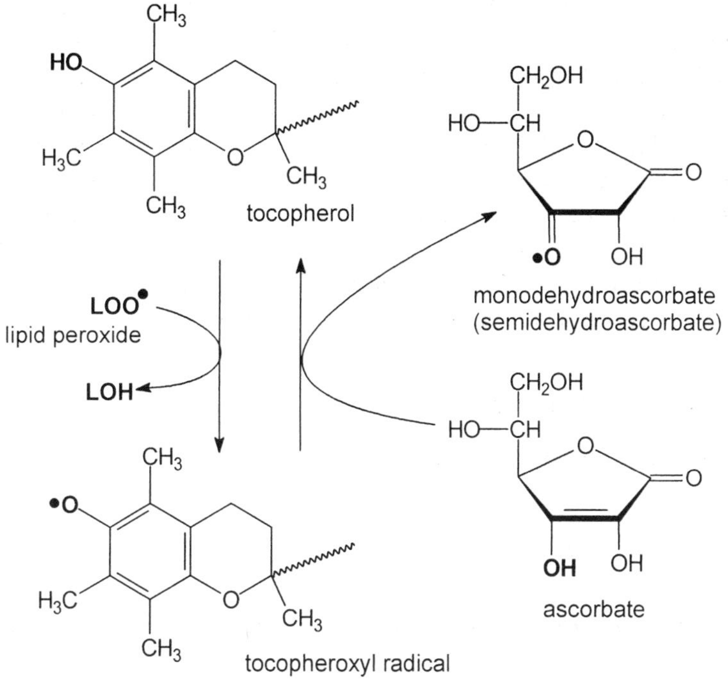

FIGURE 7.17 *The antioxidant role of vitamin E.*

the tocopheroxyl radical reacts with ascorbate (vitamin C) at the surface of the cell or lipoprotein, regenerating tocopherol and forming the stable monodehydroascorbate radical.

There is epidemiological evidence that intakes of vitamin E higher than those required to prevent deficiency, and probably higher than can be achieved from normal diets, may have significant protective action against the development of atherosclerosis and cardiovascular disease (see Figure 7.2), and possibly some forms of cancer. However, intervention trials with vitamin E supplements have been disappointing, with little evidence of decreased mortality from cardiovascular disease among people taking supplements.

7.4.3.4 Carotenes

A variety of carotenes, including both those that are precursors of vitamin A and those that are not (section 11.2.2), can act as radical trapping antioxidants under conditions of low oxygen tension.

As discussed in sections 7.2.4 and 7.2.5, there is epidemiological evidence from a variety of studies that high blood levels of carotene are associated with low incidence of a variety of cancers. However, again the results of intervention studies have been disappointing; in two major trials there was an increase in the incidence of lung cancer among people taking supplements of β-carotene (section 7.2.6).

7.4.3.5 Vitamin C

It was noted above (section 7.2.3.3) that vitamin C can act at the surface of cells or lipoproteins to reduce the tocopheroxyl radical back to tocopherol, forming the stable monodehydroascorbate radical. Vitamin C can also react with superoxide and hydroxyl radicals:

$$\text{ascorbate} + {}^{\bullet}O_2^- + H^+ \rightarrow H_2O_2 + \text{monodehydroascorbate}$$

$$\text{ascorbate} + {}^{\bullet}OH + H^+ \rightarrow H_2O + \text{monodehydroascorbate}$$

As shown in Figure 7.18, the resultant monodehydroascorbate can then undergo enzymic reduction back to ascorbate or a non-enzymic reaction between 2 mol of monodehydroascorbate to yield ascorbate and dehydroascorbate. Dehydroascorbate may then either be reduced to ascorbate or be oxidized to diketogulonate.

Although ascorbate has a protective role in the reactions shown above, it can also be a source of oxygen radicals, and hence potentially damaging:

$$\text{ascorbate} + O_2 \rightarrow {}^{\bullet}O_2^- + \text{monodehydroascorbate}$$

$$\text{ascorbate} + Cu^{2+} \rightarrow Cu^+ + \text{monodehydroascorbate}$$

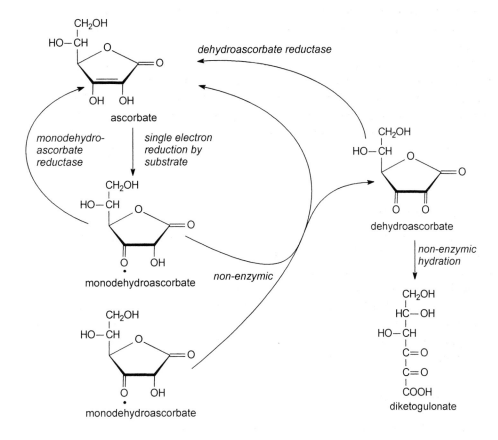

FIGURE 7.18 *Metabolism of the monodehydroascorbate radical to non-radical products.*

$$Cu^+ + H_2O_2 \rightarrow Cu^{2+} + {}^\bullet OH + OH^-$$

However, it is unlikely that high intakes of vitamin C will result in significant radical formation, as once intake rises above about 100–120 mg/day the vitamin is excreted quantitatively in the urine.

7.4.3.6 Non-nutrient antioxidants

A number of other compounds that are not nutrients but are formed in the body as normal metabolites also provide protection against radical damage. Such compounds include uric acid (the end-product of the metabolism of the purines) and the coenzyme ubiquinone (section 3.3.1.2). The latter is sometimes marketed as vitamin Q, but it can be synthesized in the body, and there is no evidence that it is a dietary essential or that an increase above the amount that is normally present in tissues confers any benefit.

In addition to these protective nutrients and normal metabolites, a wide variety of compounds that are naturally present in plant foods also have antioxidant action. These are mainly polyphenols, which are capable of forming stable radicals that persist long enough to undergo reaction to non-radical products. However, they are also potentially capable of undergoing non-enzymic redox cycling, leading to increased formation of oxygen radicals.

7.5 Other protective non-nutrients in foods

Some non-nutrient compounds present in plant foods have potentially protective effects other than as antioxidants. The actions of these compounds include:

- inhibition of cholesterol synthesis or absorption, which is potentially beneficial with respect to atherosclerosis;
- decreased metabolic activation and/or increased conjugation and excretion of potentially carcinogenic compounds;
- anti-oestrogenic actions that may be beneficial with respect to hormone-dependent cancer of the breast and uterus.

Collectively, these potentially protective non-nutrients in plant foods are known as phytochemicals or phytoceuticals. They are not classified as nutrients because they do not have a clear function in the body, and deficiency does not lead to any specific lesions. Nevertheless, they are important in the diet, and provide a sound basis for increasing intake of fruits and vegetables, quite apart from the beneficial effects of increased intake of non-starch polysaccharides, vitamins and minerals and reduced intake of fat (and especially saturated fat).

7.5.1 INHIBITION OF CHOLESTEROL ABSORPTION OR SYNTHESIS

Plant sterols (such as β-sitosterol, which differs from cholesterol in the structure of the side-chain) and stanols (which differ from sterols in having a saturated B-ring; see Figure 4.13) inhibit the absorption of cholesterol from the small intestine. As discussed in section 4.3.2.1, in addition to about 500 mg of dietary cholesterol, about 2 g of cholesterol is secreted each day in the bile. Almost all of this is normally reabsorbed; any inhibition of cholesterol absorption is therefore likely to have a more marked hypocholesterolaemic effect than might be expected simply by considering the dietary intake. A number of products, such as margarine, yoghurts and cream, that contain plant sterols and/or stanol esters have been marketed.

The rate-limiting step of cholesterol synthesis is the reduction of hydroxy-

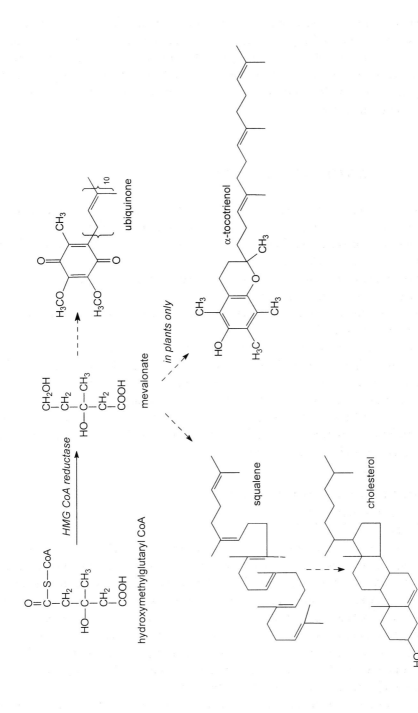

FIGURE 7.19 *Compounds synthesized from mevalonate that inhibit cholesterol synthesis by inhibition of hydroxymethylglutaryl CoA (HMG CoA) reductase.*

methylglutaryl CoA to mevalonic acid, catalysed by hydroxymethylglutaryl (HMG) CoA reductase. Cholesterol acts to repress synthesis of HMG CoA reductase, and so do a number of other compounds derived from mevalonic acid, as shown in Figure 7.19. Such compounds include:

- Plant sterols and stanols (see Figure 4.13), which are absorbed to a limited extent.
- The tocotrienol vitamers of vitamin E, which have an unsaturated side-chain. This means that the tocotrienols, although they have low vitamin activity (sections 11.4.1 and 11.4.3.1), may have a quite different protective effect with respect to atherosclerosis.
- Squalene, which is the last non-cyclic intermediate in cholesterol synthesis. Almost uniquely among foods, olive oil is rich in squalene. Studies of the effects of fatty acids on plasma cholesterol in the 1950s and 1960s showed a cholesterol-raising effect of saturated fatty acids, and a cholesterol-lowering action of polyunsaturated fatty acids (see Figure 7.10), with monounsaturated fatty acids being neutral. In most of these studies the source of monounsaturated fatty acids was rape-seed (canola) oil. However, studies in the 1980s and 1990s using olive oil as the source of monounsaturated fatty acids showed a cholesterol-lowering effect. It is not clear whether this was due to the presence of oleic acid (C18:1 ω9) or whether the high squalene content of olive oil was responsible.

7.5.2 INHIBITION OF CARCINOGEN ACTIVATION AND INCREASED CONJUGATION OF ACTIVATED METABOLITES

Foreign compounds (and a number of endogenous metabolites, including steroid hormones) undergo two stages of metabolism before excretion:

- Phase I metabolism is metabolic activation, leading to the introduction of reactive groups. Many such reactions involve hydroxylation catalysed by cytochromes of the P_{450} family.
- Phase II metabolism is conjugation of these reactive groups with glucuronic acid, amino acids or sulphate to increase water solubility and permit urinary excretion.

Although phase I metabolism is considered to be catabolic, and part of the inactivation of steroid hormones, it also results in the production of active carcinogens from a number of otherwise inactive compounds.

A number of compounds present in fruits and vegetables either inhibit phase I metabolism or activate phase II metabolism, or both.

7.5.2.1 Allyl sulphur compounds

Onions, leeks, garlic and other *Allium* species synthesize cysteine sulphoxide derivatives (allyl sulphur compounds) as a mechanism of protection against attack by pests. When the plant cells are damaged, the enzyme alliinase is released. It catalyses a series of reactions to form thiosulphinates, and a variety of organic mono-, di- and trisulphates and thiols. In onions the major product is thiopropanal-S-oxide, a potent lachrymator.

These allyl sulphur compounds lower the activity of microsomal cytochrome P$_{450}$ by three different mechanisms:

- They act as substrates, and inhibit the enzyme by mechanism-dependent (suicide) inhibition (section 2.3.4.1).
- They antagonize the induction of cytochrome P$_{450}$ by ethanol.
- They cause down-regulation of translation of mRNA, with no effect on transcription.

They also cause increased clearance of potential carcinogens and metabolites, by induction of glutathione S-transferases.

7.5.2.2 Glucosinolates

Glucosinolates (Figure 7.20) occur in brassicas (cabbage, cauliflower, broccoli, sprouts) and some other Cruciferae. The enzyme myrosinase in vacuoles in the plant cell is released when cells are damaged; it catalyses cleavage of glucosinolates to yield a variety of isothiocyanates, thiocyanates and nitriles plus the aglycone. Intestinal bacteria have a similar enzyme, so glucosinolates from cooked vegetables yield similar products.

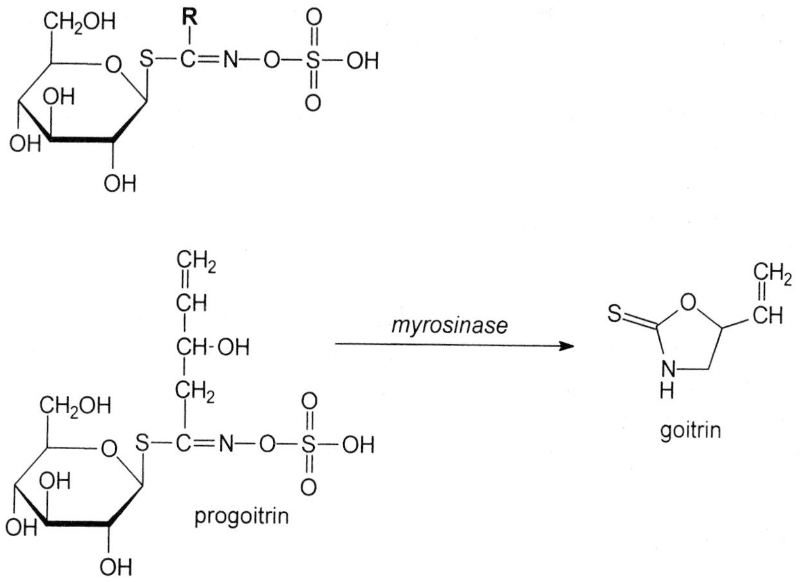

FIGURE 7.20 *The glucosinolinates.*

Like the allyl sulphur compounds in *Allium* spp., the aglycones of glucosinolates lower the activity of microsomal cytochrome P_{450} by:

- direct enzyme inhibition;
- down-regulation of enzyme synthesis – it is not known whether this is at the level of transcription or translation.

They also increase the clearance of potential carcinogens and metabolites by:

- induction of glutathione *S*-transferases;
- induction of quinone reductase.

There is a potential hazard associated with excessive consumption of brassicas – a number of the glucosinolates have a goitrogenic action, reducing synthesis of the thyroid hormones (section 11.15.3.3). Two mechanisms are involved:

- Thiocyanate (SCN^-) competes with iodide for tissue uptake; it is goitrogenic when iodine intakes are low.
- Oxazolidine-2-thiones (e.g. progoitrin; see Figure 7.20) inhibit thyroxine synthesis by inhibition of iodination of monoiodotyrosine to di-iodotyrosine. They are goitrogenic regardless of iodine nutritional status.

Goitre is a well-known problem in cattle fed on brassicas, but there is no evidence of reduced thyroid hormone status in people consuming, for example 150 g sprouts per day for several weeks. It is, however, noteworthy that iodine-deficiency goitre was a problem in The Netherlands (a country that cannot be considered to be upland, over limestone soil or inland, the usual criteria for iodine deficiency; section 11.15.3.3) until the introduction of iodide enrichment of flour at the beginning of the twentieth century. The traditional Dutch diet included a considerable amount of sauerkraut (fermented cabbage) – to such an extent that during the sixteenth and seventeenth centuries, when seafarers from most countries suffered from scurvy (vitamin C deficiency; section 11.14.3) during long voyages of exploration, the Dutch mariners did not.

7.5.2.3 Bioflavonoids

The bioflavonoids are a variety of compounds (> 4000 are known) in all plants; most occur as glycosides (with a variety of sugars) and are hydrolysed to aglycones by digestive enzymes. They serve both to protect plants against attack and also as the pigments of many plants. They were at one time considered to be vitamins (vitamin P), although there is no evidence that they are dietary essentials, then during the 1970s were considered to be mutagens and carcinogens, because, as shown in Figure 7.21, they are polyphenols and can undergo redox cycling with the production of

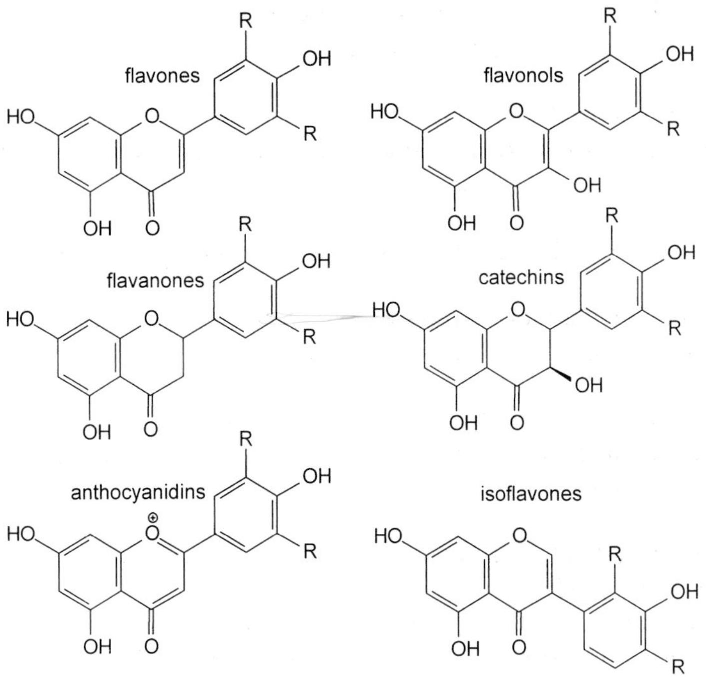

FIGURE 7.21 *The bioflavonoids.*

oxygen radicals. Since the 1990s they have been considered as potentially protective antioxidants because they can form relatively stable radicals that persist long enough to undergo reaction to non-radical products.

The bioflavonoids are also inhibitors of phase I reactions and activators of phase II reactions. In addition, they can form inactive complexes with a number of carcinogens.

Epidemiological evidence suggests a beneficial effect of a high intake of bioflavonoids with respect to cardiovascular disease (accounting for perhaps 8% of the international variation in coronary heart disease). However, despite the actions noted above, there is no epidemiological evidence of a negative association with cancer. Intakes of bioflavonoids are estimated to be around 23 mg/day, of which almost half comes from tea; onions, apples and red wine are also good sources.

7.5.3 PHYTO-OESTROGENS

A number of compounds that are widely distributed in plants as glycosides and other conjugates have weak oestrogenic action, although they are not chemically steroids. As shown in Figure 7.22, what they have in common is that all have two hydroxyl groups that are in the same position relative to each other as the hydroxyl groups in oestradiol, so that they bind to oestradiol receptors (section 10.4). The amounts present in plants are increased in response to microbial and insect attack, suggesting that

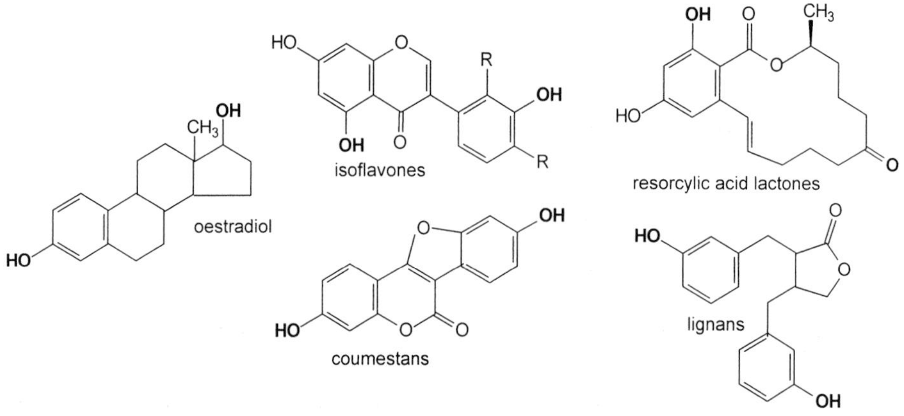

FIGURE 7.22 *Phyto-oestrogens – compounds that have two hydroxyl groups in the correct orientation to bind to the oestradiol receptor (see also section 10.4).*

they function as antimicrobial or antifungal agents in plants. Legumes, and especially soya beans, are rich sources.

The phyto-oestrogens produce typical and reproducible oestrogen responses in animals, with an oestrogenic activity 1/500–1/1000 of that of oestradiol. They may be agonistic or antagonistic to oestradiol when both are present at the target tissue (isoflavones are mainly antagonistic, lignans are mainly agonistic). They compete with oestradiol for receptor binding (section 10.4), but the phyto-oestrogen–receptor complex does not undergo normal activation, so it has only a weak effect on the hormone response element of DNA.

Phyto-oestrogens also reduce circulating free oestradiol because they increase sex hormone-binding globulin synthesis in liver – more hormone is bound to globulin, and therefore less is available for uptake into target tissues. Vegetarians have higher levels of circulating sex hormone-binding globulin than do omnivores.

It is noteworthy that in Japan, where the traditional diet contains relatively large amounts of phyto-oestrogens from soya bean products, there is a low incidence of cancer of the breast and prostate, as well as an unexpectedly low incidence of osteoporosis (despite the lower peak bone density of Japanese women compared with European or American women; see section 11.15.1.1). Although some prospective and case–control studies show a protective effect of soya bean consumption with respect to breast cancer, others do not.

There is a clear correlation between adiposity and breast cancer, which is almost certainly due to synthesis of oestradiol in adipose tissue; enterolactone and some of the other flavonoid phyto-oestrogens inhibit aromatase and will therefore reduce synthesis of oestradiol in adipose tissue.

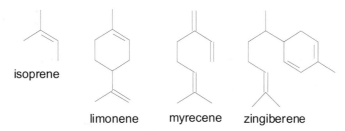

FIGURE 7.23 *Some potentially protective isoprenoids.*

7.5.4 MISCELLANEOUS ACTIONS OF PHYTOCHEMICALS

Salicylates are irreversible inhibitors of cyclo-oxygenase, and hence inhibit the synthesis of thromboxane A_2 and have an anticoagulant action. They occur in many fruits (and red wine) in amounts similar to the dose of aspirin recommended to prevent excessive blood clotting in patients at risk of thrombosis.

The allyl sulphur compounds (section 7.5.2.1) in garlic inhibit platelet coagulation, and again have a potentially beneficial effect with respect to thrombosis.

Terpenes such as limonene (in peel oil of citrus fruits and aromatic oils of caraway, dill, etc.), myrecene (in nutmeg) and zingiberine (in ginger) are polyisoprene derivatives (see Figure 7.23). They inhibit isoprenylation of the P21-*ras* oncogene product; isoprenylation is essential for action of the ras protein, which is known to be associated with pancreatic cancer.

Genistein (but not other phyto-oestrogens) inhibits cell proliferation by inhibiting the tyrosine kinase activity of the epithelial growth factor receptor.

Additional resources

PowerPoint presentation 7 on the CD.
Self-assesment exercise 7 on the CD.

PROBLEM 7.1 : *Healthy elderly people eating the wrong foods*

The guidelines for a prudent diet (section 7.3) can be summarized as:

- fat to provide 30% of energy;
- saturated fat to provide 10% of energy (one-third of total fat);
- sucrose to provide 10% of energy.

A study of healthy elderly people (aged 70–75) in Roskilde, Denmark, found that:

- 5% of them received more than 50% of energy from fat;
- 22% had an intake of more than 50% of their fat as saturated fat;
- 90% received more than 10% of energy from sugar;
- 46% of the men were smokers.

What explanation can you suggest to explain these results?

PROBLEM 7.2: *Adverse effects of lowering serum cholesterol*

Figure 7.9 shows a clear relationship between elevated serum cholesterol and risk of premature death from coronary heart disease. Table 7.4 shows the results of a meta-analysis of trials of various interventions to lower serum cholesterol.

Can you account for the disappointing results of the intervention trials?

TABLE 7.4 *Relative mortality in cholesterol-lowering intervention trials*

	Relative mortality
Cardiovascular disease	0.85
All causes	1.07
Cancer (only in drug trials)	1.43
Not illness related	1.76

From data reported by Muldoon MF *et al.* (1990) *British Medical Journal* 301: 309–314.

PROBLEM 7.3: *Adverse effects of carotene supplements*

Figures 7.5 and 7.6 suggest very strongly that β-carotene is protective against a variety of cancers. However, the results of a multimillion-dollar intervention trial, shown in Figure 7.7, showed an increase in lung and other cancers among people taking β-carotene supplements.

Can you account for the discrepancy between the epidemiological studies and the intervention trial?

PROBLEM 7.4: *Adverse effects of vitamin E supplements*

Figure 7.2 suggests very strongly that a high plasma level of vitamin E is protective against coronary heart disease. Table 7.5 shows the results of the Cambridge Heart Anti-Oxidant Study.

Can you account for the discrepancy between the epidemiological study and the intervention trial?

TABLE 7.5 *Myocardial infarction and mortality in the Cambridge Heart Anti-Oxidant Study*

	Placebo (%)	**Vitamin E supplements (%)**	**Relative risk**
Non-fatal myocardial infarction	4.23	1.35	0.32
Fatal myocardial infarction	1.35	1.74	1.29
All-cause mortality	2.69	3.48	1.29

From data reported by Stephens NG *et al.* (1996) *Lancet* 347: 781–786.

CHAPTER 8

Protein–energy malnutrition – problems of undernutrition

If the intake of metabolic fuels is lower than is required for energy expenditure, the body's reserves of fat, carbohydrate (glycogen) and protein are used to meet energy needs. Especially in lean people, who have relatively small reserves of body fat, there is a relatively large loss of tissue protein when food intake is inadequate. As the deficiency continues, so there is an increasingly serious loss of tissue, until eventually essential tissue proteins are catabolized as metabolic fuels – a process that obviously cannot continue for long.

Objectives

After reading this chapter you should be able to:

- explain what is meant by protein–energy malnutrition and differentiate between marasmus and kwashiorkor;
- explain why marasmus can be considered to be the predictable outcome of prolonged negative energy balance;
- describe the groups of people in developed countries who are at risk of protein–energy malnutrition;
- describe the features of cachexia and explain how it differs from marasmus;
- describe the features of kwashiorkor and explain how it differs from marasmus.

8.1 *Problems of deficiency*

Human beings have evolved in a hostile environment in which food has always been scarce. It is only in the last half-century, and only in Western Europe, North America and Australasia, that there is a surplus of food. Food is still desperately short in much of Africa, Asia and Latin America. Even without all too frequent droughts, floods and other disasters there is scarcely enough food produced world-wide to feed all the people of the world.

As shown in Figure 8.1, world food production has more than kept pace with population growth over the last four decades, so that most countries now have more food available per head of population than in the 1960s. This is total food potentially available, and does not take account of wastage and spoilage. It is noteworthy that there is still a twofold difference in food energy available per head of population between the USA (16 MJ/day) and Bangladesh (8 MJ/day).

Despite the advances in food production during the second half of the twentieth century, up to 300 million people are at risk from protein–energy malnutrition in developing countries. More importantly, as shown in Figures 8.2 and 8.3, the world population will increase from the present 6.25 billion to 8 billion by 2021, and most of this increase will be in less developed countries. It is extremely unlikely that food production can be increased to the same extent.

Deficiency of individual nutrients is also a major problem. The total amount of food may be adequate to satisfy hunger, but the quality of the diet is inadequate:

- Vitamin A deficiency (section 11.2.4) is the single most important cause of childhood blindness in the world, with some 14 million pre-school children showing clinical signs of deficiency and 190 million people at risk of deficiency.
- Iron deficiency anaemia affects many millions of women in both developing and developed countries (section 11.15.2.3).
- Deficiency of iodine affects many millions of people living in upland areas over limestone soil; in some areas of central Africa, Brazil and the Himalayas more than 90% of the population may have goitre due to iodine deficiency (section 11.15.3.3). Where children are iodine deficient both *in utero* and post-natally, the result is severe intellectual impairment – goitrous cretinism.
- While deficiencies of vitamin A, iron and iodine are priority targets for the World Health Organization (WHO), deficiency of vitamins B_1 (section 11.6.3) and B_2 (section 11.7.3) continues to be a major problem in large areas of Asia and Africa, and selenium deficiency (section 11.15.2.5) is a significant problem in large regions of China, and elsewhere.

Deficiency of other vitamins and minerals also occurs, and can be an important cause of ill-health. Sometimes this is the result of an acute exacerbation of a marginal food shortage, as in the outbreaks of the niacin deficiency disease pellagra reported in east and southern Africa during the 1980s (section 11.8.4); sometimes it is a problem

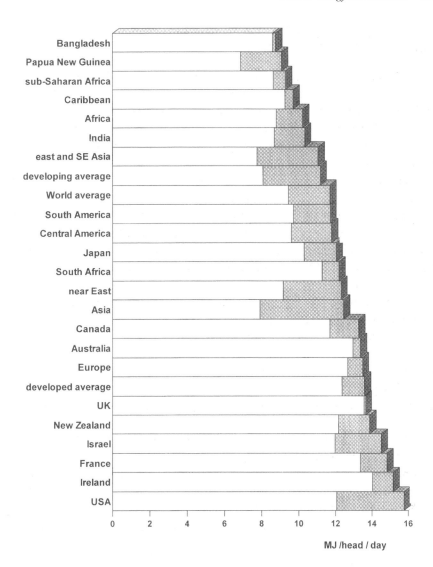

FIGURE 8.1 *Food available per head of population in various countries, 1961 (clear bars) and the increase in 1998 (shaded areas). From United Nations Food and Agriculture Organization data.*

of immigrant populations living in a new environment, where familiar foods are not readily available and foods that are available are unfamiliar.

8.2 *Protein–energy malnutrition*

The terms *protein–energy malnutrition* and *protein–energy deficiency* are widely used to mean a general lack of food, as opposed to specific deficiencies of vitamins or minerals

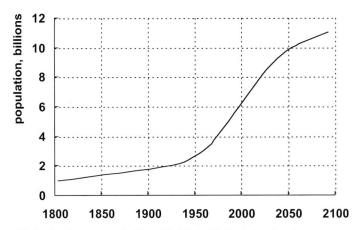

FIGURE 8.2 *World population growth. From World Health Organization data.*

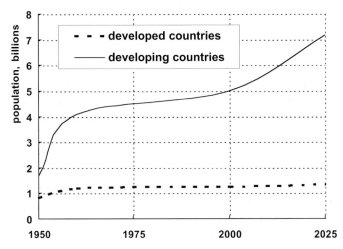

FIGURE 8.3 *Population growth in developed and developing countries. From World Health Organization data.*

(discussed in Chapter 11). However, the problem is one not of protein deficiency, but rather a deficiency of metabolic fuels. Indeed, there may be a relative excess of protein, in that protein which might be used for tissue protein replacement, or for growth in children, is being used as a fuel because of the deficiency of total food intake.

This was demonstrated in a series of studies in India in the early 1980s. Children whose intake of protein was just adequate were given additional carbohydrate (as sugary drinks). They showed an increase in growth and the deposition of new body protein. This was because their previous energy intake was inadequate, despite an adequate intake of protein. Increasing their intake of metabolic fuel both spared dietary protein for the synthesis of tissue proteins and also provided an adequate energy source to meet the high energy cost of protein synthesis (section 9.2.3.3). The body's first requirement, at all times, is for an adequate source of metabolic fuels. Only when

TABLE 8.1 *Classification of protein-energy malnutrition by body mass index*

BMI	
20–25	Acceptable/desirable range
17–18.4	Moderate protein–energy malnutrition
16–17	Moderately severe protein-energy malnutrition
< 16	Severe protein–energy malnutrition

BMI = weight (kg)/height^2 (m).

energy requirements have been met can dietary protein be used for tissue protein synthesis.

The severity of protein–energy malnutrition in adults can be assessed from the body mass index (the ratio of weight (in kg)/height^2 (in m); section 6.1.1), as shown in Table 8.1.

There are two extreme forms of protein–energy malnutrition:

- *Marasmus* can occur in both adults and children and occurs in vulnerable groups of the population in developed countries as well as in developing countries.
- *Kwashiorkor* affects only children and has been reported only in developing countries. The distinguishing feature of kwashiorkor is that there is fluid retention, leading to oedema.

Protein–energy malnutrition in children can therefore be classified by both the deficit in weight compared with what would be expected for age and also the presence or absence of oedema, as shown in Table 8.2. The most severely affected group, and therefore the priority group for intervention, are those suffering from marasmic kwashiorkor – they are both severely undernourished and also oedematous.

8.3 *Marasmus*

Marasmus is a state of extreme emaciation; the name is derived from the Greek μαρασμοσ for wasting. It is the predictable outcome of prolonged negative energy balance with severe depletion of all energy reserves in the body.

TABLE 8.2 *Classification of protein–energy malnutrition in children*

	No oedema	**Oedema**
60–80% of expected weight for age	Underweight	Kwashiorkor
< 60% of expected weight for age	Marasmus	Marasmic kwashiorkor

Not only have the body's fat reserves been exhausted, but there is wastage of muscle as well, and as the condition progresses there is loss of protein from the heart, liver and kidneys, although as far as possible essential tissue proteins are protected. As discussed in section 9.2.3.3, protein synthesis is energy expensive, and in marasmus there is a considerable reduction in the rate of protein synthesis, although catabolism continues at the normal rate (section 9.1.1). The amino acids released by the catalysis of tissue proteins are used as a source of metabolic fuel and as substrates for gluconeogenesis to maintain a supply of glucose for the brain and red blood cells (section 5.7).

As a result of the reduced synthesis of proteins, there is a considerable impairment of the immune response, so that undernourished people are more at risk from infections that those who are adequately nourished. Diseases that are minor childhood illnesses in developed countries can often prove fatal to undernourished children in developing countries. Measles is commonly cited as the cause of death among children in developing countries, although it would invariably be more correct to give the true cause of death as malnutrition – infection is simply the last straw.

One of the proteins secreted by the liver that is most severely affected by protein–energy malnutrition is the plasma retinol-binding protein, which transports vitamin A from liver stores to tissues where it is required (section 11.2.2.2). As the synthesis of retinol-binding protein is reduced, so there are increasing signs of vitamin A deficiency, although there may be adequate reserves of the vitamin in the liver. Without the binding protein, liver reserves cannot be transported to the tissues where they are required. It is quite common for signs of vitamin A deficiency to be associated with protein–energy malnutrition, but supplements of vitamin A have no effect, as the problem is in the transport and utilization of the vitamin. Nevertheless, as discussed in section 11.2.4, dietary deficiency of vitamin A is also a serious problem in many developing countries and further impairs immune responses.

A more serious effect of protein–energy malnutrition is impairment of cell proliferation in the intestinal mucosa (section 4.1). The villi are shorter than usual, and in severe cases the intestinal mucosa is almost flat. This results in a considerable reduction in the surface area of the intestinal mucosa, and hence a reduction in the absorption of such nutrients as are available from the diet. As a result, diarrhoea is a common feature of protein–energy malnutrition. Thus, not only does the undernourished person have an inadequate intake of food, but the absorption of what is available is impaired, so making the problem worse.

8.3.1 CAUSES OF MARASMUS AND VULNERABLE GROUPS OF THE POPULATION

In developing countries, the causes of marasmus are either a chronic shortage of food or the more acute problem of famine, where there will be very little food available at all. All too frequently, famine comes on top of a long-term shortage of food, so its effects are all the more rapid and serious.

A lack of food is unlikely to be a problem in developed countries, although the most socially and economically disadvantaged in the community are at risk of hunger and perhaps even protein–energy undernutrition in extreme cases. Two factors may cause marasmus in developed countries: disorders of appetite and impairment of the absorption of nutrients.

8.3.1.1 Disorders of appetite: anorexia nervosa and bulimia

As discussed in section 6.2.1, there is considerable pressure on people in Western countries to be slim. We are bombarded with more or less well- or ill-informed articles about obesity in magazines and newspapers and on radio and TV; many of the fashion models and media stars who provide role models for young people are extremely thin.

While obesity is indeed a serious health problem (see section 6.2.2), one effect of the propaganda is to put considerable pressure on people to reduce their body weight, even if they are within the acceptable and healthy weight range. In some cases this pressure may be a factor in the development of anorexia nervosa – a major psychological disturbance of appetite and eating behaviour. The group most at risk are adolescent girls, although similar disturbances of eating behaviour can occur in older women and (more rarely) in adolescent boys and men.

The main feature of anorexia nervosa is a refusal to eat – with the obvious result of very considerable weight loss. Despite all evidence and arguments to the contrary, the anorectic subject is convinced that she is overweight and restricts her eating very severely. Dieting becomes the primary focus of her life. She has a preoccupation with, and often a considerable knowledge of, food, and frequently has a variety of stylized compulsive behaviour patterns associated with food. As a part of her pathological obsession with thinness, the anorectic subject frequently takes a great deal of strenuous exercise, often exercising to exhaustion in solitude. She will go to extreme lengths to avoid eating, and frequently when forced to eat will induce vomiting soon afterwards. Many anorectics also make excessive use of laxatives.

Surprisingly, many anorectic people are adept at hiding their condition, and it is not unknown for the problem to remain unnoticed, even in a family setting. Food is played with, but little or none is actually eaten; excuses are frequently made to leave the table in the middle of the meal, perhaps on the pretext of going into the kitchen to prepare the next course.

Some anorectic subjects also exhibit a further disturbance of eating behaviour – bulimia or binge eating. After a period of eating little or nothing, they suddenly eat an extremely large amount of food (40 MJ or more in a single meal, compared with an average daily requirement of 8–12 MJ), frequently followed by deliberate induction of vomiting and heavy doses of laxatives. This is followed by a further prolonged period of anorexia.

Bulimia also occurs in the absence of anorexia nervosa – a person of normal weight will consume a very large amount of food (commonly 40–80 MJ over a period of a few hours), again followed by induction of vomiting and excessive use of laxatives. In severe cases such binges may occur five or six times a week.

Anorexia nervosa and bulimia are psychological problems, and require sensitive specialist treatment. It is not simply a matter of persuading the patient to eat. One theory is that the root cause of the problem, at least in adolescent girls, is a reaction to the physical changes of puberty. By refusing food, the girl believes that she can delay or prevent these changes. To a considerable extent this is so. Breast development slows down or ceases as the energy balance becomes more negative and, as body weight falls below about 45 kg, menstruation ceases.

It is estimated that about 2% of adolescent girls go through at least a short phase of anorexia. In most cases it is self-limiting and normal eating patterns are re-established as the emotional crises of adolescence resolve. Other people may require specialist counselling and treatment, and in an unfortunate few problems of eating behaviour persist into adult life.

8.3.1.2 Malabsorption

Any clinical condition that impairs the absorption of nutrients from the intestinal tract will lead to undernutrition, although the intake is apparently adequate. The problem is one of digestion and/or absorption of the food.

Obviously, major intestinal surgery will result in a reduction in the amount of intestine available for the digestion and absorption of nutrients. In this case, the problem is known in advance, and precautionary measures can be taken: a period of intravenous feeding, to supplement normal food intake, and careful counselling by a dietitian, so as to ensure adequate nutrient intake despite the problems.

A variety of infectious diseases can cause malabsorption and diarrhoea. In many cases, this lasts only a few days and so has no long-term consequences. However, a number of intestinal parasites can cause long-lasting diarrhoea and damage to the intestinal mucosa, leading to malnutrition if the infection remains untreated for too long.

8.3.1.3 Food intolerance and allergy

It was noted in section 4.4.3.2 that relatively large peptides derived from dietary proteins can be absorbed intact, and these can stimulate the production of antibodies – this is the basis of food allergy. Allergic reactions to foods may include dermatitis, eczema and urticaria, asthma, allergic rhinitis, muscle pain, rheumatoid arthritis and migraine, as well as effects on the gastrointestinal tract. All of these are likely to impair the sufferer's appetite, and hence may contribute to undernutrition. There can be serious damage to the intestinal mucosa, leading to severe malabsorption, and hence malnutrition despite an apparently adequate intake of food. One of the best understood such conditions is coeliac disease.

Coeliac disease is an allergy to one specific protein in wheat – the gliadin fraction of wheat gluten. The result is a considerable loss of intestinal mucosa and flattening of the intestinal villi, so that the appearance of the intestine is similar to that seen in marasmus. This reduction in the absorptive surface of the intestine leads to persistent fatty diarrhoea (steattorhoea) and a failure to absorb nutrients. The result is undernutrition; although the intake of food is apparently adequate, there is inadequate digestion and absorption of nutrients. Severe emaciation can occur in patients with untreated coeliac disease.

Once the diagnosis is established, and the immediate problems of undernutrition have been dealt with, treatment is relatively simple – avoidance of all wheat and rye-based products. In practice, this is less easy than it sounds – apart from the obvious foods, such as bread and pasta, wheat flour is used in a great many food products. There is therefore a need for counselling from a dietitian, and careful reading of labels for lists of ingredients. A number of products have the symbol of the Coeliac Society on the label, to show that they are known to be free from gluten and therefore safe for patients to eat.

A number of other intolerances or allergic reactions to foods can also lead to similar persistent diarrhoea, loss of intestinal mucosa and hence malnutrition. The problem of disaccharide intolerance was discussed in section 4.2.2.2. In general, once the offending food has been identified, the patient's condition has stabilized and body weight has been restored, continuing treatment is relatively easy, although avoidance of some common foods may provide significant problems.

It is the identification of the offending food that poses the greatest problem and frequently calls for lengthy investigations, maintaining the patient on a very limited range of foods then gradually introducing additional foods until the offending item is identified.

Patients with food intolerances or allergies are generally extremely ill after they have eaten the offending food, and this may persist for several days. Even after the offending foods have been identified, and the patient's condition has been stabilized, there may be continuing problems of appetite and eating behaviour.

8.4 *Cachexia*

Patients with advanced cancer, human immunodeficiency virus (HIV) infection and acquired immune deficiency syndrome (AIDS) and a number of other chronic diseases are frequently undernourished. Physically they show all the signs of marasmus, but there is considerably more loss of body protein than occurs in starvation. The condition is called cachexia, from the Greek καχεξιο for 'in a poor condition'). A number of factors contribute to the problem:

- The patients are extremely sick, and because of this their wish to eat may be impaired.
- Many of the drugs used in chemotherapy can cause nausea, loss of appetite and alteration of the senses of taste and smell (section 1.3.3.1), so that foods that were appetizing are now either unappetizing or even aversive.

- Chemotherapy and radiotherapy inhibit cell division; this leads to reduced cell proliferation in the intestinal mucosa, and hence malabsorption (section 8.3.1.2).
- There is a considerable increase in basal metabolic rate, to the extent that patients are described as being hypermetabolic. Even a mild fever causes an increase in basal metabolic rate of about 13% per degree Celsius increase in body temperature.
- The secretion of cytokines, including tumour necrosis factor (also known as cachectin), in response to infection and cancer increases the rate of breakdown of tissue protein. This is a major difference from marasmus, in which protein synthesis is reduced but catabolism in unaffected.

A number of factors account for the increase in metabolic rate in cachexia:

- Many tumours metabolize glucose anaerobically to release lactate. This is then used for gluconeogenesis in the liver – as discussed in section 5.4.1.2, there is a net cost of six ATP for each mole of glucose cycled between lactate and glucose in this way, and hence there has to be an increased rate of metabolism on the liver. Figure 8.4 shows the increase in glucose cycling in patients with advanced cancer.
- There is increased stimulation of uncoupling proteins (section 3.3.1.4), leading to thermogenesis and hence increased oxidation of metabolic fuels.
- There is futile cycling of lipids. Hormone sensitive lipase in adipose tissue (section 10.5.1) is activated by a small proteoglycan produced by tumours that cause cachexia (but not by those that do not). This results in liberation of fatty acids from adipose tissue, and re-esterification to triacylglycerols (which are exported in VLDL; section 5.6.2.2) in the liver. As discussed in section 5.6.1.2, esterification of fatty acids to triacylglycerol is an energy-expensive process.

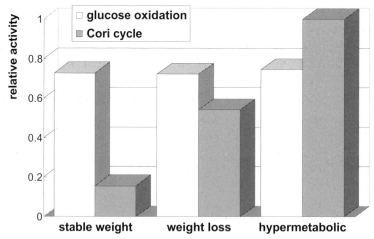

FIGURE 8.4 *Glucose cycling in patients with cancer cachexia. From data reported by Holroyde CP et al. (1975)* Cancer Research *35: 3710–3714.*

Both decreased synthesis and accelerated catabolism contribute to the loss of tissue protein.

- There is a considerable depletion of individual amino acids, resulting in an incomplete mixture of amino acids available for protein synthesis (section 9.1.2.2):
  - many tumours have a high requirement for glutamine and leucine;
  - there is increased utilization of alanine and other amino acids as a result of the stimulation of gluconeogenesis by tumour necrosis factor;
  - interferon-γ induces indoleamine dioxygenase and depletes tissue pools of tryptophan.
- Tumour necrosis factor causes increased protein catabolism. It increases both expression of ubiquitin and the activity of the ubiquitin-dependent proteolysis system (section 9.1.1.1).
- The proteoglycan produced by tumours that cause cachexia also stimulates protein catabolism – in this case the mechanism is unknown.

8.5 *Kwashiorkor*

Kwashiorkor was first described in Ghana, in west Africa, in 1932 – the word is the Ghanaian name for the condition. In addition to the wasting of muscle tissue, loss of intestinal mucosa and impaired immune responses seen in marasmus, children with kwashiorkor show a number of characteristic features which distinguish this disease:

- Fluid retention and hence severe oedema, associated with a decreased concentration of plasma proteins. The puffiness of the limbs, due to the oedema, masks the severe wasting of arm and leg muscles.
- Enlargement of the liver. This is due to the accumulation of abnormally large amounts of fat in the liver, to the extent that, instead of its normal reddish-brown colour, the liver is pale yellow when examined at post-mortem or during surgery. The metabolic basis for this fatty infiltration of the liver is not known. It is the enlargement of the liver that causes the paradoxical 'pot-bellied' appearance of children with kwashiorkor; together with the oedema, they appear, from a distance, to be plump, yet they are starving;
- Characteristic changes in the texture and colour of the hair. This is most noticeable in African children; instead of tightly curled black hair, children with kwashiorkor have sparse, wispy hair, which is less curled than normal, and poorly pigmented – it is often reddish or even grey.
- A sooty, sunburn-like skin rash.
- A characteristic expression of deep misery.

8.5.1 FACTORS IN THE AETIOLOGY OF KWASHIORKOR

The underlying cause of kwashiorkor is an inadequate intake of food, as is the case for marasmus. Kwashiorkor traditionally affects children aged between of 3 and 5 years. In many societies a child continues to suckle until about this age, when the next child is born. As a result, the toddler is abruptly weaned, frequently onto very unsuitable food. In some societies, children are weaned onto a dilute gruel made from whatever is the local cereal; in others the child may be fed on the water in which rice has been boiled – it may look like milk, but has little nutritional value. Sometimes the child is given little or no special treatment but has to compete with the rest of the family for its share from the stew-pot. A small child has little chance of getting an adequate meal under such conditions, especially if there is in any case not much food for the whole family.

There is no satisfactory explanation for the development of kwashiorkor rather than marasmus. At one time it was believed that it was due to a lack of protein, with a more or less adequate intake of energy. However, analysis of the diets of children suffering from kwashiorkor shows clearly that this is not so. Furthermore, children who are protein deficient have a slower rate of growth, and are therefore stunted (section 9.1.2.1); as shown in Figure 8.5, children with kwashiorkor are less stunted that those with marasmus. Finally, many of the signs of kwashiorkor, and especially the oedema, begin to improve early in treatment, when the child is still receiving a low-protein diet (section 8.5.2).

Very commonly, an infection precipitates kwashiorkor in children whose nutritional status is inadequate, even if they are not yet showing signs of malnutrition. Indeed, paediatricians in developing countries expect an outbreak of kwashiorkor a few months after an outbreak of measles.

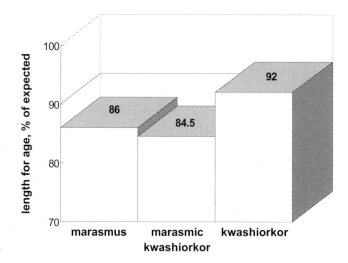

FIGURE 8.5 *Stunting of growth in kwashiorkor, marasmus and marasmic kwashiorkor.*

The most likely precipitating factor is that, superimposed on general food deficiency, there is a deficiency of the antioxidant nutrients such as zinc, copper, carotene and vitamins C and E (section 7.4.3). As discussed in section 7.4.2.2, the respiratory burst in response to infection leads to the production of oxygen and halogen radicals as part of the cytotoxic action of stimulated macrophages. The added oxidant stress of an infection may well trigger the sequence of events that leads to the development of kwashiorkor.

8.5.2 REHABILITATION OF MALNOURISHED CHILDREN

The intestinal tract of the malnourished patient is in a very poor state. This means that the child is not able to deal at all adequately with a rich diet, or a large amount of food. Rather, treatment begins with small frequent feeding of liquids – a dilute sugar solution for the first few days, followed by diluted milk, and then full-strength milk. This may be achieved by use of a nasogastric tube, so that the dilute solution can be provided at a slow and constant rate throughout the day and night. Where such luxuries are not available, the malnourished infant is fed from a teaspoon, a few drops at a time, more or less continually.

Once the patient has begun to develop a more normal intestinal mucosa (when the diarrhoea ceases), ordinary foods can gradually be introduced. Recovery is normally rapid in children, and they soon begin to grow at a normal rate.

Additional resources

PowerPoint presentation 8 on the CD.
Self-assessment exercise 8 on the CD.

Problem 8.1: Arthur N

Arthur is a 75-year-old man, 170 cm tall and weighing 50 kg. He has advanced cancer, and has lost 2 kg body weight over the last 4 weeks.

What is his body mass index? Is it within the desirable range?

His mean skinfold thickness is 1.9 mm, suggesting that he has negligible reserves of adipose tissue, and he shows considerable wasting of muscle, so we can assume that most of his weight loss is muscle. The composition of muscle is: 79% water, 17% protein (at 17 kJ/g) and 3% fat (at 37 kJ/g).

What was his overall energy deficit over the last 4 weeks (total energy deficit and average/day)?

For his age and body weight, BMR would be expected to be between 4.7 and 4.9 MJ/day. His BMR was determined by measuring oxygen consumption with a respirometer; regardless of the fuel being oxidized, 1 L of oxygen is equivalent to 20 kJ. His oxygen consumption was 11.2 L/h. What is his BMR (in MJ/day)?

Assuming the mean BMR for his age and weight = 4.8 MJ/day, what is his daily energy deficit now?

How much intravenous glucose would be required daily to restore energy balance and prevent further weight loss? (energy yield of glucose = 16 kJ/g).

What volume of 5% glucose would be required?

CHAPTER 9

Protein nutrition and metabolism

The need for protein in the diet was demonstrated early in the nineteenth century, when it was shown that animals which were fed only on fats, carbohydrates and mineral salts were unable to maintain their body weight and showed severe wasting of muscle and other tissues. It was known that proteins contain nitrogen (mainly in the amino groups of their constituent amino acids; section 6.4.1), and methods of measuring total amounts of nitrogenous compounds in foods and excreta were soon developed.

Objectives

After reading this chapter you should be able to:

- explain what is meant by the terms nitrogen balance and dynamic equilibrium;
- describe the processes involved in tissue protein catabolism;
- explain the basis for current recommendations for protein intake and for essential and non-essential amino acids;
- explain what is meant by protein nutritional value or quality, and why it is of little importance in most diets;
- describe the processes involved in protein synthesis, outline the flow of information from DNA to RNA to protein, and explain the energy cost of protein synthesis;
- describe and explain the pathways by which the amino nitrogen of amino acids is metabolized and explain the importance of transamination;
- describe and explain the metabolism of ammonia, and the synthesis of urea;
- describe the metabolic fates of the carbon skeletons of amino acids.

9.1 *Nitrogen balance and protein requirements*

Figure 9.1 shows an overview of protein metabolism; in addition to the dietary intake of about 80 g of protein, almost the same amount of endogenous protein is secreted into the intestinal lumen. There is a small faecal loss equivalent to about 10 g of protein per day; the remainder is hydrolysed to free amino acids and small peptides, and absorbed (section 4.4.3). The faecal loss of nitrogen is partly composed of undigested dietary protein, but the main contributors are intestinal bacteria and shed mucosal cells, which are only partially broken down, and the protective mucus secreted by intestinal mucosal goblet cells (see Figure 4.2). Mucus is especially resistant to enzymic hydrolysis, and contributes a considerable proportion of inevitable losses of nitrogen, even on a protein-free diet.

There is only a small pool of free amino acids in the body, in equilibrium with proteins that are being catabolized and synthesized. A small proportion of the amino acid pool is used for synthesis of a wide variety of specialized metabolites (including hormones and neurotransmitters, purines and pyrimidines). An amount of amino acids equivalent to that absorbed is oxidized, with the carbon skeletons being used for gluconeogenesis (sections 5.7 and 9.3.2) or as metabolic fuels, and the nitrogen being excreted mainly as urea (section 9.3.1.4).

The state of protein nutrition, and the overall state of body protein metabolism, can be determined by measuring the dietary intake of nitrogenous compounds and

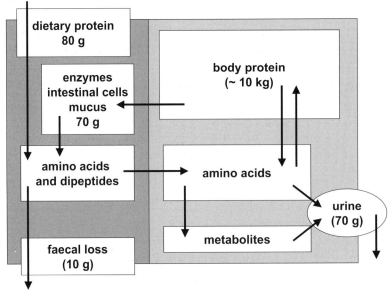

FIGURE 9.1 *An overview of protein metabolism.*

the output of nitrogenous compounds from the body. Although nucleic acids also contain nitrogen (section 9.2.1), protein is the major dietary source of nitrogenous compounds, and measurement of total nitrogen intake gives a good estimate of protein intake. Nitrogen constitutes 16% of most proteins, and therefore the protein content of foods is calculated on the basis of mg N × 6.25, although for some foods with an unusual amino acid composition other factors are used.

The output of N from the body is largely in the urine and faeces, but significant amounts may also be lost in sweat and shed skin cells – and in longer-term studies the growth of hair and nails must be taken into account. Obviously, any loss of blood or tissue will also involve a loss of protein. Although the intake of nitrogenous compounds is mainly protein, the output is mainly urea (section 9.3.1.4), though small amounts of a number of other products of amino acid metabolism are also excreted, as shown in Table 9.1.

The difference between intake and output of nitrogenous compounds is known as nitrogen balance. Three states can be defined:

- An adult in good health and with an adequate intake of protein excretes the same amount of nitrogen each day as is taken in from the diet. This is nitrogen balance or nitrogen equilibrium: intake = output and there is no change in the total body content of protein.
- In a growing child, a pregnant woman or someone recovering from protein loss, the excretion of nitrogenous compounds is less than the dietary intake – there is a net retention of nitrogen in the body and an increase in the body content of protein. This is positive nitrogen balance: intake > output and there is a net gain in total body protein.
- In response to trauma or infection (section 9.1.2.2) or if the intake of protein is inadequate to meet requirements, there is net a loss of nitrogen from the body – the output is greater than the intake. This is negative nitrogen balance: intake < output and there is a loss of body protein.

TABLE 9.1 *Average daily excretion of nitrogenous compounds in the urine*

Urea	10–35 g	150–600 mol	Depends on the intake of protein
Ammonium	340–1200 mg	20–70 mmol	Depends on the state of acid–base balance
Amino acids, peptides and conjugates	1.3–3.2 g	–	
Protein	< 60 mg	–	Significant proteinuria indicates kidney damage
Uric acid	250–750 mg	1.5–4.5 mmol	Major product of purine metabolism
Creatinine	Male 1.8 g	Male 16 mmol	Depends on muscle mass
	Female 1.2 g	Female 10 mmol	
Creatine	< 50 mg	< 400 mmol	Higher levels indicate muscle catabolism

9.1.1 Dynamic equilibrium

The proteins of the body are continually being broken down and replaced. As shown in Table 9.2, some proteins (especially enzymes that have a role in controlling metabolic pathways) may turn over within a matter of minutes or hours; others last for longer before they are broken down, perhaps days or weeks. Some proteins only turn over very slowly – for example the connective tissue protein collagen is broken down and replaced so slowly that it is almost impossible to measure the rate – perhaps half of the body's collagen is replaced in a year.

This continual breakdown and replacement is dynamic equilibrium. Superficially, there is no change in body protein. In an adult there is no detectable change in the amount of protein in the body from one month to the next. Nevertheless, if an isotopically labelled amino acid is given, the process of turnover can be followed. As shown in Figure 9.2, the label rapidly becomes incorporated into newly synthesized proteins, and is gradually lost as the proteins are broken down. The rate at which the label is lost from any one protein depends on the rate at which that protein is broken down and replaced; the time for the labelling to fall to half its peak is the half-life of that protein.

Protein breakdown occurs at a more or less constant rate throughout the day, and an adult catabolizes and replaces some 3–6 g of protein per kilogram body weight per day. Turnover is also important in growing children, who synthesize considerably more protein per day than the net increase in body protein. Even children recovering from severe protein–energy malnutrition (see Chapter 8), and increasing their body protein rapidly, still synthesize 2–3 times more protein per day than the net increase.

Although an adult may be in overall nitrogen balance, this is the average of periods of negative balance in the fasting state and positive balance in the fed state. As discussed

TABLE 9.2 *Half-lives of some proteins*

Protein	Half-life
Ornithine decarboxylase	11 minutes
Lipoprotein lipase	1 hours
Tyrosine transaminase	1.5 hours
Phosphoenolpyruvate carboxykinase	2 hours
Tryptophan oxygenase	2 hours
HMG CoA reductase	3 hours
Glucokinase	12 hours
Alanine transaminase	0.7–1 days
Glucokinase	1.25 days
Serum albumin	3.5 days
Arginase	4–5 days
Lactate dehydrogenase	16 days
Adult collagen	300 days
Infant collagen	1–2 days and 150 days

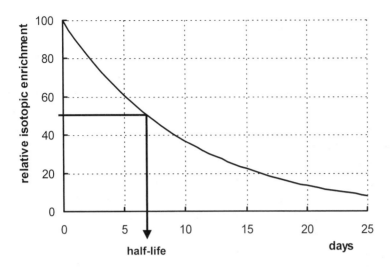

FIGURE 9.2 *Determination of the half-life of body proteins using* ^{15}*N-labelled amino acids.*

in section 9.2.3.3, protein synthesis is energy expensive, and in the fasting state the rate of synthesis is lower than that of protein catabolism. There is a loss of tissue protein, which provides amino acids for gluconeogenesis (section 5.7). In the fed state, when there is an abundant supply of metabolic fuel, the rate of protein synthesis increases and exceeds that of breakdown, so that what is observed is an increase in tissue protein, replacing that which was lost in the fasting state.

As discussed in section 8.3, even in severe undernutrition, the rate of protein breakdown remains more or less constant, while the rate of replacement synthesis falls, as a result of the low availability of metabolic fuels. It is only in cachexia (section 8.4) that there is increased protein catabolism as well as reduced replacement synthesis.

9.1.1.1 Mechanisms involved in tissue protein catabolism

The catabolism of tissue proteins is obviously a highly regulated process; as shown in Table 9.1, different proteins are catabolized (and replaced) at very different rates. Three different mechanisms are involved in the process:

- *Lysosomal cathepsins* are proteases with a broad range of specificity, leading to complete hydrolysis of proteins to free amino acids. They hydrolyse proteins that have entered the cell by phagocytosis and are also involved in the hydrolysis of cell proteins after cell death, when they are released into the cytosol. In addition, a number of intracellular proteins contain the sequence Lys-Phe-Glu-Arg-Gly, which targets them for uptake into the lysosomes, where they undergo hydrolysis.
- *Calpain* is a protease with a broad specificity for hydrophobic amino acids, resulting in partial proteolysis. It has a calcium-dependent regulatory subunit and is inhibited by a second protein, calstatin, so its activity in the cell is regulated. Both proteins

turn over relatively rapidly, and there is an increase in the amount of mRNA for both proteins in the cell during fasting and starvation – this seems to be the result of increased gene expression in order to maintain a constant amount of both proteins despite the reduction in overall protein synthesis.

- *The ubiquitin–proteasome system* catalyses ATP-dependent proteolysis. It is important in both protein turnover and antigen processing.
  - Ubiquitin is a small peptide (M_r 8,500) that forms a covalent bond from the carboxy terminus to the ε-amino of lysine residues in target proteins – this is an ATP-dependent process, and multiple molecules of ubiquitin are attached to target proteins. It is not known what targets proteins for ubiquitination; at least four different ubiquitin-transferring enzymes are known.
  - The proteasome (also known as the multifunctional protease) is a multi-subunit complex that accounts for about 1% of the total soluble protein of cells. There are at least five types of subunit with specificity for esters of hydrophobic, basic and acidic amino acids.

9.1.2 PROTEIN REQUIREMENTS

It is the continual catabolism of tissue proteins that creates the requirement for dietary protein. Although some of the amino acids released by breakdown of tissue proteins can be re-used, most are metabolized, by pathways which are discussed in section 9.3, yielding intermediates that can be used as metabolic fuels and for gluconeogenesis (section 5.7) and urea (section 9.3.1.4), which is excreted. This means that there is a need for dietary protein to replace losses even in an adult who is not growing. In addition, relatively large amounts of protein are lost from the body in mucus, enzymes and other proteins, which are secreted into the gastrointestinal tract and are not completely digested and reabsorbed.

Current estimates of protein requirements are based on studies of the amount required to maintain nitrogen balance. If the intake is not adequate to replace the protein that has been broken down, then there is negative nitrogen balance – a greater output of nitrogen from the body than the dietary intake. Once the intake is adequate to meet requirements, nitrogen balance is restored. The proteins that have been broken down can be replaced, and any surplus intake of protein can be used as a metabolic fuel.

Such studies show that for adults the average daily requirement is 0.6 g of protein per kilogram body weight. Allowing for individual variation, the reference intake (section 11.1.1) is 0.75 g/kg body weight, or 50 g/day for a 65 kg adult. Average intakes of protein by adults in developed countries are considerably greater than requirements, of the order of 80–100 g/day. The reference intake of protein is sometimes called the safe level of intake, meaning that it is safe and (more than) adequate to meet requirements, not implying that there is any hazard from higher levels of intake.

Protein requirements can also be expressed as a proportion of energy intake. The energy yield of protein is 17 kJ/g, and the reference intake of protein represents some 7–8% of energy intake. In Western countries protein provides 14–15% of energy intake.

It is unlikely that adults in any country will suffer from protein deficiency if they are eating enough food to meet their energy requirements. As shown in Figure 9.3, the major dietary staples that are generally considered as sources of carbohydrate also provide significant amounts of protein. Even among people in Western countries who eat meat, fish and eggs (which are generally regarded as rich protein sources) about 25% of protein intake comes from cereals and cereal products, with an additional 10% from fruit and vegetables.

Only cassava, yam and possibly rice provide insufficient protein (as a percentage of energy) to meet adult requirements. The shortfall in protein provided by a diet based on yam or rice would be made up by small amounts of other foods that are sources of protein – this may be either small amounts of meat and fish or legumes and nuts, which are rich vegetable sources of protein. With diets based largely on cassava there is a more serious problem in meeting protein requirements.

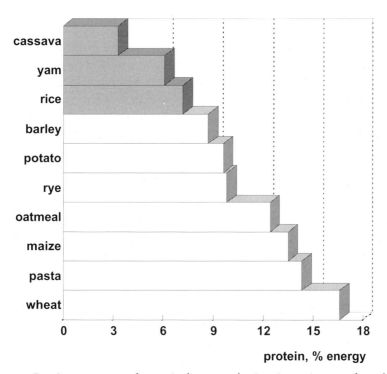

FIGURE 9.3 *Protein as percentage of energy in dietary staples. Protein requirements of an adult are met when the diet provides 7–8% of energy from protein. Of the major dietary staples, only cassava, yam and (marginally) rice fail to provide this much protein.*

9.1.2.1 Protein requirements of children

Because children are growing, and increasing the total amount of protein in the body, they have a proportionally greater requirement than adults. A child should be in positive nitrogen balance while he or she is growing. Even so, the need for protein for growth is relatively small compared with the requirement to replace proteins which are turning over. Table 9.3 shows protein requirements at different ages. Children in Western countries consume more protein than is needed to meet their requirements, but in developing countries protein intake may well be inadequate to meet the requirement for growth.

A protein-deficient child will grow more slowly than one receiving an adequate intake of protein – this is stunting of growth. As discussed in section 8.2, the protein–energy deficiency diseases, marasmus and kwashiorkor, result from a general lack of food (and hence metabolic fuels), not a specific deficiency of protein.

9.1.2.2 Protein losses in trauma and infection – requirements for convalescence

One of the metabolic reactions to a major trauma, such as a burn, a broken limb or surgery, is an increase in the net catabolism of tissue proteins. As shown in Table 9.4, apart from the loss of blood associated with injury, as much as 750 g of protein (about 6–7% of the total body content) may be lost over 10 days. Even prolonged bed rest results in a considerable loss of protein, because there is atrophy of muscles that are not used. Muscle protein is catabolized as normal, but without the stimulus of exercise it is not completely replaced.

This protein loss is mediated by the hormone cortisol, which is secreted in response to stress, and the cytokines that are secreted in response to trauma; four mechanisms are involved:

- Tryptophan dioxygenase and tyrosine transaminase. This results in depletion of the tissue pools of these two amino acids, leaving an unbalanced mixture of amino acids that cannot be used for protein synthesis (section 9.2.3).
- In response to cytokine action there is an increase in metabolic rate, leading to an increased rate of oxidation of amino acids as metabolic fuel, so reducing the amount available for protein synthesis.
- Cytokines cause an increase in the rate of protein catabolism, as occurs in cachexia (section 8.4).
- A variety of plasma proteins synthesized in increased amount in response to cytokine action (the so-called acute-phase proteins) are richer in two amino acids, cysteine and threonine, than most tissue proteins. This leads to depletion of tissue pools of these two amino acids, again leaving an unbalanced mixture of amino acids that cannot be used for protein synthesis.

The lost protein has to be replaced during recovery, and patients who are

TABLE 9.3 *Reference nutrient intakes for protein*

Age	Recommended protein intake (g/day)
4–6 months	1.85
7–9 months	1.65
10–12 months	1.50
1–1.5 years	1.20
1.5–2 years	1.20
2–3 years	1.15
3–4 years	1.10
4–5 years	1.10
5–6 years	1.00
6–7 years	1.00
7–8 years	1.00
8–9 years	1.00
9–10 years	1.00
Males	
10 years	1.00
11 years	1.00
12 years	1.00
13 years	1.00
14 years	0.95
15 years	0.95
16 years	0.90
17 years	0.90
Adult	0.75
Females	
10 years	1.00
11 years	1.00
12 years	0.95
13 years	0.95
14 years	0.90
15 years	0.90
16 years	0.80
17 years	0.80
Adult	0.75

Source: FAO/WHO/UNU (1985) Energy and protein requirements. Report of a Joint FAO/WHO/UNU Expert Consultation. *WHO Technical Report Series* 724, Geneva.

convalescing will be in positive nitrogen balance. However, this does not mean that a convalescent patient requires a diet that is richer in protein than usual. As discussed in section 9.1.2, average protein intakes are twice requirements; a normal diet will provide adequate protein to permit replacement of the losses due to illness and hospitalization.

TABLE 9.4 *Protein losses (g) over 10 days after trauma or infection*

	Tissue loss	Blood loss	Catabolism	Total
Fracture of femur	–	200	700	900
Muscle wound	500–750	150–400	750	1350–1900
35% burns	500	150–400	750	1400–1650
Gastrectomy	20–180	20–10	625–750	645–850
Typhoid fever	–	–	675	685

From data reported by Cuthbertson DP (1964), in *Human Protein Metabolism*, Vol. II, Munro HN and Allison JB (eds), New York, Academic Press, pp. 373–414.

9.1.3 ESSENTIAL AMINO ACIDS

Early studies of nitrogen balance showed that not all proteins are nutritionally equivalent. More of some is needed to maintain nitrogen balance than others. This is because different proteins contain different amounts of the various amino acids (section 4.4.1). The body's requirement is not simply for protein, but for the amino acids which make up proteins, in the correct proportions to replace the body proteins.

As shown in Table 9.5, the amino acids can be divided into two main groups, with each group further subdivided:

- The nine essential or indispensable amino acids, which cannot be synthesized in the body. If one of these is lacking or provided in inadequate amount, then regardless of the total intake of protein it will not be possible to maintain nitrogen balance, as there will not be an adequate amount of the amino acid for protein synthesis.
  - Two amino acids, cysteine and tyrosine, can be synthesized in the body, but only from essential amino acid precursors – cysteine from methionine and tyrosine from phenylalanine. The dietary intakes of cysteine and tyrosine thus affect the requirements for methionine and phenylalanine – if more of either is provided in the diet, then less will have to be synthesized from the essential precursor.
  - For premature infants, and possibly also for full-term infants, a tenth amino acid is essential – arginine. Although adults can synthesize adequate amounts of arginine to meet their requirements, the capacity for arginine synthesis is low in infants and may not be adequate to meet the requirements for growth.
- The non-essential or dispensable amino acids, which can be synthesized from metabolic intermediates, as long as there is enough total protein in the diet. If one of these amino acids is omitted from the diet, nitrogen balance can still be maintained.
- Only three amino acids, alanine, aspartate and glutamate, can be considered to be truly dispensable; they are synthesized from common metabolic intermediates (pyruvate, oxaloacetate and α-ketoglutarate respectively; section 9.3.1.2).

TABLE 9.5 *Essential and non-essential amino acids*

Essential	Essential precursor	Non-essential	Semi-essential
Histidine		Alanine	Arginine
Isoleucine		Aspartate	Asparagine
Leucine		Glutamate	Glutamine
Lysine			Glycine
Methionine	Cysteine		Proline
Phenylalanine	Tyrosine		Serine
Threonine			
Tryptophan			
Valine			

- The remaining amino acids are generally considered as non-essential, but under some circumstances the requirement may outstrip the capacity for synthesis:
  - A high intake of compounds that are excreted as glycine conjugates will increase the requirement for glycine considerably.
  - In response to severe trauma there is an increased requirement for proline for collagen synthesis for healing,
  - In surgical trauma and sepsis the requirement for glutamine increases significantly – a number of studies have shown considerably improved healing after major surgery if additional glutamine is provided.

The requirements for essential amino acids for growth (expressed as proportion of total protein intake) are higher than the requirement to maintain N balance in adults, and younger children, with a faster growth rate, have a higher requirement for essential amino acids as a proportion of total protein than do older children with a lower rate of growth. Table 9.6 shows various estimates of essential amino acid requirements and the 'reference pattern' of the amount of each amino acid that should ideally be present per gram of dietary protein.

Early studies of essential amino acid requirements were based on the amounts required to maintain nitrogen balance in young adults. Interestingly, for reasons that are not clear, these relatively short-term studies did not show any requirement for histidine. More recent studies have measured the rate of whole-body protein turnover using isotopically labelled amino acids. These have shown that the maximum rate of protein turnover is achieved with intakes of the essential amino acids some threefold higher than are required to maintain nitrogen balance. What is not clear is whether the maximum rate of protein turnover is essential, or even desirable.

9.1.3.1 Protein quality and complementation

A protein that contains at least as much of each of the essential amino acids as is required will be completely useable for tissue protein synthesis, whereas one that is

TABLE 9.6 *Estimates of essential amino acids requirements and reference pattern for adults*

| | WHO/FAO (1973) | | FAO/WHO/ UNU (1985) | | Protein turnover require- ment (mg/kg bw) | Amino acid oxidation require- ment (mg/kg bw) |
	Require- ment (mg/kg bw)	Pattern (mg/g protein)	Require- ment (mg/kg bw)	Pattern (mg/g protein)		
Histidine	0	0	8–12	16	–	–
Isoleucine	10	18	10	13	38	–
Leucine	14	25	14	19	65	66
Lysine	12	22	12	16	70	50
Methionine + cysteine	13	24	13	17	27	22
Phenylalanine + tyrosine	14	25			65	–
Threonine	7	13	7	9	35	25
Tryptophan	3.5	6.5	3.5	5	10	–
Valine	10	18	10	13	40	33

Sources: WHO/FAO (1973) Energy and protein requirements: Report of a joint FAO/WHO ad hoc expert committee. *WHO Technical Reports Series* 522, WHO, Geneva. FAO/WHO/UNU (1985) Energy and protein requirements. Report of a Joint FAO/WHO/UNU Expert Consultation. *WHO Technical Report Series* 724, Geneva. Young VR, Bier DM and Pellett PL (1989) *American Journal of Clinical Nutrition* 50: 80–92. Young VR (1994) *Journal of Nutrition* 124: 1517–1523S.

relatively deficient in one or more of the essential amino acids will not. More of such a protein will be required to maintain nitrogen balance or growth.

The limiting amino acid of a protein is that essential amino acid which is present in lowest amount relative to the requirement. In cereal proteins the limiting amino acid is lysine, while in animal and most other vegetable proteins it is methionine. (Correctly, the sum of methionine plus cysteine, as cysteine is synthesized from methionine and the presence of cysteine lowers the requirement for methionine.)

The nutritional value or quality of individual proteins depends on whether or not they contain the essential amino acids in the amounts that are required. A number of different ways of determining protein quality have been developed:

- Biological value (BV) is the proportion of absorbed protein retained in the body. A protein that is completely useable (e.g. egg and human milk) has a BV of 0.9–1; meat and fish have a BV of 0.75–0.8, wheat protein 0.5 and gelatine (which completely lacks tryptophan) a BV of 0.

- Net protein utilization (NPU) is the proportion of dietary protein that is retained in the body (i.e. it takes account of the digestibility of the protein). By convention it is measured at 10% dietary protein, at which level the protein synthetic mechanism of the animal can utilize all of the protein so long as the balance of essential amino acids is correct.

- Protein efficiency ratio (PER) is the gain in weight of growing animals per gram of protein eaten.
- Relative protein value (RPV) is the ability of a test protein, fed at various levels of intake, to support nitrogen balance, compared with a standard protein.
- Chemical score is based on chemical analysis of the protein; it is the amount of the limiting amino acid compared with the amount of the same amino acid in egg protein (which is completely useable for tissue protein synthesis). Protein score (or amino acid score) uses a reference pattern of amino acid requirements as the standard.

Although protein quality is important when considering individual dietary proteins, it is not particularly relevant when considering total diets, because different proteins are limited by different amino acids, and have a relative excess of other essential amino acids. This means that the result of mixing different proteins in a diet is to give an unexpected increase in the nutritional value of the mixture. Wheat protein is limited by lysine and has a protein score of 0.6; pea protein is limited by methionine and cysteine and has a protein score of 0.4. A mixture of equal amounts of these two individually poor-quality proteins has a protein score of 0.82 – as high as that of meat.

The result of this complementation between proteins that might individually be of low quality means that most diets have very nearly the same protein quality, regardless of the quality of individual protein sources. The average Western diet has a protein score of 0.73, while the poorest diets in developing countries, with a restricted range of foods, and very little milk, meat or fish, have a protein score of 0.6.

9.2 *Protein synthesis*

The information for the amino acid sequence of each of the 30–50,000 different proteins in the body is contained in the DNA in the nucleus of each cell. As required, a working copy of the information for an individual protein (the gene for that protein) is transcribed, as messenger RNA (mRNA), and this is then translated during protein synthesis on the ribosomes. Both DNA and RNA are linear polymers of nucleotides. In RNA the sugar is ribose, whereas in DNA it is deoxyribose.

9.2.1 THE STRUCTURE AND INFORMATION CONTENT OF DNA

As shown in Figure 9.4, DNA is a linear polymer of nucleotides. It consists of a backbone of alternating deoxyribose and phosphate units, with the phosphate groups forming links from carbon-3 of one sugar to carbon-5 of the next. The bases of the nucleotides project from this sugar–phosphate backbone. There are of two strands of

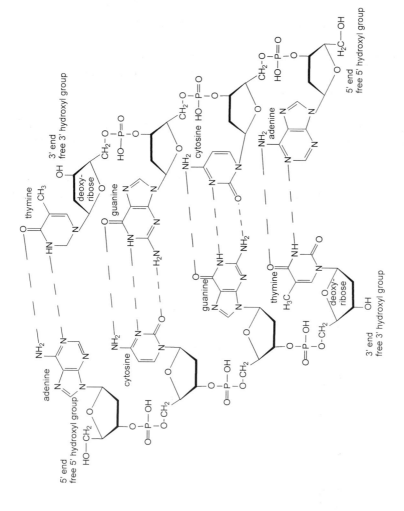

FIGURE 9.4 *The structure of DNA.*

deoxyribonucleotides, held together by hydrogen bonds between a purine (adenine or guanine) and a pyrimidine (thymine or cytosine): adenine forms two hydrogen bonds to thymine, and guanine forms three hydrogen bonds to cytosine.

The double strand coils into a helix, the so-called 'double helix' (Figure 9.5). The two strands of a DNA molecule run in opposite directions – one strand has a 3'-hydroxyl group at the end and on the complementary strand there is a free 5'-hydroxyl group. The information of DNA is always read from the 3' end towards the 5' end.

Only about 10% of the DNA in a human cell carries information for the 30–50,000 genes which make up the human genome. The remainder is made up of:

- Control regions, which promote or enhance the expression of individual genes, and include regions which respond to hormones and other factors which control gene expression (section 10.4), as well as sites for the initiation and termination of DNA replication.
- Spacer regions, both between and within genes, which carry no translatable message but serve to link those regions that do carry a translatable message. When such regions occur within a gene sequence, they are called introns.
- Pseudo-genes, which seem to be genes that have undergone mutation in our evolutionary past and are now untranslatable. Presumably, these are a reminder of evolutionary history.

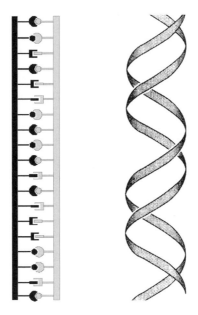

FIGURE 9.5 *The structure of DNA – hydrogen bonding between bases and coiling of the chains to form the double helix.*

9.2.1.1 The genetic code

It is difficult at first sight to understand how a code made up of only four letters (A, G, C, and T) can carry the information which must be contained in the nucleus of the cell, for the 21 different amino acids that make up the 30–50,000 different proteins which are to be synthesized. The answer is that the bases are read in groups of three, not singly. Since each group of three can contain any one of the four bases in each position, there are 64 possible combinations. This means that four bases give a code consisting of 64 words. Each group of three nucleotides is a codon – a single unit of the genetic code.

While 64 codons might not seem much to carry complex information, there is a need for only 22 codons. The information which has to be coded for in DNA is the sequence of the 21 amino acids in proteins, together with a code for the end of the message.

As can be seen from the genetic code (transcribed to RNA) in Tables 9.7 and 9.8, most amino acids are coded for by more than one codon. This provides a measure of protection against mutations – in many cases a single base change in a codon will not affect the amino acid that is incorporated into the protein, and therefore will have no functional significance.

TABLE 9.7 *The genetic code, showing the codons in mRNA*

Amino acid	Abbreviation	Codon(s)
Alanine	Ala	GCU GCC GCA GCG
Arginine	Arg	CGU CGC CGA CGG AGA AGG
Asparagine	Asn	AAU AAC
Aspartic acid	Asp	GAU GAC
Cysteine	Cys	UGU UGC
Glutamic acid	Glu	GAA GAG
Glutamine	Gln	CAA CAG
Glycine	Gly	GGU GGC GGA GGG
Histidine	His	CAU CAG
Isoleucine	Ile	AUU AUC AUA
Leucine	Leu	UUA UUG CUU CUC CUA CUG
Lysine	Lys	AAA AUG
Methionine	Met	AUG
Phenylalanine	Phe	UUU UUC
Proline	Pro	CCU CCC CCA CCG
Serine	Ser	UCU UCC UCA UCG AGU AGC
Threonine	Thr	ACU ACC ACA ACG
Tryptophan	Trp	UGG
Tyrosine	Tyr	UAU UAC
Valine	Val	GUU GUC GUA GUG
Stop		UAA UAG UGA*

*UGA also codes for selenocysteine in a specific context.

TABLE 9.8 *The genetic code, showing the codons in mRNA*

First base	Second base				Third base
	U	**C**	**A**	**G**	
U	Phe	Ser	Tyr	Cys	U
U	Phe	Ser	Tyr	Cys	C
U	Leu	Ser	Stop	Stop*	A
U	Leu	Ser	Stop	Trp	G
C	Leu	Pro	His	Arg	U
C	Leu	Pro	His	Arg	C
C	Leu	Pro	Gln	Arg	A
C	Leu	Pro	Gln	Arg	C
A	Ile	Thr	Asn	Ser	U
A	Ile	Thr	Asn	Ser	C
A	Ile	Thr	Lys	Arg	A
A	Met	Thr	Lys	Arg	G
G	Val	Ala	Asp	Gly	U
G	Val	Ala	Asp	Gly	C
G	Val	Ala	Glu	Gly	A
G	Val	Ala	Glu	Gly	G

*UGA also codes for selenocysteine in a specific context.

Three codons (UAA, UAG and UGA) do not code for amino acids, but act as stop signals to show the end of the message to be translated and so terminate protein synthesis.

UGA also codes for the selenium analogue of cysteine, selenocysteine (section 11.15.2.5). It is normally read as a stop codon, but in the presence of a specific sequence in the untranslated region of mRNA it is read as coding for selenocysteine.

9.2.2 RIBONUCLEIC ACID (RNA)

In RNA the sugar is ribose, rather than deoxyribose as in DNA, and RNA contains the pyrimidine uracil where DNA contains thymine. There are three main types of RNA in the cell:

- Messenger RNA (mRNA) is synthesized in the nucleus, as a copy of one strand of DNA (the process of transcription; section 9.2.2.1). After some editing of the message, it is transferred into the cytosol, where it binds to ribosomes. The information carried by the mRNA is then translated into the amino acid sequence of the protein.
- Ribosomal RNA (rRNA) is part of the structure of the ribosomes on which protein is synthesized (section 9.2.3.2).
- Transfer RNA (tRNA) provides the link between mRNA and the amino acids required for protein synthesis on the ribosome (section 9.2.3.1).

9.2.2.1 Transcription to form messenger RNA (mRNA)

In the transcription of DNA to form mRNA a part of the desired region of DNA is uncoiled, and the two strands of the double helix are separated. A complementary copy of one DNA strand is then synthesized by binding the complementary nucleotide triphosphate to the each base of DNA in turn, followed by condensation to form the phosphodiester link between ribose moieties.

Transcription control sites in DNA include start and stop messages and promoter and enhancer sequences. The main promoter region for any gene is about 25 bases before (upstream of) the beginning of the gene to be transcribed. It acts as a signal that what follows is a gene to be transcribed.

Enhancer and promoter regions may be found further upstream of the message, downstream or sometimes even in the middle of the message. The function of these regions, and of hormone response elements (section 10.4), is to increase the rate at which the gene is transcribed.

The first step in the transcription of a gene is to uncoil that region of DNA from its associated proteins, so as to allow the various enzymes involved in transcription to gain access to the DNA. RNA polymerase moves along the DNA strand which is to be transcribed, and matches complementary ribonucleotide triphosphates one at a time to the bases in the DNA. Adenine in DNA is matched by guanosine triphosphate, guanine by adenosine triphosphate and thymine by cytosine triphosphate. However, cytidine in DNA is matched by uridine triphosphate – RNA contains uridine rather than thymidine as in DNA.

There are three steps in the processing of the initial transcript formed by RNA polymerase before it is exported from the nucleus as messenger RNA:

- The 5′ end of the RNA is blocked by the formation of the unusual base 7-methylguanosine triphosphate. This is called the 'cap' and has a role in the initiation of protein synthesis (section 92.3.2). The 5′ end of the RNA is the first to be synthesized, and the cap is added before transcription has been completed.
- A tail of between up to 250 adenosine residues (the poly-A tail) is added to the 3′ end of the RNA, after the termination codon.

The introns that have been copied from DNA, which do not carry information for protein synthesis, are excised, and the remaining coding regions (exons) are spliced together to form messenger RNA (mRNA), which is exported into the cytosol.

9.2.3 TRANSLATION OF mRNA – THE PROCESS OF PROTEIN SYNTHESIS

The process of protein synthesis consists of translating the message carried by the sequence of bases on mRNA into amino acids, and then forming peptide bonds between the amino acids to form a protein. This occurs on the ribosome and requires a variety of enzymes, as well as specific transfer RNA (tRNA) molecules for each amino acid.

9.2.3.1 Transfer RNA (tRNA)

The key to translating the message carried by the codons on mRNA into amino acids is transfer RNA (tRNA). There are 56 different types (species) of tRNA in the cell. They all have the same general structure, RNA twisted into a clover-leaf shape, and consisting of some 70–90 nucleotides. About half the bases in tRNA are paired by hydrogen bonding, which maintains of the shape of the molecule. The 3′ and 5′ ends of the molecule are adjacent to each other as a result of this folding.

The different species of tRNA have many regions in common with each other, and all have a –CCA tail at the 3′ end, which reacts with the amino acid. Two regions are important in providing the specificity of the tRNA species:

- The anticodon, a sequence of three bases at the base of the clover-leaf. The bases in the anticodon are complementary to the bases of the codon of mRNA, and each species of tRNA binds specifically to one codon or, in some cases, two closely related codons for the same amino acid.
- The region at the 5′ end of the molecule, which again contains a base sequence specific for the amino acid, and hence repeats the information contained in the anticodon.

Amino acids bind to activating enzymes (amino acyl-tRNA synthetases), which recognize both the amino acid and the appropriate tRNA molecule. The first step is reaction between the amino acid and ATP, to form amino acyl AMP, releasing pyrophosphate. The amino acyl AMP then reacts with the –CCA tail of tRNA to form amino acyl-tRNA, releasing AMP.

The specificity of these enzymes is critically important to the process of translation. Each enzyme recognizes only one amino acid but will bind and react with all the various tRNA species that carry an anticodon for that amino acid. Mistakes are extremely rare. The easiest possible mistake would be the attachment of valine to the tRNA for isoleucine, or vice versa, because of the close similarity between the structures of these two amino acids (see Figure 4.18). However, it is only about once in every 3,000 times that this mistake occurs. Amino acyl-tRNA synthetases have a second active site that checks that the correct amino acid has been attached to the tRNA and, if this is found not to be the case, hydrolyses the newly formed bond, releasing tRNA and the amino acid.

9.2.3.2 Protein synthesis on the ribosome

The subcellular organelle concerned with protein synthesis is the ribosome. This consists of two subunits, composed of RNA with a variety of associated proteins. The ribosome permits the binding of the anticodon region of amino acyl tRNA to the codon on mRNA, and aligns the amino acids for formation of peptide bonds. As shown in Figure 9.6, the ribosome binds to mRNA, and has two tRNA binding sites. One, the P site, contains the growing peptide chain, attached to tRNA, while the other, the A site, binds the next amino acyl tRNA to be incorporated into the peptide chain.

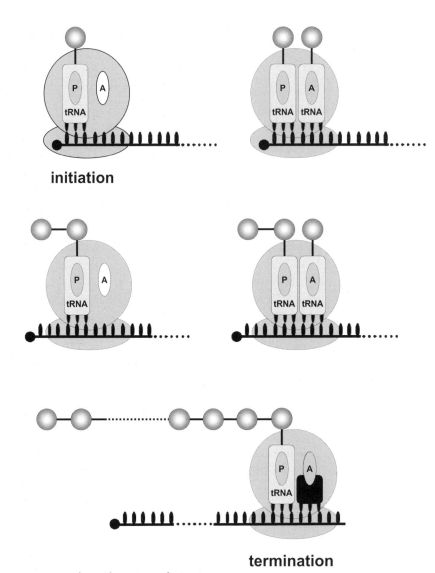

initiation

termination

FIGURE 9.6 *Ribosomal protein synthesis.*

The first codon of mRNA (the initiation codon) is always AUG, the codon for methionine. This means that the amino terminus of all newly synthesized proteins is methionine, although this may well be removed in post-translational modification of the protein (section 9.2.3.4).

An initiator methionine tRNA forms a complex with the small ribosomal subunit, then together with a variety of initiation factors (enzymes and other proteins) binds to the initiator codon of mRNA, and finally to a large ribosomal subunit, to form the complete ribosome. The 5′ cap of mRNA is important for this process, as it marks the position of the initiator codon. AUG is the only codon for methionine, and anywhere else in mRNA it binds the normal methionine tRNA. It is only immediately adjacent to the cap that AUG binds the initiator methionine tRNA.

After the ribosome has been assembled, with the initiator tRNA bound at the P site and occupying the AUG initiator codon, the next amino acyl tRNA binds to the A site of the ribosome, with its anticodon bound to the next codon in the sequence.

The methionine is released from the initiator tRNA at the P site, and forms a peptide bond to the amino group of the amino acyl tRNA at the A site of the ribosome. The initiator tRNA is then released from the P site, and the growing peptide chain, attached to its tRNA, moves from the A site to the P site. As the peptide chain is attached to tRNA, which occupies a codon on the mRNA, this means that as the peptide chain moves from the A site to the P site, so the whole assembly moves one codon along the mRNA.

As the growing peptide chain moves from the A site to the P site, and the ribosome moves along the mRNA chain, so the next amino acyl tRNA occupies the A site, covering its codon. The growing peptide chain is transferred from the tRNA at the P site, forming a peptide bond to the amino acid at the A site. Again the free tRNA at the P site is released, and the growing peptide, attached to tRNA, moves from the A site to the P site, moving one codon along the mRNA as it does so.

The stop codons (UAA, UAG and UGA) are read not by tRNA but by protein release factors. These occupy the A site of the ribosome and hydrolyse the peptide–tRNA bond. This releases the finished protein from the ribosome. As the protein leaves, so the two subunits of the ribosome separate, and leave the mRNA; they are now available to bind another initiator tRNA and begin the process of translation over again.

Just as several molecules of RNA polymerase can transcribe the same gene at the same time, so several ribosomes translate the same molecule of mRNA at the same time. As the ribosomes travel along the ribosome, so each has a longer growing peptide chain than the one following. Such assemblies of ribosomes on a molecule of mRNA are called polysomes.

Termination and release of the protein from the ribosome requires the presence of a stop codon and the protein release factors. However, protein synthesis can also come to a halt if there is not enough of one of the amino acids bound to tRNA. In this case, the growing peptide chain is not released from the ribosome, but remains, in arrested development, until the required amino acyl tRNA is available. This means that if the intake of one of the essential amino acids is inadequate then, once supplies are exhausted, protein synthesis will come to a halt.

9.2.3.3 The energy cost of protein synthesis

The minimum estimate of the energy cost of protein synthesis is four ATP equivalents per peptide bond formed, or 2.8 kJ per gram of protein synthesized:

• Formation of the amino acyl tRNA requires the formation of amino acyl AMP, with the release of pyrophosphate, which again breaks down to yield phosphate. Hence, for each amino acid attached to tRNA there is a cost equivalent to 2 mol of ATP being hydrolysed to ADP plus phosphate.

- The binding of each amino acyl tRNA to the A site of the ribosome involves the hydrolysis of GTP to GDP plus phosphate, which is equivalent to the hydrolysis of ATP to ADP plus phosphate.
- Movement of the growing peptide chain from the A site of the ribosome to the P site again involves the hydrolysis of ATP to ADP plus phosphate.

If allowance is made for the energy cost of active transport of amino acids into cells, the cost of protein synthesis is increased to 3.6 kJ/g. Allowing for the nucleoside triphosphates required for mRNA synthesis gives a total cost of 4.2 kJ per gram of protein synthesized.

In the fasting state, when the rate of protein synthesis is relatively low, about 8% of total energy expenditure (i.e. about 12% of the basal metabolic rate) is accounted for by protein synthesis. After a meal, when the rate of protein synthesis increases, it may account for 12–20% of total energy expenditure.

9.2.3.4 Post-translational modification of proteins

Proteins that are to be exported from the cell, or are to be targeted into mitochondria, are synthesized with a hydrophobic signal sequence of amino acids at the amino terminus to direct them through the membrane. This is removed in the process of post-translational modification. Many other proteins have regions removed from the amino or carboxy terminus during post-translational modification, and the initial (amino-terminal) methionine is removed from most newly synthesized proteins.

Many proteins contain carbohydrates and lipids, covalently bound to amino acid side-chains. Others contain covalently bound cofactors and prosthetic groups, such as vitamins and their derivatives, metal ions or haem. Again the attachment of these non-amino acid parts of the protein is part of the process of post-translational modification to form the active protein.

Some proteins contain unusual amino acids for which there is no codon and no tRNA. These are formed by modification of the protein after translation is complete. Such amino acids include:

- Methylhistidine in the contractile proteins of muscle.
- Hydroxyproline and hydroxylysine in the connective tissue proteins. The formation of hydroxyproline and hydroxylysine requires vitamin C as a cofactor. This explains why wound healing, which requires new synthesis of connective tissue, is impaired in vitamin C deficiency (section 11.14.3). See Problem 9.3 for the role of vitamin C in synthesis of hydroxyproline and hydroxylysine.
- Interchain links in collagen and elastin, formed by the oxidation of lysine residues. This reaction is catalysed by a copper-dependent enzyme, and copper deficiency

leads to fragility of bones and loss of the elasticity of connective tissues (section 11.15.2.2).

- γ-Carboxyglutamate in several of the blood clotting proteins, and in osteocalcin in bone. The formation of γ-carboxyglutamate requires vitamin K (section 11.15.2). See Problem 9.2 for the role of vitamin K in synthesis of γ-carboxyglutamate.

9.3 *The metabolism of amino acids*

An adult has a requirement for a dietary intake of protein because there is continual oxidation of amino acids as a source of metabolic fuel and for gluconeogenesis in the fasting state. In the fed state, amino acids in excess of immediate requirements for protein synthesis are oxidized. Overall, for an adult in nitrogen balance, the total amount of amino acids being metabolized will be equal to the total intake of amino acids in dietary proteins.

Amino acids are also required for the synthesis of a variety of metabolic products, including:

- purines and pyrimidines for nucleic acid synthesis;
- haem, synthesized from glycine;
- the catecholamine neurotransmitters, dopamine, noradrenaline and adrenaline, synthesized from tyrosine;
- the thyroid hormones thyroxine and tri-iodothyronine, synthesized from tyrosine (section 11.15.3.3);
- melanin, the pigment of skin and hair, synthesized from tyrosine;
- the nicotinamide ring of the coenzymes NAD and NADP, synthesized from tryptophan (section 11.8.2);
- the neurotransmitter serotonin (5-hydroxytryptamine), synthesized from tryptophan.
- The neurotransmitter histamine, synthesized from histidine;
- the neurotransmitter GABA (γ-aminobutyrate) synthesized from glutamate (see Figure 5.19);
- carnitine (section 5.5.1), synthesized from lysine and methionine;
- creatine (section 3.2.3.1), synthesized from arginine, glycine and methionine;
- the phospholipid bases ethanolamine and choline (section 4.2.1.3), synthesized from serine and methionine. Acetyl choline functions as a neurotransmitter;
- taurine, synthesized from cysteine.

In general, the amounts of amino acids required for synthesis of these products are small compared with the requirement for maintenance of nitrogen balance and protein turnover.

9.3.1 METABOLISM OF THE AMINO NITROGEN

The initial step in the metabolism of amino acids is the removal of the amino group (–NH$_2$), leaving the carbon skeleton of the amino acid. Chemically, these carbon skeletons are ketoacids (more correctly, they are oxo-acids). A ketoacid has a –C=O group in place of the HC–NH$_2$ group of an amino acid; the metabolism of ketoacids is discussed in section 9.3.2.

9.3.1.1 Deamination

Some amino acids can be directly oxidized to their corresponding ketoacids, releasing ammonia: the process of deamination (Figure 9.7). There is a general amino acid oxidase which catalyses this reaction, but it has a low activity.

There is an active D-amino acid oxidase in the kidneys, which acts to deaminate, and hence detoxify, the small amounts of D-amino acids that arise from bacterial proteins. The ketoacids resulting from the action of D-amino acid oxidase on D-amino acids can undergo transamination (section 9.3.1.2) to yield the L-isomers. This means that, at least to a limited extent, D-amino acids can be isomerized and used for protein synthesis. Although there is evidence from experimental animals that D-isomers of (some of) the essential amino acids can be used to maintain nitrogen balance, there is little information on utilization of D-amino acids in human beings.

Four amino acids are deaminated by specific enzymes:

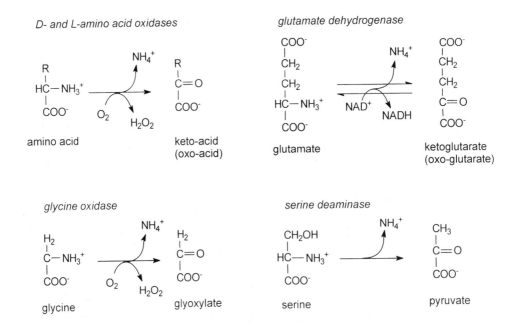

FIGURE 9.7 *Deamination of amino acids.*

- Glycine is deaminated to its ketoacid, glyoxylic acid, and ammonium ions by glycine oxidase.
- Glutamate is deaminated to ketoglutarate and ammonium ions by glutamate dehydrogenase.
- Serine is deaminated and dehydrated to pyruvate by serine deaminase (sometimes called serine dehydratase).
- Threonine is deaminated and dehydrated to oxobutyrate by threonine deaminase.

9.3.1.2 Transamination

Most amino acids are not deaminated, but undergo the process of transamination. The amino group of the amino acid is transferred onto the enzyme, leaving the ketoacid. In the second half of the reaction, the enzyme transfers the amino group onto an acceptor, which is a different ketoacid, so forming the amino acid corresponding to that ketoacid. The acceptor for the amino group at the active site of the enzyme is pyridoxal phosphate, the metabolically active coenzyme derived from vitamin B_6 (section 11.9.2), forming pyridoxamine phosphate as an intermediate in the reaction. The reaction of transamination is shown in Figure 9.8, and the ketoacids corresponding to the amino acids in Table 9.9.

Transamination is a reversible reaction, so that if the ketoacid can be synthesized in the body, so can the amino acid. The essential amino acids (section 9.1.3) are those for which the only source of the ketoacid is the amino acid itself. Three of the ketoacids listed in Table 9.9 are common metabolic intermediates; they are the precursors of the three amino acids that can be considered to be completely dispensable, in that there is no requirement for them in the diet (section 9.1.3):

- pyruvate – the ketoacid of alanine;
- α-ketoglutarate – the ketoacid of glutamate;
- oxaloacetate – the ketoacid of aspartate.

The reversibility of transamination has been exploited in the treatment of patients in renal failure. The traditional treatment was to provide them with a very low-protein diet, so as to minimize the total amount of urea that has to be excreted (section 9.3.1.4). However, they still have to be provided with the essential amino acids. If they are provided with the essential ketoacids, they can synthesize the corresponding essential amino acids by transamination, so reducing yet further their nitrogen burden. The only amino acid for which this is not possible is lysine – the ketoacid corresponding to lysine undergoes rapid non-enzymic condensation to pipecolic acid, which cannot be metabolized further.

If the acceptor ketoacid in a transamination reaction is α-ketoglutarate, then glutamate is formed, and glutamate can readily be oxidized back to α-ketoglutarate, catalysed by glutamate dehydrogenase, with the release of ammonia. Similarly, if the acceptor ketoacid is glyoxylate, then the product is glycine, which can be oxidized

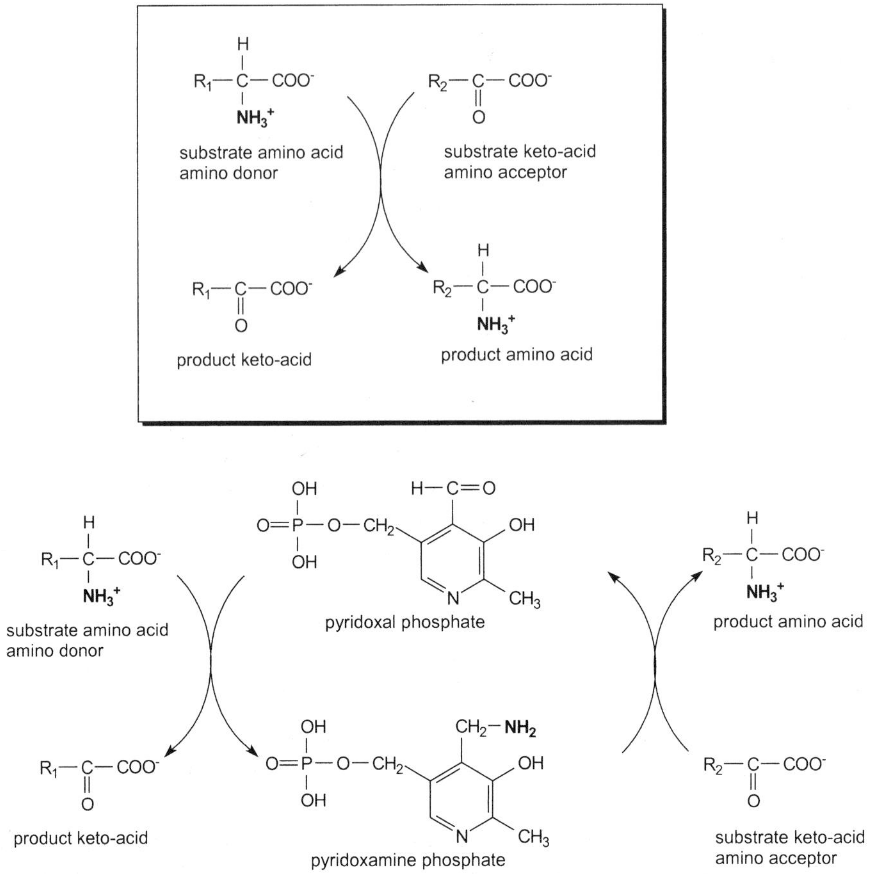

FIGURE 9.8 *Transamination of amino acids.*

back to glyoxylate and ammonia, catalysed by glycine oxidase. Thus, by means of a variety of transaminases, and using the reactions of glutamate dehydrogenase and glycine oxidase, all of the amino acids can, indirectly, be converted to their ketoacids and ammonia (Figure 9.9). Aspartate can also act as an intermediate in the indirect deamination of a variety of amino acids, as shown in Figure 9.12.

9.3.1.3 The metabolism of ammonia

The deamination of amino acids (and a number of other reactions in the body) results in the formation of ammonium ions. Ammonium is highly toxic. The normal plasma concentration is less than 50 μmol/L; an increase to 80–100 μmol/L (far too little to have any detectable effect on plasma pH) results in disturbance of consciousness, and in patients whose blood ammonium rises above about 200 μmol/L ammonia intoxication leads to coma and convulsions, and may be fatal.

TABLE 9.9 *Transamination products of the amino acids*

Amino acid	Ketoacid
Alanine	Pyruvate
Arginine	α-Keto-γ-guanidoacetate
Aspartic acid	Oxaloacetate
Cysteine	β-Mercaptopyruvate
Glutamic acid	α-Ketoglutarate
Glutamine	α-Ketoglutaramic acid
Glycine	Glyoxylate
Histidine	Imidazolepyruvate
Isoleucine	α-Keto-β-methylvalerate
Leucine	α-Ketoisocaproate
[Lysine*	α-Keto-ε-aminocaproate $\rightarrow$ pipecolic acid]
Methionine	S-Methyl-β-thiol lα-oxopropionate
Ornithine	Glutamic-γ-semialdehyde
Phenylalanine	Phenylpyruvate
Proline	γ-Hydroxypyruvate
Serine	Hydroxypyruvate
Threonine	α-Keto-β-hydroxybutyrate
Tryptophan	Indolepyruvate
Tyrosine	*p*-Hydroxyphenylpyruvate
Valine	α-Ketoisovalerate

*The ketoacid formed by transamination of lysine undergoes spontaneous cyclization.

At any time, the total amount of ammonium to be transported around the body, and eventually excreted, is greatly in excess of the toxic level. What happens is that, as it is formed, ammonium is metabolized, mainly by the formation of glutamate from α-ketoglutarate, and then glutamine from glutamate, in a reaction catalysed by glutamine synthetase, as shown in Figure 9.10. Glutamine is transported in the bloodstream to the liver and kidneys.

It is the formation of glutamate from α-ketoglutarate that explains the neurotoxicity of ammonium; as ammonium concentrations in the nervous system rise, the reaction of glutamate dehydrogenase depletes the mitochondrial pool of α-ketoglutarate, resulting in impairment of the activity of the citric acid cycle (section 5.4.4), and so impairing energy-yielding metabolism.

In the kidneys, some glutamine is hydrolysed to glutamate (which remains in the body) and ammonium, which is excreted in the urine to neutralize excess acid excretion.

9.3.1.4 The synthesis of urea

In the liver, ammonium arising from either the hydrolysis of glutamine or the reaction of adenosine deaminase (section 9.3.1.5) is the substrate for synthesis of urea, the main nitrogenous excretion product. The cyclic pathway for urea synthesis is shown

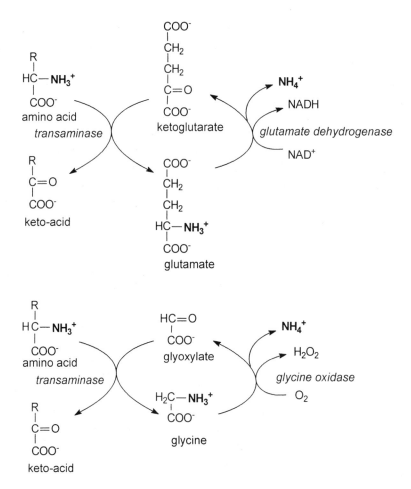

FIGURE 9.9 *Transdeamination of amino acids – transamination linked to oxidative deamination.*

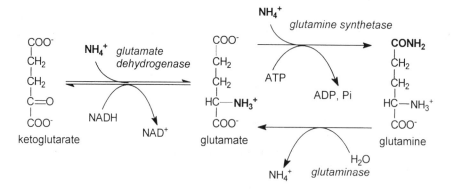

FIGURE 9.10 *The synthesis of glutamate and glutamine from ammonium, and hydrolysis of glutamine by glutaminase.*

in Figure 9.11. The key compound is ornithine, which acts as a carrier on which the molecule of urea is built up. At the end of the reaction sequence, urea is released by the hydrolysis of arginine, yielding ornithine to begin the cycle again. Some urea is retained in the distal renal tubules, where it has an important role in maintaining an osmotic gradient for the resorption of water.

The total amount of urea synthesized each day is several-fold higher than the amount that is excreted. Urea diffuses readily from the bloodstream into the large intestine, where it is hydrolysed by bacterial urease to carbon dioxide and ammonium. Much of the ammonium is reabsorbed and used in the liver for the synthesis of glutamate and glutamine, and then a variety of other nitrogenous compounds. Studies with ^{15}N urea show that a significant amount of label is found in essential amino acids. This may reflect intestinal bacterial synthesis of amino acids, or it may reflect the reversibility of the transamination of essential amino acids.

The urea synthesis cycle is also the pathway for the synthesis of the amino acid arginine. Ornithine is synthesized from glutamate, and then undergoes the reactions shown in Figure 9.11 to form arginine. Although the whole pathway of urea synthesis occurs only in the liver, the sequence of reactions leading to the formation of arginine also occurs in the kidneys, and the kidneys are the main source of arginine in the body.

The precursor for ornithine synthesis is *N*-acetylglutamate, which is also an obligatory activator of carbamyl phosphate synthetase. This provides a regulatory mechanism – if *N*-acetylglutamate is not available for ornithine synthesis (and hence there would be impaired activity of the urea synthesis cycle), then ammonium is not incorporated into carbamyl phosphate. This can be a cause of hyperammonaemia in a variety of metabolic disturbances that lead to either a lack of acetyl CoA for *N*-acetyl glutamate synthesis or an accumulation of propionyl CoA, which is a poor substrate for, and hence an inhibitor of, *N*-acetylglutamate synthetase.

9.3.1.5 Incorporation of nitrogen in biosynthesis

Amino acids are the only significant source of nitrogen for synthesis of nitrogenous compounds such as haem, purines and pyrimidines. Three amino acids are especially important as nitrogen donors:

- Glycine is incorporated intact into purines, haem and other porphyrins, and creatine (section 3.2.3.1).
- Glutamine; the amide nitrogen is transferred in an ATP-dependent reaction, replacing an oxo-group in the acceptor with an amino group.
- Aspartate undergoes an ATP- or GTP-dependent condensation reaction with an oxo-group, followed by cleavage to release fumarate.

As shown in Figure 9.12, reactions in which aspartate acts as a nitrogen donor in this way result in a net gain of ATP, as the fumarate is hydrated to malate, then oxidized to oxaloacetate, which is then available to undergo transamination to aspartate.

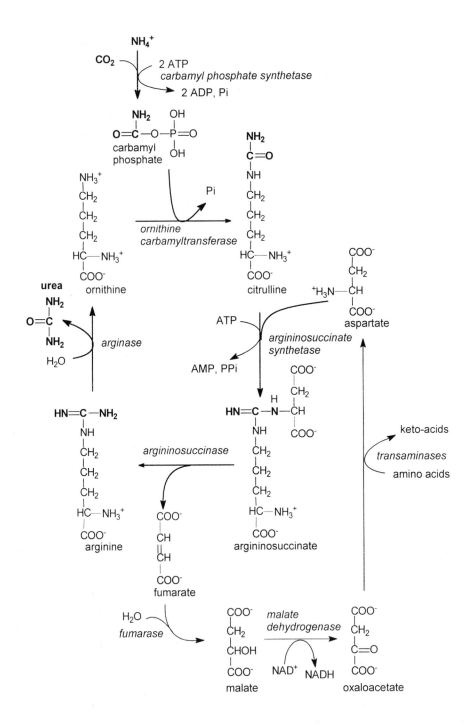

FIGURE 9.11 *The synthesis of urea.*

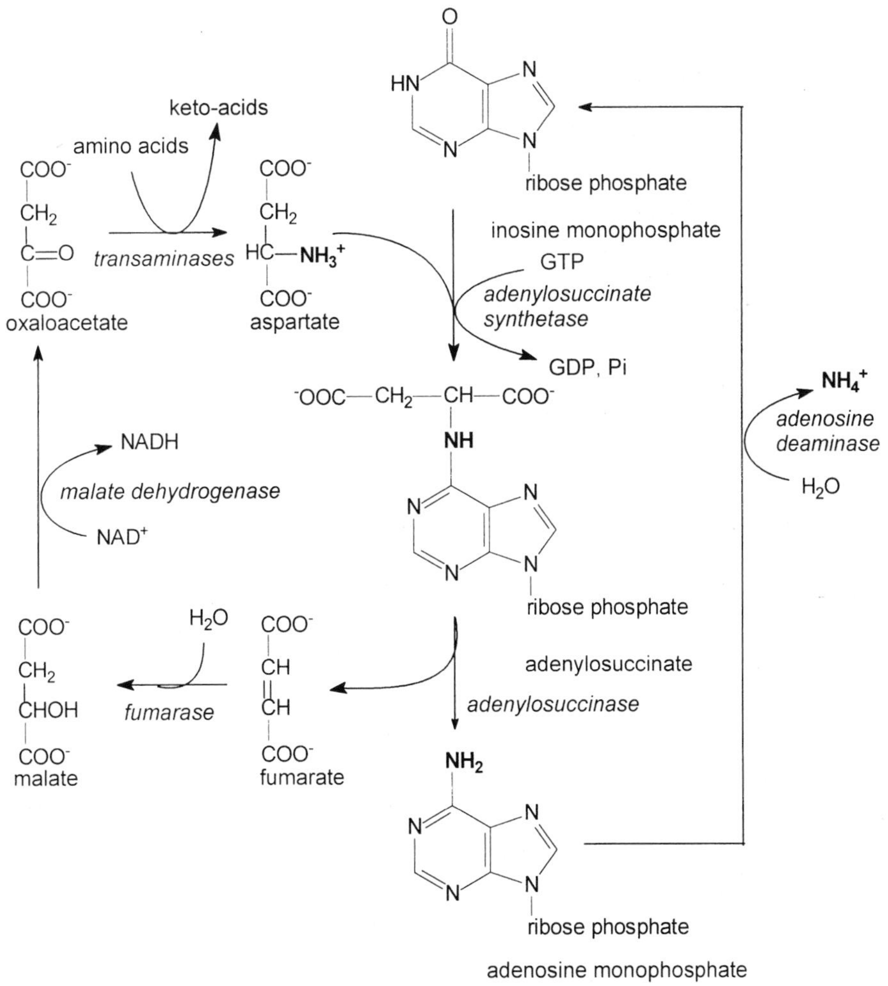

FIGURE 9.12 *The role of aspartate as a nitrogen donor in synthetic reactions, and of adenosine deaminase as a source of ammonium ions.*

Adenosine deaminase converts adenosine monophosphate back to inosine monophosphate, liberating ammonia. This sequence of reactions thus provides a pathway for the deamination of a variety of amino acids, linked to transamination, similar to those shown in Figure 9.9 for transamination linked to glutamate dehydrogenase or glycine oxidase.

9.3.2 THE METABOLISM OF AMINO ACID CARBON SKELETONS

Acetyl CoA and acetoacetate arising from the carbon skeletons of amino acids may be used for fatty acid synthesis (section 5.6.1) or be oxidized as metabolic fuel, but cannot be utilized for the synthesis of glucose (gluconeogenesis; section 5.7). Amino acids that yield acetyl CoA or acetoacetate are termed ketogenic.

By contrast, those amino acids that yield intermediates that can be used for gluconeogenesis are termed glucogenic. As shown in Table 9.10, only two amino acids are purely ketogenic: leucine and lysine. Three others yield both glucogenic fragments and either acetyl CoA or acetoacetate: tryptophan, isoleucine and phenylalanine.

The principal substrate for gluconeogenesis is oxaloacetate, which undergoes the reaction catalysed by phosphoenolpyruvate carboxykinase to yield phosphoenolpyruvate, as shown in Figure 5.31. The onward metabolism of phosphoenolpyruvate to glucose is essentially the reverse of glycolysis shown in Figure 5.10.

The points of entry of amino acid carbon skeletons into central metabolic pathways are shown in Figure 5.20. Those that give rise to ketoglutarate, succinyl CoA, fumarate or oxaloacetate can be regarded as directly increasing the tissue pool of citric acid cycle intermediates, and hence permitting the withdrawal of oxaloacetate for gluconeogenesis.

Those amino acids that give rise to pyruvate also increase the tissue pool of oxaloacetate, as pyruvate is carboxylated to oxaloacetate in the reaction catalysed by pyruvate carboxylase (section 5.7).

Gluconeogenesis is an important fate of amino acid carbon skeletons in the fasting state, when the metabolic imperative is to maintain a supply of glucose for the central nervous system and red blood cells. However, in the fed state the carbon skeletons of

TABLE 9.10 *Metabolic fates of the carbon skeletons of amino acids*

	Glucogenic intermediates	Ketogenic intermediates
Alanine	Pyruvate	—
Glycine → serine	Pyruvate	—
Cysteine	Pyruvate	—
Tryptophan	Pyruvate	Acetyl CoA
Arginine → ornithine	α-Ketoglutarate	—
Glutamine → glutamate	α-Ketoglutarate	—
Proline → glutamate	α-Ketoglutarate	—
Histidine → glutamate	α-Ketoglutarate	—
Methionine	Propionyl CoA	—
Isoleucine	Propionyl CoA	Acetyl CoA
Valine	Succinyl CoA	—
Asparagine → aspartate	Oxaloacetate	—
Aspartate	Oxaloacetate *or* fumarate	—
Phenylalanine → tyrosine	Fumarate	Acetoacetate
Leucine	—	Acetoacetate *and* acetyl CoA
Lysine		Acetyl CoA

amino acids in excess of requirements for protein synthesis will mainly be used for formation of acetyl CoA for fatty acid synthesis, and storage as adipose tissue triacylglycerol.

Additional resources

PowerPoint presentation 9 on the CD.
Self-assessment quiz 9 on the CD.
Simulation program Nitrogen Balance on the CD.
Simulation program Urea Synthesis on the CD.

Problem 9.1: Amino acid output by muscle in the fasting state

In the fasting state, the liver releases glucose into the circulation, as a metabolic fuel for the central nervous system and red blood cells. Some of this glucose arises from the breakdown of liver glycogen, but much arises by gluconeogenesis from amino acids. These amino acids are mainly derived from the breakdown of muscle protein. Note that, although muscle contains a large amount of glycogen, this cannot be released as glucose because muscle lacks glucose 6-phosphatase.

The lower part of Figure 9.13 shows the results of experiments in which the artery supplying the leg muscle and the femoral vein were both cannulated in a group of fasting healthy volunteers. Plasma free amino acids were measured, and the results

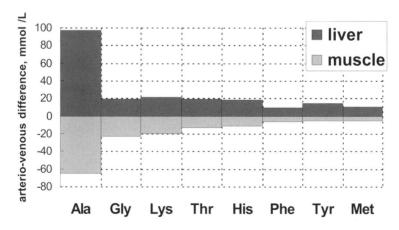

FIGURE 9.13 *Arteriovenous differences in amino acids across the liver (arterio-hepatic venous difference) and skeletal muscle (arterio-femoral venous difference). A positive arteriovenous difference means uptake of amino acids by the tissue; a negative difference means output of amino acids by the tissue. From data reported by Felig P and Wahren J (1974)* Federation Proceedings 33: 1092–1097.

TABLE 9.11 *Approximate amino acid content of muscle protein*

	mg amino acid **N** per g total **N**
Alanine	370
Glycine	330
Lysine	590
Threonine	280
Histidine	170
Phenylalanine	250
Tyrosine	230
Methionine	170

are shown as the arteriovenous difference. A negative value represents a net output of the amino acid from muscle.

The upper part of Figure 9.13 shows the arteriohepatic venous difference in plasma amino acids in the same subjects, and hence the uptake or release of amino acids by the liver. Although the results are not shown, there was also a net output of glucose by the liver.

Table 9.11 shows the approximate amino acid composition of muscle protein. Can you account for the difference between the amino acid output from muscle and the amino acid composition of muscle proteins?

Problem 9.2: A problem of bleeding cows and chickens, rat poison and patients with thrombosis

During the 1920s a new disease of cattle involving fatal bleeding appeared over a wide area of prairie land in North America. It was eventually traced to feeding the animals on hay made from sweet clover (*Melilotus alba* and *M. officinalis*), which had 'mysteriously gone bad'. After eating the hay, the animals suffered a gradual decline in the clotting power of the blood (over about 15 days), followed by the development of internal haemorrhage which was generally fatal after 30–50 days. The disease was caused only by feeding the animals on spoilt sweet clover hay, and is commonly called 'sweet clover disease'. It could be treated by removing the spoilt hay from the animals' diet and transfusing them with blood freshly drawn from normal healthy animals.

What conclusions can you draw from these observations?

The addition of oxalate or citrate to blood will chelate calcium ions, and prevent clotting. Addition of a solution of calcium chloride to oxalated normal plasma results in rapid clotting; addition of calcium chloride to oxalated plasma from calves with sweet clover disease did not result in clotting.

What conclusions can you draw from this observation?

Partially purified prothrombin was prepared from blood of either healthy animals or those with sweet clover disease and tested on blood from an affected animal – the results are shown in Table 9.12.

What conclusions can you draw from these results?

The toxin present in spoiled sweet clover hay was identified as bis-hydroxycoumarin (dicoumarol; see Figure 11.10); it is formed by the oxidation of coumarin, which is naturally present in sweet clover. Once dicoumarol was available in adequate amounts, its mode of action could be investigated; early studies showed that there was a dose-dependent impairment of blood clotting, but with a latent period of 12–24 hours before any effect became apparent.

What conclusions can you draw from this observation?

Why do you think it was that dicoumarol was adopted for use in low doses to reduce blood clotting in patients at risk of thrombosis and as a rat poison in relatively high doses.

Further research at the University of Wisconsin resulted in the synthesis of a variety of compounds related to dicoumarol that were more potent as rat poisons and had fewer side-effects in human beings. The most successful of these compounds was called warfarin (from the initials of the Wisconsin Alumnus Research Fund, which supported the research – see Figure 11.10); it is still the most widely used anticoagulant in clinical use and the most commonly used rodenticide.

In 1929, Dam and co-workers in Copenhagen fed chickens on a fat-free diet and reported the development of subcutaneous and intramuscular haemorrhages, as well as impaired blood clotting. They went on to demonstrate a fat-soluble compound in vegetables, grains and animal liver that would normalize blood clotting when fed to deficient chickens. They proposed the name vitamin K (section 11.5) for this new nutrient, and defined a unit of biological activity as that amount required per kilogram body weight on three successive days to normalize blood clotting in a deficient animal.

Why do you think the response to vitamin K in deficient animals takes several days to develop?

In 1952, an army recruit attempted suicide by taking rat poison containing warfarin. On admission to hospital he had numerous subcutaneous haemorrhages and was suffering from nose-bleeds. His prothrombin time was 54 seconds, compared with a normal value of 14 seconds. *(The prothrombin time is the time taken for the formation of a fibrin clot in citrated plasma after the addition of calcium ions and thromboplastin to activate*

TABLE 9.12 *Clotting time of blood from a calf affected by sweet clover disease when treated with the prothrombin fraction from a normal animal or an affected animal*

	Prothrombin fraction prepared from plasma of			
	Normal calf		**Affected calf**	
Volume added (mL)	0.5	1.0	2.5	0.5
Time to clot (min)	60	45	20	> 360

From data reported by Roderick LM (1931) *American Journal of Physiology* 96: 413–425.

the extrinsic clotting system.) He was given 20 mg vitamin K intravenously daily for 10 days, when he recovered, with a normal prothrombin time.

What does this suggest about the way in which warfarin affects blood clotting?

In animals treated with warfarin it is possible to isolate a protein that reacts with antiserum to prothrombin, but has no biological activity. During warfarin treatment, the concentration of this abnormal, inactive, prothrombin in plasma increases, and that of active prothrombin decreases. The abnormal prothrombin is less negatively charged than normal prothrombin, and does not migrate so rapidly towards the anode on electrophoresis. The addition of calcium ions to a sample of normal prothrombin reduces its electrophoretic mobility but has no effect on the electrophoretic mobility of the abnormal prothrombin. Feeding high intakes of vitamin K to warfarin-treated animals normalizes their blood clotting and leads to disappearance of the abnormal prothrombin and reappearance of active prothrombin with normal calcium-binding capacity.

What conclusions can you draw from these results?

The results of studies of the synthesis of prothrombin in the post-mitochondrial supernatant fraction from liver of vitamin K-deficient rats incubated with vitamin K added *in vitro* are shown in Table 9.13.

What conclusions can you draw from these results?

A novel amino acid is present in prothrombin that is not present in the abnormal prothrombin (now called preprothrombin) formed in vitamin K deficiency or on treatment with warfarin – γ-carboxyglutamate (abbreviated to Gla; see Figure 11.11). There are 10 Gla residues in the amino-terminal region of active prothrombin, and these form a binding site for four calcium ions.

All of the codons for amino acids are known. How does γ-carboxyglutamate become incorporated into prothrombin? What is the likely role of vitamin K in this process?

It has been known for some years that vitamin K must be reduced to its hydroquinone for activity in prothrombin synthesis, i.e. it is the hydroquinone that is the active metabolite of the vitamin. In rats treated with warfarin and given [14]C-

TABLE 9.13 *Prothrombin synthesis by post-mitochondrial supernatant fraction from liver of vitamin K-deficient rats*

Incubation conditions	Relative prothrombin activity (%)
No vitamin K	7 ± 1
+ 20 µg/mL vitamin K	100
+ 20 µg/mL vitamin K + cycloheximide	94 ± 1
+ 20 µg/mL vitamin K + 2-chlorophytylmenaquinone	18 ± 1
+ 20 µg/mL vitamin K + warfarin	87 ± 3
+ 20 µg/mL vitamin K, anaerobic	0

From data reported by Shah DV and Suttie JW (1974) *Biochemical and Biophysical Research Communications* 60: 1397–1402.

labelled vitamin K more than 50% of the radioactivity was found in a new compound, vitamin K epoxide, which has the biological activity of vitamin K in deficient animals. A very small amount is present in the liver of normal animals.

Can you propose the sequence of reactions which vitamin K undergoes in the synthesis of prothrombin?

Which step is likely to be inhibited by warfarin?

Can you explain why it is that high intakes of vitamin K will overcome the inhibition of prothrombin synthesis caused by warfarin?

The classical way of assessing vitamin K nutritional status was by determination of prothrombin time. Can you suggest a more sensitive way of detecting marginal vitamin K deficiency?

Problem 9.3: Vitamin C and collagen synthesis

Clinically, scurvy (section 11.14.3) is characterized by fragility of the blood vessel walls and small subcutaneous haemorrhages around hair follicles (petechial haemorrhages), as well as inflammation of the gums and loss of the dental cement (and hence loss of teeth) and poor healing of wounds. In advanced cases there is intense deep bone pain, and there may be degenerative changes in the heart, leading to cardiac emergency. In some cases there are also mood changes (indeed, *scurvy* is the old English word for ill-tempered). It was known from the studies of Lind in 1757 that fresh orange and lemon juice would prevent or cure scurvy; studies during the early part of the twentieth century identified the protective or curative factor as ascorbic acid or vitamin C (see Figure 11.28).

Studies in the 1940s showed that in vitamin C deficiency there was poor healing of wounds, and the scar tissue was weak with little collagen present. The results of studies of the formation of collagen in granulomatous tissue from guinea pigs at different levels of vitamin C nutrition in response to subcutaneous injection of carrageenan are shown in Table 9.14.

What conclusions can you draw from these results?

TABLE 9.14 *Percentage composition of granulatomous tissue in vitamin C-deficient guinea pigs after subcutaneous injection of carageenan*

	Control animals	Vitamin C-deficient animals
Collagen	11.6 ± 0.64	2.3 ± 0.14
Water	66.0	85.0

From data reported by Robertson WvB and Schwartz B (1953) *Journal of Biological Chemistry* 201: 689–696.

Isolated fibroblasts synthesize and secrete collagen. If they are incubated in the presence of low vitamin C, they secrete only a very small amount of collagen, and a soluble, gelatine-like protein accumulates in the rough endoplasmic reticulum. Similarly, incubation of fibroblasts under anaerobic conditions, or in the presence of iron-chelating compounds, also prevents the secretion of normal collagen and the accumulation of the soluble gelatine-like protein in the rough endoplasmic reticulum.

What conclusions can you draw from these observations?

One of the characteristic features of collagen is its relatively high content of hydroxyproline (Hyp). Table 9.15 shows the incorporation of radioactivity into guinea pig granuloma tissue incubated with [^{14}C]proline or [^{14}C]hydroxyproline.

What conclusions can you draw from these results?

Figure 9.14 shows the incorporation of [^{14}C]proline into proline and hydroxyproline in a cell-free system from chick embryos.

What conclusions can you draw from these results?

Table 9.16 shows the incorporation of [^{3}H]proline into hydroxyproline in collagen formed by granuloma tissue from control and vitamin C-deficient (scorbutic) guinea pigs, and Table 9.17 the effects of various inhibitors of transcription and translation on the stimulation by ascorbate of proline hydroxylation in mouse fibroblasts in culture.

What conclusions can you draw from these results?

Prolyl hydroxylase has been purified. It requires ascorbate, molecular oxygen and iron (Fe^{2+}) for activity. There is no change in the redox state of the iron during the reaction. In addition, with the purified enzyme there is an absolute requirement for α-ketoglutarate for activity. Table 9.18 shows the disappearance of ketoglutarate and appearance of hydroxyproline on incubation of purified prolyl hydroxylase.

What is the approximate ratio of ketoglutarate utilised/hydroxyproline formed?

What conclusions can you draw from these results?

Studies with ^{18}O$_2$ showed that one atom of oxygen is incorporated into hydroxyproline and the other into succinate formed by oxidative decarboxylation of ketoglutarate.

What conclusions can you draw from these results?

There is oxidation of ascorbate during the hydroxylation of proline, but very much less than 1 mol of ascorbate is oxidized per mol of hydroxyproline or succinate formed,

TABLE 9.15 *Incorporation of radioactivity into collagen from [^{14}C]proline and [^{14}C]hydroxyproline*

	Tissue incubated with	
Radioactivity (dpm/μmol) in	**[^{14}C]Proline**	**[^{14}C]Hydroxyproline**
Free amino acids in tissue	2400	3500
Hydroxyproline in collagen	465	2.3*

In samples maintained at 4 °C there was apparent incorporation of 2–2.5 dpm/μmol into hydroxyproline.

From data reported by Green NM and Lowther DA (1959) *Biochemical Journal* 71: 55–66.

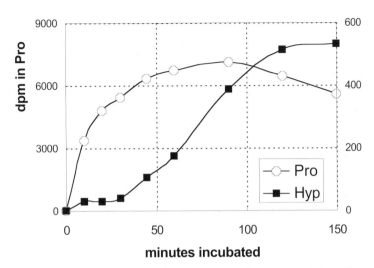

FIGURE 9.14 *Incorporation of label from {^{14}C}proline into proline and hydroxyproline in proteins synthesized by a cell-free system. From data reported by Peterkovsky B and Udenfriend S (1963)* Journal of Biological Chemistry *38: 3966–3977.*

TABLE 9.16 *Incorporation of radioactivity from {^{3}H}proline into hydroxyproline in collagen formed by granuloma tissue from control and vitamin C-deficient (scorbutic) guinea pigs*

	Radioactivity (dpm) in hydroxyproline in tissue from	
Incubation time (min)	Control animals	Vitamin C-deficient animals
30	2400	100
60	5070	150
120	8700	360

From data reported by Stone N and Meister A (1962) *Nature* 194: 555–557.

TABLE 9.17 *The effects of various inhibitors of transcription and translation on the stimulation by ascorbate of proline hydroxylation in mouse fibroblasts in culture*

	Hydroxyproline dpm per mg protein
No addition	27,700
+ 2.5 × 10^{-4} mol/L ascorbate	58,800
+ Actinomycin D, then ascorbate 15 minutes later	58,700
+ Puromycin, then ascorbate 15 minutes later	62,900
+ Cycloheximide, then ascorbate 15 minutes later	65,100

From data reported by Stassen FLH, Cardinale GJ and Udenfriend S (1973) *Proceedings of the National Academy of Sciences of Sciences of the USA* 70: 1090.

TABLE 9.18 *The disappearance of α-ketoglutarate and appearance of hydroxyproline during incubation of purified prolyl hydroxylase*

α-Ketoglutarate (nmol)			
Initial	**Remaining**	**Utilized**	**Proline hydroxylated (nmol)**
15.1	1.3	?	13.7
31.6	3.2	?	28.2
46.0	8.0	?	40.1
64.6	16	?	47.7

From data reported by Rhoads RE and Udenfriend S (1968) *Proceedings of the National Academy of Sciences of the USA* 60: 1473.

or of O_2 consumed. Figure 9.15 shows the hydroxylation of proline-containing peptides by purified prolyl hydroxylase in the presence and absence of ascorbate. The upper graph shows the results for incubation over 1 minute; during the first 10 seconds the enzyme catalyses hydroxylation of ∼30 mol of proline per mole of enzyme in the absence of ascorbate. The lower graph shows the results of incubation over 5 minutes,

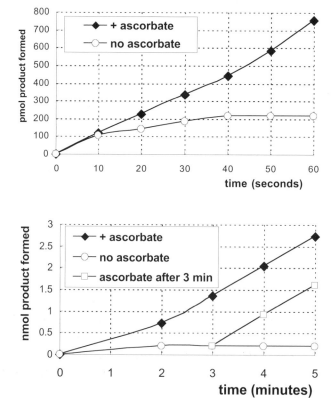

FIGURE 9.15 *Activity of purified prolyl hydroxylase incubated with and without ascorbate. From data reported by Myllylä R et al. (1978)* Biochemical and Biophysical Research Communications *83: 441–448.*

as well as the addition of ascorbate to the ascorbate-free incubation after 3 minutes. After 2 minutes' incubation without added ascorbate the protein-bound iron had been oxidized from Fe^{2+} to Fe^{3+}, and was reduced back to Fe^{2+} on addition of ascorbate.

What conclusions can you draw from these results? Can you explain the role of ascorbate in proline hydroxylation ?

Problem 9.4: an experiment with ^{13}C- and ^{15}N-labelled urea

The first enzyme to be crystallized (and hence the first evidence that enzymes are proteins) was urease, which catalyses the hydrolysis of urea to ammonium and carbon dioxide. The original preparation of urease was from plant material, but the enzyme is also known to occur in a number of bacteria. In this study, a group of volunteers were given an intravenous infusion of 20 mmol urea labelled with both ^{13}C and ^{15}N and their urinary excretion of label was measured over 24 hours. Complete recovery of the label in urine would amount to 40 mmol ^{15}N and 20 mmol ^{13}C. The results are shown in column 2 of Table 9.19. The experiment was repeated a week later, after they had received the antibiotic neomycin for 4 days to sterilize the gut; these results are shown in column 3.

What conclusions can you draw from these results?

TABLE 9.19 *Recovery of label in urine after intravenous infusion of 20 mmol labelled with ^{13}C and ^{15}N*

Recovery (mmol/24 h)	Initial study	After neomycin
Total urine N	609	613
Total urea	500	497
Total urine ^{15}N	34	39
Total urine ^{13}C	0.5	19.5
Urea ^{15}N	29	39
Urea ^{13}C	< 0.1	19.5

Problem 9.5: Angela P

At the age of 28 weeks Angela was admitted to the accident and emergency department of her local hospital in a coma, having suffered a convulsion after feeding. She had a mild infection and slight fever at the time. Since birth she had been a sickly child, and had frequently vomited and become drowsy after feeding. She was bottle fed, and at one time cows' milk allergy was suspected, although the problems persisted when she was fed on a soya-milk substitute.

On admission she was mildly hypoglycaemic, ketotic and her plasma pH was 7.29. Analysis of a blood sample showed normal levels of insulin but considerable hyperammonaemia (plasma ammonium ion concentration 500 μmol/L; reference range 40–80 μmol/L). She responded well to intravenous glucose infusion and enteral administration of lactulose, regaining consciousness, although she showed poor muscle tone.

A liver biopsy sample was taken, and the activity of the enzymes of urea synthesis (see Figure 9.11) were determined and compared with activities in post-mortem liver samples from six infants of the same age. The results are shown in Table 9.20. She remained well on a high-carbohydrate, low-protein diet for several days, although the poor muscle tone and muscle weakness persisted. A second liver biopsy sample was taken after 4 days and the activity of the enzymes determined again.

TABLE 9.20 *Activity of enzymes of the urea synthesis cycle in liver biopsy samples from Angela P on admission and after 4 days on a high-carbohydrate, low-protein diet, compared with activities in post-mortem samples from six infants of the same age*

	Amount of product formed (μmol /min per mg protein)		
	Angela P		
	On admission	**After 4 days**	**Control**
Carbamyl phosphate synthetase	0.337	1.45	1.30 ± 0.40
Ornithine carbamyltransferase	29.0	28.6	18.1 ± 4.9
Argininosuccinate synthetase	0.852	0.75	0.49 ± 0.09
Argininosuccinase	1.19	0.95	0.64 ± 0.15
Arginase	183	175	152 ± 56

TABLE 9.21 *Metabolism of $\{^{13}C\}$propionate*

	Angela	**Mother**	**Father**	**Control**
Per cent recovered in $^{13}CO_2$ over 3 hours	1.01	32.6	33.5	65 ± 5
dpm fixed per mg fibroblast protein over 30 minutes	5.0	230	265	561 ± 45

TABLE 9.22 *Liver and muscle carnitine*

Amount (μmol/g wet weight tissue)	Liver		Muscle	
	Angela P	**Control**	**Angela P**	**Control**
Total carnitine	0.23	0.83 ± 0.26	1.56	2.29 ± 0.75
Free carnitine	0.05	0.41 ± 0.17	0.29	1.62 ± 0.67
Short-chain acylcarnitine	0.16	0.37 ± 0.20	1.16	0.58 ± 0.32
Long-chain acylcarnitine	0.01	0.05 ± 0.02	0.11	0.09 ± 0.03

Her very low-protein diet was continued, but in order to ensure an adequate supply of essential amino acids for growth she was fed a mixture of the ketoacids of threonine, methionine, leucine, isoleucine and valine. After each feed she again became abnormally drowsy and markedly ketotic, with significant acidosis. Her plasma ammonium ion concentration was within the normal range, and a glucose tolerance test was normal, with a normal increase in insulin secretion after glucose load.

High-pressure liquid chromatography of her plasma revealed an abnormally high concentration of propionic acid (24 μmol/L; reference range 0.7–3.0 μmol/L). Urine analysis showed considerable excretion of methylcitrate (1.1 μmol per milligram of creatinine), which is not normally detectable. She was also excreting a significant amount of short-chain acyl-carnitine (mainly propionyl carnitine) – 28.6 μmol/24 h, compared with a reference range of 5.7 ± 3.5 μmol/24 h.

The metabolism of a test dose of [^{13}C]propionate given by intravenous infusion was determined in Angela, her parents and a group of control subjects; skin fibroblasts were cultured and the activity of propionyl CoA carboxylase was determined by incubation with propionate and $NaH^{14}CO_3$, followed by acidification and measurement of the radioactivity in products. The results are shown in Table 9.21.

The results of measuring carnitine in the first liver biopsy sample and in a muscle biopsy sample gave the results shown in Table 9.22.

What conclusions can you draw from these results? Can you explain the biochemical basis of Angela's condition?

CHAPTER **10**

The integration and control of metabolism

There is an obvious need to regulate metabolic pathways within individual cells, so as to ensure that catabolic and biosynthetic pathways are not attempting to operate at the same time. There is also a need to integrate and coordinate metabolism throughout the body, so as to ensure a steady provision of metabolic fuels and to control the extent to which different fuels are used by different tissues.

Objectives

After reading this chapter you should be able to:
- explain what is meant by instantaneous, fast and slow mechanisms of metabolic control;
- describe and explain allosteric regulation of enzyme activity;
- describe and explain the regulation of glycolysis and explain what is meant by substrate cycling and why it is important;
- describe and explain the hormonal control of glycogen synthesis and utilization;
- describe and explain the role of G-proteins and second messengers in signal transduction in response to fast-acting hormones and explain how there is amplification of the hormone signal;
- describe and explain the mechanisms involved in response to slow-acting hormones and explain how there is amplification of the hormone signal;

- describe and explain hormonal control of the fed and fasting states and hormonal control of adipose tissue and liver metabolism;
- describe and explain the factors involved in the selection of fuels for muscle activity under different conditions;
- describe and explain the metabolic derangements in diabetes mellitus and their biochemical basis.

10.1 *Patterns of metabolic regulation*

The rate at which different pathways operate is controlled by changes in the activity of key enzymes. In general, the first reaction unique to a given pathway or branch of a pathway will be the one most subject to regulation, although the activities of other enzymes are also regulated. The enzymes that exert the greatest control over flux (flow of metabolites) through a pathway are often those that catalyse essentially unidirectional reactions, i.e. those for which the substrates and products are far from thermodynamic equilibrium.

Within any one cell the activities of regulatory enzymes may be controlled by two mechanisms that act instantaneously:

- the availability of substrates;
- inhibition or activation by accumulation of precursors, end-products or intermediates of a pathway.

On a whole-body basis, metabolic regulation is achieved by the actions of hormones. A hormone is released from the organ (endocrine gland) in which it is synthesized in response to a stimulus such as the blood concentration of metabolic fuels, circulates in the bloodstream and acts only on target cells that have receptors for that hormone. In addition, locally acting hormones (sometimes called paracrine agents) are secreted into the interstitial fluid (rather than the bloodstream) by cells that are close to target cells. Other compounds secreted by cells act on the secretory cells themselves – these are known as autocrine agents.

There are two types of response to hormones:

- Fast responses due to changes in the activity of existing enzymes as a result of covalent modification of the enzyme protein. Fast-acting hormones activate cell-surface receptors, leading to the release of a second messenger inside the cell. The second messenger then acts directly or indirectly to activate an enzyme that catalyses the covalent modification of the target enzymes.
- Slow responses due to changes in the rate of synthesis of enzymes. Slow-acting hormones activate intracellular receptors that bind to regulatory regions of DNA and increase or decrease the rate of transcription of one or more genes.

Regardless of the mechanism by which a hormone acts to regulate a pathway, there are three key features of hormonal regulation:

- tissue selectivity, determined by whether or not the tissue contains receptors for the hormone;
- amplification of the hormone signal;
- a mechanism to terminate or reverse the hormone action as its secretion decreases.

10.2 *Intracellular regulation of enzyme activity*

As discussed in section 2.3.3, the rate at which an enzyme catalyses a reaction increases with increasing concentration of substrate, until the enzyme is more or less saturated. This means that an enzyme that has a high K_m relative to the usual concentration of its substrate will be sensitive to changes in substrate availability. By contrast, an enzyme that has a low K_m relative to the usual concentration of its substrate will act at a more or less constant rate regardless of changes in substrate availability.

The availability of substrate may be regulated by uptake from the bloodstream – for example, muscle and adipose tissue only take up glucose to any significant extent in response to insulin. In the absence of insulin the glucose transporters are in intracellular vesicles; in response to insulin these vesicles migrate to the cell surface and fuse with the cell membrane, revealing active glucose transporters. Similarly, fatty acid oxidation is controlled by the availability of fatty acyl CoA in the mitochondrial matrix, and this is regulated by the activity of carnitine palmitoyl transferase (section 5.5.1).

10.2.1 ALLOSTERIC MODIFICATION OF THE ACTIVITY OF REGULATORY ENZYMES

Allosteric regulation of enzyme activity is due to reversible, non-covalent, binding of effectors to regulatory sites, leading to a change in the conformation of the active site. This may result in either increased catalytic activity (allosteric activation) or decreased catalytic activity (allosteric inhibition). Enzymes that are subject to allosteric regulation are usually multiple subunit proteins.

Many enzymes that are subject to allosteric regulation have two interconvertible conformations:

- A relaxed (R) form, which binds substrates well, and therefore has high catalytic activity. Allosteric activators bind to, and stabilize, the active R form of the enzyme.
- A tense (T) form, which binds substrates poorly and therefore has low catalytic activity. Allosteric inhibitors bind to, and stabilize, the less active T form of the enzyme.

Compounds that act as allosteric inhibitors are commonly end-products of the pathway, and this type of inhibition is known as end-product inhibition. The decreased rate of enzyme activity results in a lower rate of formation of a product that is present is adequate amounts.

Compounds that act as allosteric activators of enzymes are often precursors of the pathway, so this is a mechanism for feed-forward activation, increasing the activity of a controlling enzyme in anticipation of increased availability of substrate.

As discussed in section 2.3.3.3, enzymes that consist of multiple subunits frequently display cooperativity between the subunits, so that binding of substrate to the active site of one subunit leads to conformational changes that enhance the binding of substrate to the other active sites of the complex. This again is allosteric activation of the enzyme, in this case by the substrate itself. The activity of such cooperative enzymes is more sharply dependent on the concentration of substrate than is the case for enzymes that do not show cooperativity.

As shown in Figure 10.1, an allosteric activator of an enzyme that shows substrate cooperativity acts by decreasing that cooperativity, so that the enzyme has a greater activity at a low concentration of the substrate than would otherwise be the case. Conversely, an allosteric inhibitor of a cooperative enzyme acts by increasing the cooperativity, so that the enzyme has less activity at a low concentration of substrate than it would in the absence of the inhibitor.

10.2.2 CONTROL OF GLYCOLYSIS — THE ALLOSTERIC REGULATION OF PHOSPHOFRUCTOKINASE

The reaction catalysed by phosphofructokinase in glycolysis, the phosphorylation of fructose 6-phosphate to fructose 1,6-bisphosphate (see Figure 5.10), is essentially

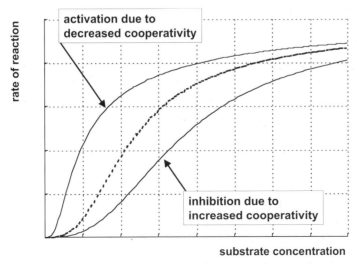

FIGURE 10.1 *Allosteric inhibition and activation of an enzyme showing subunit cooperativity.*

irreversible. In gluconeogenesis, the hydrolysis of fructose 1,6-bisphosphate is catalysed by a separate enzyme, fructose bisphosphatase. Regulation of the activities of these two enzymes determines whether the overall metabolic flux is in the direction of glycolysis or gluconeogenesis.

Inhibition of phosphofructokinase leads to an accumulation of glucose 6-phosphate in the cell, and this results in inhibition of hexokinase, which has an inhibitory binding site for its product. The result of this is a decreased rate of entry of glucose into the glycolytic pathway in tissues other than the liver, which contains glucokinase as well as hexokinase (section 5.3.1), and glucokinase is not inhibited by glucose 6-phosphate. This means that, despite inhibition of glucose utilization as a metabolic fuel, liver can take up glucose for synthesis of glycogen (section 5.6.3).

10.2.2.1 Feedback control of phosphofructokinase

Phosphofructokinase is allosterically inhibited by ATP binding at a regulatory site that is distinct from the substrate binding site for ATP. As shown in Figure 10.2, at physiological intracellular concentrations of ATP phosphofructokinase has very low activity and a more markedly sigmoid dependency on the concentration of its substrate. This can be considered to be end-product inhibition, as ATP can be considered to be an end-product of glycolysis.

When there is a requirement for increased glycolysis, and hence increased ATP production, this inhibition is relieved, and there may be a 1000-fold or higher increase in glycolytic flux in response to increased demand for ATP. However, there is less than a 10% change in the intracellular concentration of ATP. Figure 10.3 shows the inhibition of phosphofructokinase; a 10% change would not have a significant effect

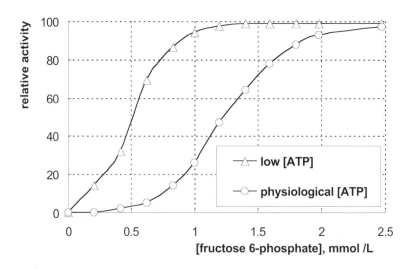

FIGURE 10.2 *The substrate dependence of phosphofructokinase at low and physiological concentrations of ATP.*

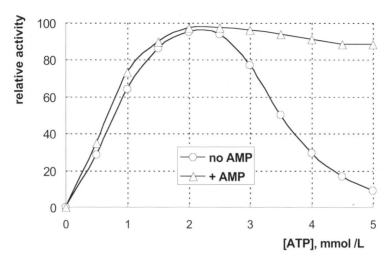

FIGURE 10.3 *The inhibition of phosphofructokinase by ATP, and relief of inhibition by 5'-AMP.*

on the activity of the enzyme. What happens is that as the concentration of ADP begins to increase, so adenylate kinase catalyses the reaction:

$$2 \times ADP \rightleftharpoons ATP + AMP$$

AMP acts as an intracellular signal that energy reserves are low and ATP formation must be increased. It binds to phosphofructokinase and both reverses the inhibition caused by ATP and increases the cooperativity between the subunits, so that the enzyme has greater affinity for fructose 6-phosphate. AMP also binds to fructose 1,6-bisphosphatase, reducing its activity.

Citrate, which can also be considered to be an end-product of glycolysis, also inhibits phosphofructokinase, by enhancing the inhibition by ATP. In muscle, creatine phosphate (section 3.2.3.1) has a similar effect. Phosphoenolpyruvate, which is synthesized in increased amounts for gluconeogenesis (section 5.7), also inhibits phosphofructokinase.

10.2.2.2 Feed-forward control of phosphofructokinase

High intracellular concentrations of fructose 6-phosphate activate a second enzyme, phosphofructokinase-2, which catalyses the synthesis of fructose 2,6-bisphosphate from fructose 6-phosphate (Figure 10.4). Fructose 2,6-bisphosphate is an allosteric activator of phosphofructokinase and an allosteric inhibitor of fructose 1,6-bisphosphatase. It thus acts to both increase glycolysis and inhibit gluconeogenesis. This is feed-forward control – allosteric activation of phosphofructokinase because there is an increased concentration of substrate available.

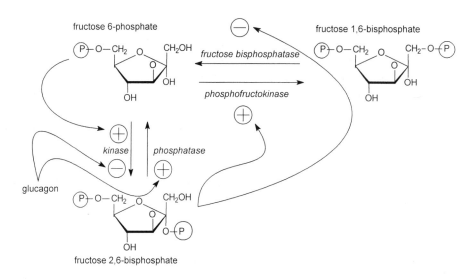

FIGURE 10.4 *The role of 2,6-fructose bisphosphate in regulation of phosphofructokinase.*

Phosphofructokinase-2 is an interesting enzyme, in that it is a single protein with two catalytic sites. One site is a kinase that catalyses the phosphorylation of fructose 6-phosphate to fructose 2,6-bisphosphate while the other is a phosphatase that catalyses the hydrolysis of fructose 2,6-bisphosphate to fructose 6-phosphate and inorganic phosphate. A single regulatory site controls the activity of the two catalytic sites in opposite directions. In response to glucagon (which stimulates gluconeogenesis and inhibits glycolysis; section 10.3), the kinase activity is decreased and the phosphatase activity increased. This results in a low concentration of fructose 2,6-bisphosphate, and hence decreased activity of phosphofructokinase and increased activity of fructose 1,6-bisphosphatase.

10.2.2.3 Substrate cycling

A priori it would seem sensible that the activities of opposing enzymes such as phosphofructokinase and fructose 1,6-bisphosphatase should be regulated in such a way that one is active and the other inactive at any time. If both were active at the same time then there would be cycling between fructose 6-phosphate and fructose 1,6-bisphosphate, with hydrolysis of ATP – a so-called futile cycle.

What is observed is that both enzymes are indeed active to some extent at the same time, although the activity of one is greater than the other, so there is a net metabolic flux. One function of such substrate cycling is thermogenesis – deliberate hydrolysis of ATP for heat production. It is not known to what extent substrate cycling can be increased to enhance thermogenesis (which is normally mediated by uncoupling of electron transport and oxidative phosphorylation; section 3.3.1.4). However, it is noteworthy that the honey bee, which does not exhibit significant substrate cycling, cannot fly in cold weather, whereas the bumble bee, which has adaptive substrate cycling, can initiate thermogenesis and so fly in cold weather.

Substrate cycling also provides a means of increasing the sensitivity and speed of metabolic regulation. The increased rate of glycolysis in response to a need for ATP for muscle contraction would imply a more or less instantaneous 1000-fold increase in phosphofructokinase activity if phosphofructokinase were inactive and fructose 1,6-bisphosphatase active. If there is moderate activity of phosphofructokinase, but greater activity of fructose 1,6-bisphosphatase, so that the metabolic flux is in the direction of gluconeogenesis, then a more modest increase in phosphofructokinase activity and decrease in fructose 1,6-bisphosphatase activity will achieve the same reversal of the direction of flux.

10.3 *Responses to fast-acting hormones by covalent modification of enzyme proteins*

A number of regulatory enzymes have a serine (or sometimes a tyrosine or threonine) residue at a regulatory site. This can undergo phosphorylation catalysed by a protein kinase, as shown in Figure 10.5. Phosphorylation may increase or decrease the activity of the enzyme. Later, the phosphate group is removed from the enzyme by phosphoprotein phosphatase, thus restoring the enzyme to its original state. These responses are not instantaneous, but they are rapid, with a maximum response within a few seconds of hormone stimulation.

The reduction in activity of pyruvate dehydrogenase in response to increased concentrations of acetyl CoA and NADH (section 10.5.2) is the result of phosphorylation. This control of enzyme phosphorylation by substrates is unusual. In most cases, the activities of protein kinases and phosphoprotein phosphatases are regulated by second messengers released intracellularly in response to fast-acting hormones binding to receptors at the cell surface. 5′-AMP, formed by the action of adenylate kinase (section 10.2.2.1) also activates a protein kinase – in this case it is acting as an intracellular messenger in response to changes in ATP availability, rather than in response to an external stimulus.

The hormonal regulation of glycogen synthesis and utilization is one of the best understood of such mechanisms. Two enzymes are involved, and obviously it is not desirable that both enzymes should be active at the same time:

*   Glycogen synthase catalyses the synthesis of glycogen, adding glucose units from UDP-glucose (section 5.6.3 and Figure 5.29).
*   Glycogen phosphorylase catalyses the removal of glucose units from glycogen, as glucose 1-phosphate (section 5.6.3.1 and Figure 5.30).

In response to insulin (secreted in the fed state) there is increased synthesis of glycogen and inactivation of glycogen phosphorylase. In response to glucagon (secreted

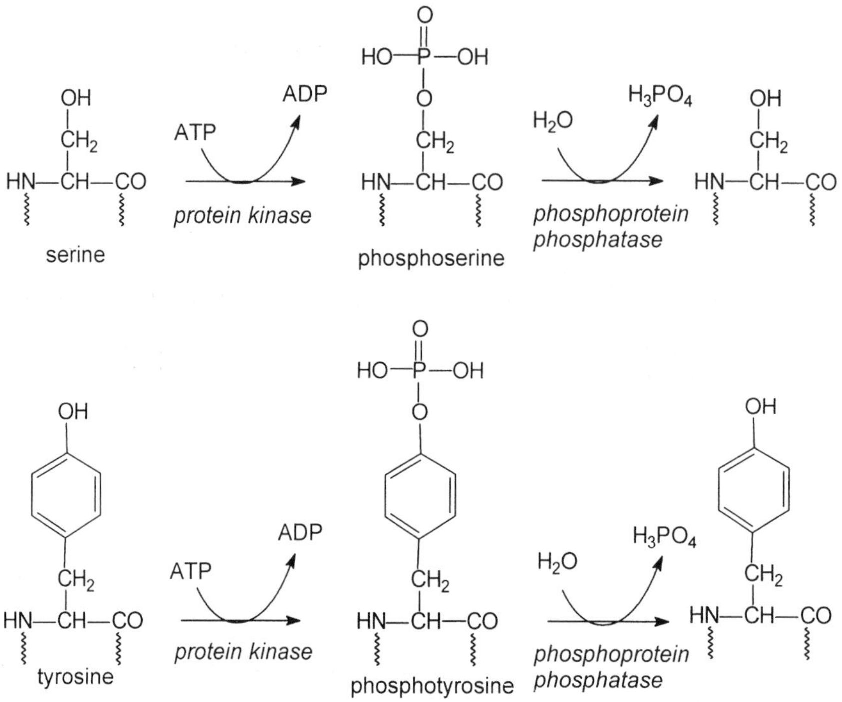

FIGURE 10.5 *Regulation of enzyme activity by phosphorylation and dephosphorylation.*

in the fasting state) or adrenaline (secreted in response to fear or fright) there is inactivation of glycogen synthase and activation of glycogen phosphorylase, permitting utilization of glycogen reserves. As shown in Figure 10.6, both effects are mediated by protein phosphorylation and dephosphorylation:

* Protein kinase is activated in response to glucagon or adrenaline:
  - Phosphorylation of glycogen synthase results in loss of activity.
  - Phosphorylation of glycogen phosphorylase results in activation of the inactive enzyme.
* Phosphoprotein phosphatase is activated in response to insulin:
  - Dephosphorylation of phosphorylated glycogen synthase restores its activity.
  - Dephosphorylation of phosphorylated glycogen phosphorylase results in loss of activity.

There is a further measure of instantaneous control by intracellular metabolites which can over-ride this hormonal regulation:

response to glucagon and adrenaline

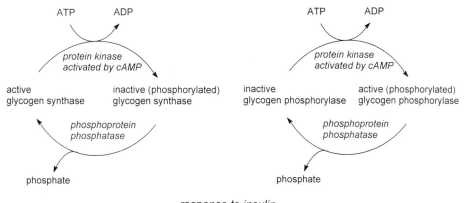

response to insulin

FIGURE 10.6 *Hormonal regulation of glycogen synthetase and glycogen phosphorylase – responses to glucagon or adrenaline and insulin.*

- Inactive glycogen synthase is allosterically activated by high concentrations of glucose 6-phosphate.
- Active glycogen phosphorylase is allosterically inhibited by ATP, glucose and glucose 6-phosphate.

10.3.1 MEMBRANE RECEPTORS AND G-PROTEINS

A cell will respond to a fast-acting hormone only if it has cell-surface receptors that bind the hormone. The receptors are transmembrane proteins; at the outer face of the membrane they have a site which binds the hormone, in the same way as an enzyme binds its substrate, by non-covalent equilibrium binding.

When the receptor binds the hormone, it undergoes a conformational change that permits it to interact with proteins at the inner face of the membrane. These are known as G-proteins because they bind guanine nucleotides (GDP or GTP). They function to transmit information from an occupied membrane receptor protein to an intracellular effector, which in turn leads to the release into the cytosol of a second messenger, ultimately resulting in the activation of protein kinases.

The G-proteins that are important in hormone responses consist of three subunits, α, β and γ. As shown in Figure 10.7, in the resting state the subunits are separate, and the α-subunit binds GDP. When the receptor at the outer face of the membrane is occupied by its hormone, it undergoes a conformational change and recruits the α-, β- and γ-subunits to form a G-protein trimer–receptor complex. The complex then reacts with GTP, which displaces the bound GDP. Once GTP has bound, the complex dissociates.

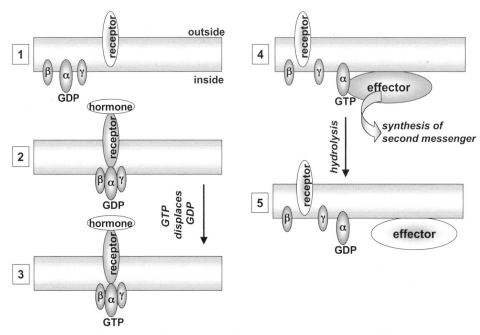

FIGURE 10.7 *The response to fast-acting (surface acting) hormones – the role of G-proteins.*

The α-subunit of the G-protein with GTP bound then binds to, and activates, the effector, which may be adenylyl cyclase (section 10.3.2), phospholipase C (section 10.3.3) or an ion transport channel in a cell membrane, resulting in release of a second messenger.

The α-subunit slowly catalyses hydrolysis of its bound GTP to GDP. As this occurs, the α-subunit–effector complex dissociates, and the effector loses its activity. The G-protein subunits are then available to be recruited by another receptor that has been activated by binding the hormone.

10.3.2 CYCLIC AMP AND CYCLIC GMP
AS SECOND MESSENGERS

One of the intracellular effectors that is activated by the (G-protein α-subunit)–GTP complex is adenylyl cyclase. This is an integral membrane protein which catalyses the formation of cyclic AMP (cAMP) from ATP (Figure 10.8). cAMP then acts as the second messenger in response to hormones such as glucagon and adrenaline. It is an allosteric activator of protein kinases. cAMP is also formed in the same way in response to a number of neurotransmitters.

As shown in Figure 10.8, phosphodiesterase catalyses the hydrolysis of cAMP to yield 5′-AMP, thus providing a mechanism for termination of the intracellular response to the hormone. Under normal conditions, 5′-AMP is then phosphorylated to ADP by the reaction of adenylate kinase – it is only under conditions of relatively low ATP

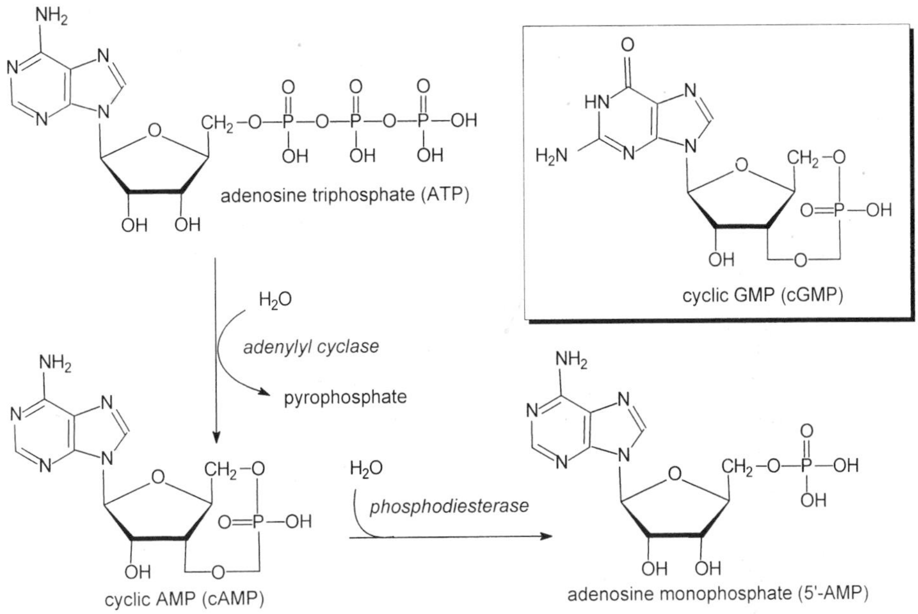

FIGURE 10.8 *Adenylyl cyclase and the formation of cyclic AMP as an intracellular second messenger. (The structure of cyclic GMP is shown in the box.)*

availability and relatively high ADP that adenylate kinase acts to form 5′-AMP as an intracellular signal (section 10.2.2.1).

Phosphodiesterase is activated in response to insulin action (which thus acts to terminate the actions of glucagon and adrenaline), and is inhibited by drugs such as caffeine and theophylline, which therefore potentiate hormone and neurotransmitter action.

In the same way as cAMP is formed from ATP by adenylyl cyclase, the guanine analogue, cGMP, can be formed from GTP by guanylyl cyclase. This may be either an integral membrane protein, like adenylyl cyclase, or a cytosolic protein. cGMP is produced in response to a number of neurotransmitters and also nitric oxide, the endothelium-derived relaxation factor that is important in vasodilatation.

10.3.2.1 Amplification of the hormone signal

The active (G-protein α-subunit)–GTP released in response to binding of 1 mol of hormone to the cell-surface receptor will activate adenylyl cyclase or guanylyl cyclase for as long as it contains GTP. The hydrolysis to yield inactive (G-protein α-subunit)–GDP occurs only relatively slowly. Therefore, a single molecule of (G-protein α-subunit)-GTP will lead to the production of many thousands of mol of cAMP or cGMP as second messenger.

There is an equilibrium between cAMP or cGMP bound to protein kinase and in free solution in the cytosol and therefore accessible to phosphodiesterase for inactivation. Each molecule of cAMP or cGMP activates a molecule of protein kinase for as long as it remains bound, resulting in the phosphorylation of many molecules of target protein.

Each enzyme molecule that has been activated by protein kinase will catalyse the reaction of many thousands of mol of substrate per second until it is dephosphorylated by phosphoprotein phosphatase.

10.3.3 INOSITOL TRISPHOSPHATE AND DIACYLGLYCEROL AS SECOND MESSENGERS

The other response to G-protein activation involves phosphatidylinositol, one of the phospholipids in cell membranes (section 4.3.1.2). As shown in Figure 10.9, phosphatidylinositol can undergo two phosphorylations, catalysed by phosphatidylinositol kinase, to yield phosphatidylinositol bisphosphate (PIP_2). PIP_2 is a substrate for phospholipase C, which is activated by the binding of (G-protein α-subunit)–GTP. The products of phospholipase C action are inositol trisphosphate (IP_3) and diacylglycerol, both of which act as intracellular second messengers.

Inositol trisphosphate opens a calcium transport channel in the membrane of the endoplasmic reticulum. This leads to an influx of calcium from storage in the endoplasmic reticulum and a 10-fold increase in the cytosolic concentration of calcium ions. Calmodulin is a small calcium-binding protein found in all cells. Its affinity for calcium is such that at the resting concentration of calcium in the cytosol (of the order of 0.1 μmol/L), little or none is bound to calmodulin. When the cytosolic concentration of calcium rises to about 1 μmol/L, as occurs in response to opening of the endoplasmic reticulum calcium transport channel, calmodulin binds 4 mol of calcium per mol of protein. When this occurs, calmodulin undergoes a conformational change, and calcium–calmodulin binds to, and activates, cytosolic protein kinases, which, in turn, phosphorylate target enzymes.

The diacylglycerol released by phospholipase C action remains in the membrane, where it activates a membrane-bound protein kinase. It may also diffuse into the cytosol, where it enhances the binding of calcium–calmodulin to cytosolic protein kinase.

Inositol trisphosphate is inactivated by further phosphorylation to inositol tetrakisphosphate (IP_4), and the diacyl glycerol is inactivated by hydrolysis to glycerol and fatty acids.

10.3.3.1 Amplification of the hormone signal

The active (G-protein α-subunit)–GTP released in response to binding of 1 mol of hormone to the cell-surface receptor will activate phospholipase C for as long as it contains GTP, and therefore, a single molecule of (G-protein α-subunit)–GTP complex will lead to the production of many thousands of mol of IP_3 and diacylglycerol as second messengers.

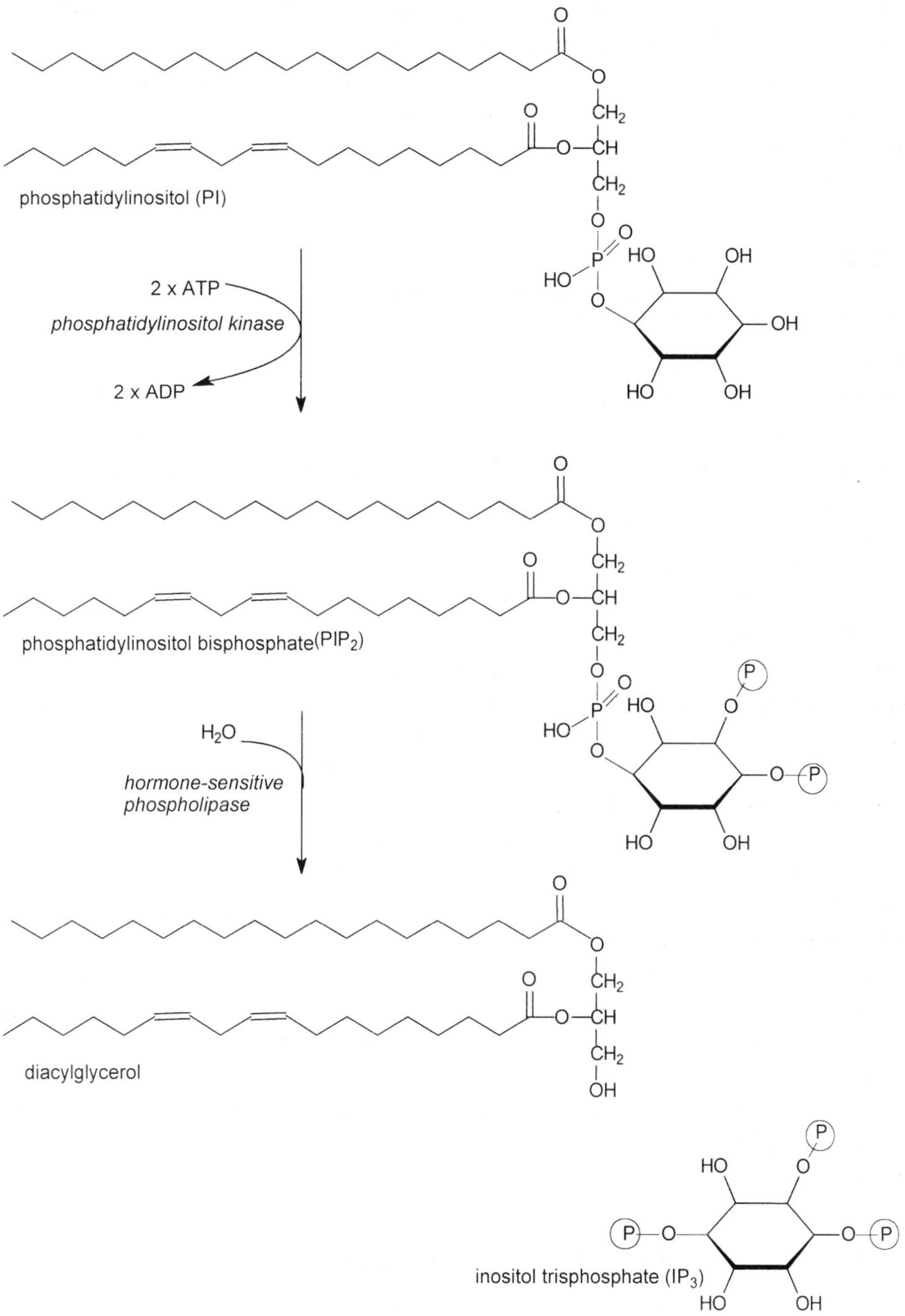

FIGURE 10.9 *Phospholipase and the formation of inositol trisphosphate and diacylglycerol as intracellular messengers.*

Each molecule of diacylglycerol will activate membrane protein kinase until it is hydrolysed (relatively slowly) by lipase, so resulting in the phosphorylation of many molecules of target protein, each of which will catalyse the metabolism of many thousands of mol of substrate per second, until it is dephosphorylated by phosphoprotein phosphatase.

Similarly, each molecule of IP_3 will continue to keep the endoplasmic reticulum calcium channel open until it is phosphorylated to inactive inositol tetrakisphosphate, thus maintaining a flow of calcium ions into the cytosol. Each molecule of calcium–calmodulin will bind to, and activate, a molecule of protein kinase for as long as the cytosol calcium concentration remains high. It is only as the calcium is pumped back into the endoplasmic reticulum that the calcium concentration falls low enough for calmodulin to lose its bound calcium and be inactivated. Again each molecule of phosphorylated enzyme will catalyse the metabolism of many thousands of mol of substrate per second, until it is dephosphorylated by phosphoprotein phosphatase.

10.3.4 THE INSULIN RECEPTOR

The insulin receptor itself is a protein kinase, which phosphorylates susceptible tyrosine residues in proteins. When insulin binds to the external part of the receptor, there is a conformational change in the whole of the protein, resulting in activation of the protein kinase region at the inner face of the membrane. This phosphorylates, and activates, cytosolic protein kinases, which, in turn, phosphorylate target enzymes, including phosphoprotein phosphatase (see Figure 10.6), cAMP phosphodiesterase (see Figure 10.8) and acetyl CoA carboxylase.

There is amplification of the response to insulin. As long as insulin remains bound to the receptor, the intracellular tyrosine kinase is active, phosphorylating, and therefore activating, many molecules of protein kinase, each of which phosphorylates many molecules of target enzyme.

A number of the receptors for growth factors have the same type of intracellular tyrosine kinase as does the insulin receptor. A mutant of the receptor for the epidermal growth factor (EGF) is permanently activated, even when not occupied by EGF. This results in continuous signalling for cell division and is one of the underlying mechanisms in cancer.

10.4 *Slow-acting hormones: changes in enzyme synthesis*

As discussed in section 9.1.1, there is continual turnover of proteins in the cell, and not all proteins are broken down and replaced at the same rate. Some are relatively stable, whereas others, and especially enzymes that are important in metabolic regulation, have short half-lives – of the order of minutes or hours. This rapid turnover means that it is possible to control metabolic pathways by changing the rate at which a key enzyme is synthesized, and hence the total amount of that enzyme in the tissue. An increase in the rate of synthesis of an enzyme is induction, while the reverse, a decrease in the rate of synthesis of the enzyme by a metabolite, is repression. A number of key enzymes in metabolic pathways are induced by their substrates, and similarly many are repressed by high concentrations of the end-products of the pathways they control.

Slow-acting hormones, including the steroid hormones such as cortisol and the sex steroids (androgens, oestrogens and progesterone), vitamin A (section 11.2.3.2), vitamin D (section 11.3.3) and the thyroid hormones (section 11.15.3.3) act by changing the rate at which the genes for individual enzymes are expressed.

The response is considerably slower than for hormones that increase the activity of existing enzyme molecules because of the need for an adequate amount of new enzyme protein to be synthesized. Similarly, the response is prolonged, as after the hormone has ceased to act there is still an increased amount of enzyme protein in the cell, and the effect will only diminish as the newly synthesized enzyme is catabolized. The time scale of action of slow-acting hormones ranges from hours to days.

As shown in Figure 10.10, the hormone enters the cell and binds to a receptor protein in the nucleus. Binding of the hormone causes a conformational change in the receptor protein and loss of a chaperone protein that is bound to the unoccupied receptor. Loss of the chaperone protein reveals a dimerization site on the receptor. The hormone–receptor complex dimerizes and undergoes activation that enables it to bind to a hormone response element on DNA, which may be some distance upstream of the gene that is regulated.

Binding of the activated hormone–receptor complex to the hormone response element acts as a signal to recruit the various transcription factors required for

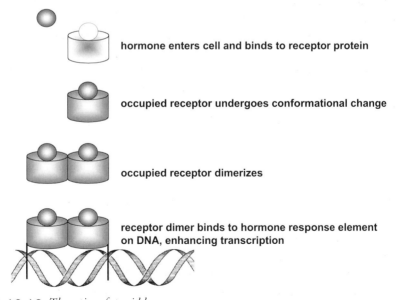

hormone enters cell and binds to receptor protein

occupied receptor undergoes conformational change

occupied receptor dimerizes

receptor dimer binds to hormone response element on DNA, enhancing transcription

FIGURE 10.10 *The action of steroid hormones.*

transcription of the gene, leading to increased synthesis of mRNA (section 9.2.2.1). Increased mRNA synthesis results in increased synthesis of the protein (section 9.2.3).

A cell will only respond to a slow-acting hormone if it synthesizes the receptor protein. The response to the same hormone in different tissues, and at different stages in development, may well be different, because only genes that are expressed in the cell will be induced. The control of gene expression by slow-acting hormones is not a matter of switching on a gene that is otherwise silent. Rather, the hormone causes an increase in the expression of a gene which is in any case being transcribed at a low rate. Similarly, the secretion of steroid hormones is not a strictly on/off affair, rather a matter of changes in the amount being secreted.

Although there is a great deal of information about the molecular mechanisms involved in initiating the responses to nuclear-acting hormones, less is known about the termination of action. It is known that vitamin B_6 (section 11.9.2) displaces hormone–receptor complexes from DNA binding, and there is good evidence that the responsiveness of target tissues to slow-acting hormones is increased in vitamin B_6 deficiency. As hormone stimulation decreases, so the newly synthesized enzymes are catabolized, as discussed in section 9.1.1.1.

10.4.1 AMPLIFICATION OF THE HORMONE SIGNAL

The amplification of the hormone signal in response to a slow-acting hormone is the result of increased synthesis of mRNA – there is increased transcription for as long as the hormone–receptor complex remains bound to the hormone response element on DNA. Each molecule of mRNA is translated many times over, leading to a considerable (albeit relatively slow) increase in the amount of enzyme protein in the cell. Each molecule of enzyme will then catalyse the metabolism of many thousands of mol of substrate per second, until it is catabolized.

10.5 *Hormonal control in the fed and fasting states*

In the fed state (see Figure 5.6), when there is an ample supply of metabolic fuels from the gut, the main processes occurring are synthesis of reserves of triacylglycerol and glycogen; glucose is in plentiful supply and is the main fuel for most tissues. By contrast, in the fasting state (see Figure 5.7) the reserves of triacylglycerol and glycogen are mobilized for use, and glucose, which is now scarce, must be spared for use by the brain and red blood cells.

As discussed in section 5.3, the principal hormones involved are insulin in the fed state and glucagon in the fasting state. Adrenaline and noradrenaline share many of the actions of glucagon, and act to provide an increased supply of metabolic fuels from triacylglycerol and glycogen reserves in response to fear or fright, regardless of whether or not fuels are being absorbed from the gut.

In liver and muscle, insulin and glucagon act to regulate the synthesis and breakdown of glycogen, as shown in Figure 10.6. They also regulate glycolysis (stimulated by insulin and inhibited by glucagon) and gluconeogenesis (inhibited by insulin and stimulated by glucagon). The result of this is that in the fed state the liver takes up and utilizes glucose, to form either glycogen or triacylglycerols, which are exported to other tissues in VLDL. By contrast, in the fasting state the liver exports glucose formed from the breakdown of both glycogen and gluconeogenesis. As discussed in section 5.5.3, in the fasting state the liver also oxidizes fatty acids and exports ketone bodies for use by other tissues.

10.5.1 HORMONAL CONTROL OF ADIPOSE TISSUE METABOLISM

As shown in Figure 10.11, insulin has three actions in adipose tissue in the fed state:

- *Stimulation of glucose uptake.* In the absence of insulin, glucose transporters in adipose tissue are in intracellular vesicles. An early response to insulin is migration of

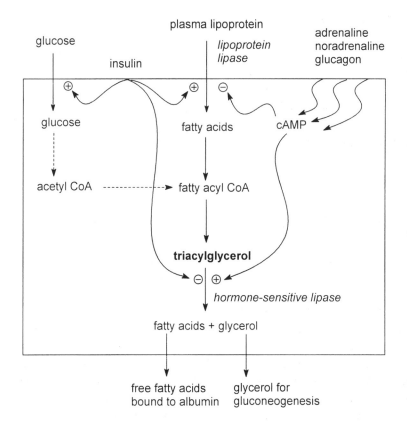

FIGURE 10.11 *Hormonal control of the synthesis and hydrolysis of triacylglycerol in adipose tissue.*

these vesicles to the cell surface, where they fuse with the cell membrane, exposing glucose transporters. This results in an increased rate of glucose uptake, and hence increased glycolysis (section 5.4.1) and increased availability of acetyl CoA for fatty acid synthesis (section 5.6.1). In the fasting state, when insulin secretion is low, little or no glucose is taken up into adipose tissue cells.

- *Activation of lipoprotein lipase at the cell surface.* As shown in Table 9.2, lipoprotein lipase has a very short half-life, of the order of 1 hour. In response to insulin acting on adipocytes there is induction of enzyme synthesis. The newly synthesized enzyme then migrates to the surface of the blood vessel endothelial walls, where it binds chylomicrons or VLDL (section 5.6.2) and catalyses the hydrolysis of triacylglycerol. The non-esterified fatty acids are mainly taken up by adipose tissue and used for synthesis of triacylglycerol.
- *Inhibition of intracellular lipase (hormone-sensitive lipase).* This reduces the hydrolysis of triacylglycerol reserves and the release of non-esterified fatty acids into the bloodstream.

cAMP, produced in response to adrenaline and noradrenaline, stimulates protein kinase. This has two actions:

- Lipoprotein lipase decreases markedly.
- Activation of intracellular hormone-sensitive lipase. This catalyses the hydrolysis of the triacylglycerol stored in adipose tissue cells, leading to release into the bloodstream of free fatty acids (which are transported bound to albumin) and glycerol, which is an important substrate for gluconeogenesis in the liver.

There is a continuous release of non-esterified fatty acids from adipose tissue. In the fed state most of the fatty acids are taken up by the liver, re-esterified to form triacylglycerol and exported in VLDL (section 5.6.2.2). This apparently futile (and ATP-expensive) cycling between lipolysis in adipose tissue and re-esterification in the liver permits increased utilization of fatty acids as fuel in muscle by increasing the rate of fatty acid uptake into muscle without the need to increase the rate of lipolysis. As discussed in section 10.6, the extent to which muscle utilizes fatty acids is determined to a considerable extent by the intensity of physical activity, rather than by their availability.

10.5.2 CONTROL OF LIPID METABOLISM IN THE LIVER

The liver synthesizes fatty acids in the fed state, and oxidizes them in the fasting state. The direction of metabolic flux (lipogenesis or lipolysis) is controlled both in response to insulin and glucagon and also by intracellular concentrations of substrates.

- In the fed state, insulin stimulates glycolysis (and inhibits gluconeogenesis), leading to increased formation of pyruvate, which results in increased formation of acetyl

CoA, and hence increased formation of citrate, which is exported to the cytosol for fatty acid synthesis (see Figure 5.27 and section 5.6.1).

• Insulin also stimulates the activity of acetyl CoA carboxylase, leading to increased formation of malonyl CoA for fatty acid synthesis (see Figure 5.27).

• In the fasting state, glucagon has the opposite actions, decreasing glycolysis (and so reducing the availability of pyruvate, acetyl CoA and hence citrate for fatty acid synthesis), increasing gluconeogenesis and decreasing the activity of acetyl CoA carboxylase.

Pyruvate dehydrogenase is inhibited in response to increased acetyl CoA, and also an increase in the NADH/NAD$^+$ ratio in the mitochondrion. The concentration of acetyl CoA will be high when β-oxidation of fatty acids is occurring, and there is no need to utilize pyruvate as a metabolic fuel. Similarly, the NADH/NAD$^+$ ratio will be high when there is an adequate amount of metabolic fuel being oxidized in the mitochondrion, so that again pyruvate is not required as a source of acetyl CoA. Under these conditions pyruvate will mainly be carboxylated to oxaloacetate for gluconeogenesis (section 5.7).

The regulation of pyruvate dehydrogenase is the result of phosphorylation of the enzyme (see Figure 10.5). Pyruvate dehydrogenase kinase is allosterically activated by acetyl CoA and NADH, and catalyses the phosphorylation of pyruvate dehydrogenase to an inactive form. Pyruvate dehydrogenase phosphatase acts constantly to dephosphorylate the inactive enzyme, so restoring its activity and maintaining sensitivity to changes in the concentrations of acetyl CoA and NADH.

As discussed in section 5.6.1, citrate leaves the mitochondria to act as a source of acetyl CoA for fatty acid synthesis only when there is an adequate amount to maintain citric acid cycle activity. As citrate accumulates in the cytosol, it acts as a feed-forward activator of acetyl CoA carboxylase, increasing the formation of malonyl CoA.

Fatty acyl CoA in the cytosol implies a high rate of fatty acid uptake from the bloodstream; fatty acyl CoA inhibits acetyl CoA carboxylase and so reduces the rate of malonyl CoA synthesis and fatty acid synthesis.

As well as being the substrate for fatty acid synthesis, malonyl CoA has an important role in controlling β-oxidation of fatty acids. Malonyl CoA is a potent inhibitor of carnitine palmitoyl transferase 1, the mitochondrial outer membrane enzyme that regulates uptake of fatty acyl CoA into the mitochondria (section 5.5.1). This means that, under conditions in which fatty acids are being synthesized in the cytosol, there will not be uptake into the mitochondria for β-oxidation. (See also section 10.6.2.1 for a discussion of the role of malonyl CoA in regulating muscle fuel selection.)

10.6 *Selection of fuel for muscle activity*

Muscle can use a variety of fuels:

- plasma glucose;
- its own reserves of glycogen;
- triacylglycerol from plasma lipoproteins;
- plasma non-esterified fatty acids;
- plasma ketone bodies;
- triacylglycerol from adipose tissue reserves within the muscle.

The selection of metabolic fuel depends on both the intensity of work being performed and also whether the individual is in the fed or fasting state.

10.6.1 THE EFFECT OF WORK INTENSITY ON MUSCLE FUEL SELECTION

Skeletal muscle contains two types of fibres:

- *Type I (red muscle) fibres.* These are also known as slow-twitch muscle fibres. They are relatively rich in mitochondria and myoglobin (hence their colour), and have a high rate of citric acid cycle metabolism, with a low rate of glycolysis. These are the fibres used mainly in prolonged, relatively moderate, work.
- *Type II (white muscle) fibres.* These are also known as fast-twitch fibres. They are relatively poor in mitochondria and myoglobin, and have a high rate of glycolysis. Type IIA fibres also have a high rate of aerobic (citric acid cycle) metabolism, whereas type IIB have a low rate of citric acid cycle activity, and are mainly glycolytic. White muscle fibres are used mainly in high-intensity work of short duration (e.g. sprinting and weight-lifting).

Intense physical activity requires rapid generation of ATP, usually for a relatively short time. Under these conditions substrates and oxygen cannot enter the muscle at an adequate rate to meet the demand, and muscle depends on anaerobic glycolysis of its glycogen reserves. As discussed in section 5.4.1.2, this leads to the release of lactate into the bloodstream, which is used as a substrate for gluconeogenesis in the liver after the exercise has finished.

Less intense physical activity is often referred to as aerobic exercise, because it involves mainly red muscle fibres (and type IIA white fibres) and there is less accumulation of lactate.

The increased rate of glycolysis for exercise is achieved in three ways:

- As ADP begins to accumulate in muscle, it undergoes a reaction catalysed by adenylate kinase: $2 \times ADP \rightleftharpoons ATP + AMP$. As discussed in section 10.2.2.1, AMP is a potent activator of phosphofructokinase, reversing the inhibition of this key regulatory enzyme by ATP, and so increasing the rate of glycolysis.

moderate exercise

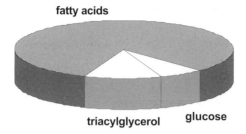

intense exercise

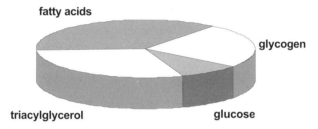

FIGURE 10.12 *Utilization of different metabolic fuels in muscle in moderate and intense exercise.*

- Nerve stimulation of muscle results in an increased cytosolic concentration of calcium ions, and hence activation of calmodulin. Calcium–calmodulin activates glycogen phosphorylase, so increasing the rate of formation of glucose 1-phosphate and providing an increased amount of substrate for glycolysis.
- Adrenaline, released from the adrenal glands in response to fear or fright, acts on cell-surface receptors, leading to the formation of cAMP, which leads to increased activity of protein kinase and increased activity of glycogen phosphorylase (see Figure 10.6).

In prolonged aerobic exercise at a relatively high intensity (e.g. cross-country or marathon running), muscle glycogen and endogenous triacylglycerol are the major fuels, with a modest contribution from plasma non-esterified fatty acids and glucose (see Figure 10.12). As the exercise continues, and muscle glycogen and triacylglycerol begin to be depleted, so plasma non-esterified fatty acids become more important.

At more moderate levels of exercise (e.g. gentle jogging or walking briskly), plasma non-esterified fatty acids provide the major fuel. This means that, for weight reduction, when the aim is to reduce adipose tissue reserves (section 6.3), relatively prolonged exercise of moderate intensity is more desirable than shorter periods of more intense exercise. More importantly for overweight people, most of the non-esterified fatty acids that are metabolized in moderate exercise are derived from abdominal rather than subcutaneous adipose tissue (section 6.2.3).

At rest, triacylglycerol from plasma lipoproteins is a significant fuel for muscle, providing 5–10% of the fatty acids for oxidation, but non-esterified fatty acids are more important in exercise.

10.6.2 MUSCLE FUEL UTILIZATION
IN THE FED AND FASTING STATES

Glucose is the main fuel for muscle in the fed state, but in the fasting state glucose is spared for use by the brain and red blood cells; glycogen, fatty acids and ketone bodies are now the main fuels for muscle.

As shown in Figure 10.13, there are five mechanisms involved in the control of glucose utilization by muscle:

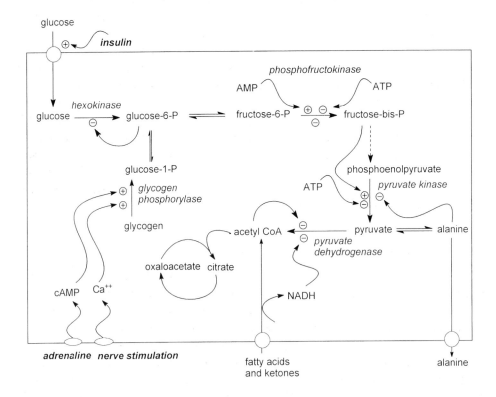

FIGURE 10.13 *Control of the utilization of metabolic fuels in muscle.*

- The uptake of glucose into muscle is dependent on insulin, as it is in adipose tissue (section 10.5.1). This means that in the fasting state, when insulin secretion is low, there will be little uptake of glucose into muscle.
- Hexokinase is inhibited by its product, glucose 6-phosphate. As shown in Figure 5.9, glucose 6-phosphate may arise either as a result of the action of hexokinase on glucose or by isomerization of glucose 1-phosphate from glycogen breakdown. The activity of glycogen phosphorylase is increased in response to glucagon in the fasting state (see Figure 10.6), and the resultant glucose 6-phosphate inhibits utilization of glucose. Because glucose transport in muscle acts by facilitated diffusion followed by metabolic trapping by phosphorylation (section 3.2.2.2), this inhibition of hexokinase will also reduce glucose uptake.
- The activity of pyruvate dehydrogenase is reduced in response to increasing concentrations of both NADH and acetyl CoA (section 10.5.2). This means that the oxidation of fatty acids and ketones will inhibit the decarboxylation of pyruvate. Under these conditions, the pyruvate that is formed from muscle glycogen by glycolysis will undergo transamination (section 9.3.1.2) to form alanine. Alanine is exported from muscle and used for gluconeogenesis in the liver (section 5.7 and Problem 9.1). Thus, although muscle cannot directly release glucose from its glycogen reserves (because it lacks glucose 6-phosphatase), muscle glycogen is an indirect source of blood glucose in the fasting state.
- If alanine accumulates in muscle, it acts as an allosteric inhibitor of pyruvate kinase, so reducing the rate at which pyruvate is formed. This end-product inhibition of pyruvate kinase by alanine is over-ridden by high concentrations of fructose bisphosphate, which acts as a feed-forward activator of pyruvate kinase.
- ATP is an inhibitor of pyruvate kinase, and at high concentrations acts to inhibit the enzyme. More importantly, ATP acts as an allosteric inhibitor of phosphofructokinase (section 10.2.2.1). This means that, under conditions in which the supply of ATP (which can be regarded as the end-product of all energy-yielding metabolic pathways) is more than adequate to meet requirements, the metabolism of glucose is inhibited.

10.6.2.1 Regulation of fatty acid metabolism in muscle

β-Oxidation of fatty acids is controlled by the uptake of fatty acids into the mitochondria – as discussed in section 5.5.1, this is controlled by the activity of carnitine acyl transferase on the outer mitochondrial membrane, and by the countertransport of acyl-carnitine and free carnitine across the inner mitochondrial membrane.

Carnitine acyl transferase activity is controlled by malonyl CoA. As discussed in section 10.5.2, in liver and adipose tissue this serves to inhibit mitochondrial uptake and β-oxidation of fatty acids when fatty acids are being synthesized in the cytosol. Muscle also has an active acetyl CoA carboxylase, and synthesizes malonyl CoA, although it does not synthesize fatty acids, and muscle carnitine acyl transferase is more sensitive to inhibition by malonyl CoA than is the enzyme in liver and adipose tissue.

Muscle also has malonyl CoA decarboxylase, which acts to decarboxylate malonyl CoA back to acetyl CoA. Acetyl CoA carboxylase and malonyl CoA decarboxylase are regulated in opposite directions by phosphorylation catalysed by a 5′-AMP-dependent protein kinase (which thus reflects the state of ATP reserves in the cell; section 10.2.2.1). Phosphorylation in response to an increase in intracellular 5′-AMP results in:

- inactivation of acetyl CoA carboxylase;
- activation of malonyl CoA decarboxylase.

This results in a rapid fall in the concentration of malonyl CoA, so relieving the inhibition of carnitine palmitoyl transferase and permitting mitochondrial uptake and β-oxidation of fatty acids in response to a fall in ATP, and hence a need for increased energy-yielding metabolism.

In the fed state, there is decreased oxidation of fatty acids in muscle as a result of increased activity of acetyl CoA carboxylase in response to insulin action.

10.7 *Diabetes mellitus – a failure of regulation of blood glucose concentration*

Diabetes mellitus is an impaired ability to regulate the concentration of blood glucose as a result of a failure of the normal control by insulin. Therefore, the plasma glucose concentration is considerably higher than normal, especially after a meal. When it rises above the capacity of the kidney to reabsorb it from the glomerular filtrate (the renal threshold, 11 mmol/L), the result is glucosuria – excretion of glucose in the urine. As a result of glucosuria, there is increased excretion of urine because of osmotic diuresis; one of the common presenting signs of diabetes is frequent urination, accompanied by excessive thirst.

The diagnosis of diabetes mellitus is by measurement of plasma glucose after an oral dose of 1 g of glucose per kilogram body weight – an oral glucose tolerance test. Figure 10.14 shows the response of plasma glucose in a control subject; there is a modest increase, and then glucose is cleared rapidly as it is taken up into liver, muscle and adipose tissue for synthesis of glycogen and fatty acids (section 5.6). In a diabetic subject, fasting plasma glucose is higher than normal, and in response to the test dose it rises considerably higher (possibly to above the renal threshold) and remains elevated for a considerable time.

There are two main types of diabetes mellitus:

- Type I diabetes (insulin-dependent diabetes mellitus, IDDM) is due to a failure to secrete insulin as a result of damage to the β-cells of the pancreatic islets resulting from viral infection or autoimmune disease. There is also a genetic susceptibility; the concordance of IDDM in monozygotic (identical) twins is about 50%. IDDM

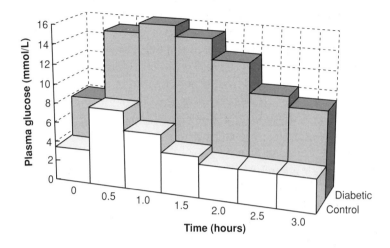

FIGURE 10.14 *The oral glucose tolerance test in control and diabetic subjects.*

commonly develops in childhood and is sometimes known as juvenile-onset diabetes. Injection of insulin and strict control of carbohydrate intake are essential for control of blood glucose.

- Type II diabetes (non-insulin-dependent diabetes mellitus, NIDDM) is due to failure of responsiveness to insulin as a result of decreased sensitivity of insulin receptors (insulin resistance). There is a clear genetic susceptibility to type II diabetes, which usually develops in middle-age, with a gradual onset, and is sometimes known as maturity-onset diabetes.

Initially, insulin secretion in response to glucose is normal or higher than normal in people with insulin resistance, and they can maintain adequate glycaemic control, although they have an impaired response to a glucose tolerance test. When the demand for insulin exceeds to the capacity of the β-islet cells of the pancreas, overt diabetes is the result.

NIDDM is more common in obese people, and especially those with abdominal rather than subcutaneous obesity (section 6.2.3). Significant weight loss can often restore normal glycaemic control without the need for any other treatment. The so-called 'metabolic syndrome' (also known as syndrome X) is the simultaneous development of insulin resistance, hypertension and hypertriglyceridaemia, all associated with (abdominal) obesity.

As NIDDM develops, control of glucose metabolism can be achieved by using oral hypoglycaemic agents, which both stimulate increased insulin secretion and enhance insulin receptor function. Increasingly, as biosynthetic human insulin has become widely available, treatment of NIDDM includes insulin injection to maintain better control over blood glucose concentration.

Acutely, diabetics are liable to coma as a result of hypo- or hyperglycaemia:

- Hypoglycaemic coma occurs if the plasma concentration of glucose falls below about 2 mmol/L, as a result of administration of insulin or oral hypoglycaemic agents without an adequate intake of carbohydrate. Strenuous exercise without additional food intake can also cause hypoglycaemia. In such cases oral or intravenous glucose is required.
- Hyperglycaemic coma develops in people with insulin-dependent diabetes because, despite an abnormally high plasma concentration of glucose, tissues are unable to utilize it in the absence of insulin. The high plasma concentration of glucose leads to elevated plasma osmolarity, which results in coma. In such cases insulin injection is required.
- Because glucose cannot be utilized, ketone bodies are synthesized in the liver (section 5.5.3). However, when the metabolism of glucose is impaired, there is little pyruvate available for synthesis of oxaloacetate to maintain citric acid cycle activity (section 5.4.4). The result is ketoacidosis together with a very high plasma concentration of glucose. In such cases insulin injection is required, as well as intravenous bicarbonate if the acidosis is severe.

In the long term, failure of glycaemic control and a persistently high plasma glucose concentration results in damage to capillary blood vessels (especially in the retina, leading to a risk of blindness), kidneys and peripheral nerves (leading to loss of sensation) and the development of cataracts in the lens of the eye and abnormal metabolism of plasma lipoproteins (which increases the risks of atherosclerosis and ischaemic heart disease). Two mechanisms have been proposed to explain these effects:

- At high concentrations, glucose can be reduced to sorbitol by aldose reductase. In tissues such as the lens of the eye and nerves, which cannot metabolize sorbitol, it accumulates, causing osmotic damage.
- As shown in Figure 10.15, glucose can react non-enzymically with free amino groups on proteins, resulting in glycation of the proteins. Glycated proteins include:
  - Collagen. This may explain the problems of arthritis experienced by many diabetic subjects, as well as the thickening of basement membranes that is associated with blood capillary and kidney damage. Diabetic retinopathy, a cause of blindness, is the result of capillary damage in the retina.
  - Apolipoprotein B. This may explain the increased risk of atherosclerosis and ischaemic heart disease associated with diabetes and poor glycaemic control.
  - α-Crystallin in the lens. This may explain the high prevalence of cataracts associated with diabetes and poor glycaemic control.
  - Haemoglobin A. Glycation of haemoglobin A (with the formation of what can be measured as haemoglobin A_{1c}) provides a sensitive means of assessing the adequacy of glycaemic control over the preceding 4–6 weeks. It provides a better index of compliance with dietary restriction than a simple spot test of plasma glucose.

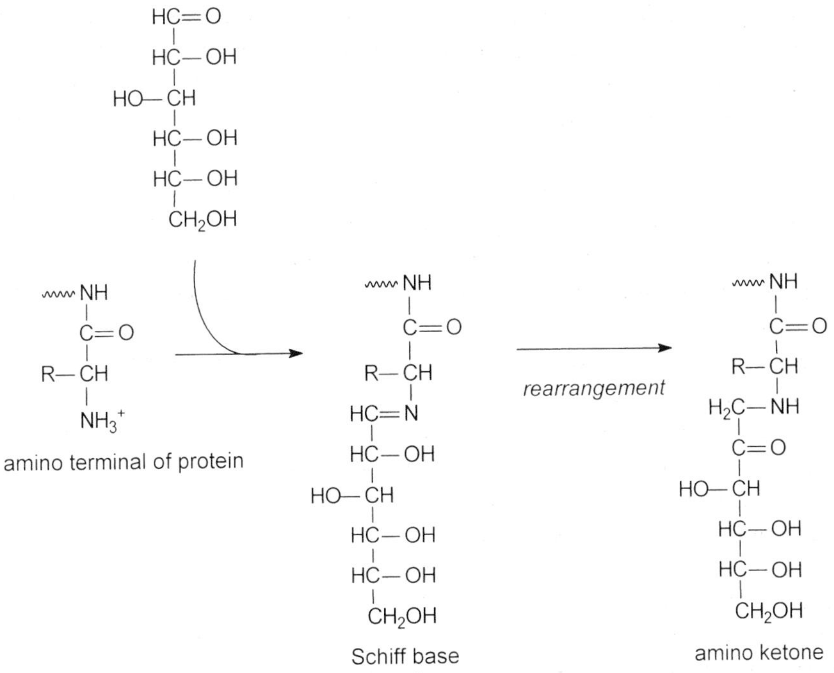

FIGURE 10.15 *Non-enzymic glycation of proteins by high concentrations of glucose in poorly controlled diabetes mellitus.*

Additional resources

PowerPoint presentation 10 on the CD
Self-assessment quiz 10 on the CD

The simulation program Radioimmunoassay on the CD lets you go through the steps that would be involved in selecting an antiserum for radioimmunoassay of a steroid hormone and use the selected antiserum to determine oestradiol in plasma samples.

Problem 10.1: Louis C

Louis was born in 1967, at term, after an uneventful pregnancy. He was a sickly infant and did not grow well. On a number of occasions his mother noted that he appeared drowsy, or even comatose, and said that there was a 'chemical, alcohol-like' smell on his breath and in his urine. The GP suspected diabetes mellitus, and sent him to the Middlesex Hospital for a glucose tolerance test, which showed clearly that he was diabetic (see Figure 10.14).

Blood samples were also taken for measurement of insulin at zero time and 1 hour after the glucose load. At this time a new method of measuring insulin was being developed, radioimmunoassay, and therefore both this and the conventional biological assay were used. The biological method of measuring insulin is to determine the uptake and metabolism of glucose in rat muscle *in vitro*. This can be performed relatively simply by measuring the radioactivity in the $^{14}CO_2$ produced after incubating samples of rat muscle with [^{14}C]glucose in the presence and absence of the patient's blood. The then newly developed method of measuring insulin involves measuring the ability of insulin to bind to anti-insulin antibodies, in competition with radioactively labelled insulin – this is radioimmunoassay, and it is generally preferred because it is possible to assay a large number of blood samples at the same time. The antibody recognizes, and binds to, the surface of the tertiary structure of the protein. The results are shown in Table 10.1.

As a part of their studies of the new radioimmunoassay for insulin, the team at the Middlesex Hospital performed gel exclusion chromatography of a pooled sample of normal serum and determined insulin in the fractions eluted from the columns both by radioimmunoassay (graph A in Figure 10.16) and by stimulation of glucose oxidation (graph B). Gel exclusion chromatography separates compounds by their molecular mass, so that larger molecules flow through the column faster, and are eluted earlier, than smaller molecules. Three molecular mass markers were used; they eluted as follows: 9000 in fraction 10, 6000 in fraction 23 and 4500 in fraction 27.

The investigators also measured insulin in the fractions eluted from the chromatography column after treatment of each fraction with trypsin. The results are shown in graph C.

After seeing the results of these studies, they subjected the same pooled serum to brief treatment with trypsin, and performed gel exclusion chromatography on the resulting sample. Again they measured insulin by radioimmunoassay (graph D) and biological assay (graph E).

What conclusions can you draw from these results?

More recently, the gene for human insulin has been cloned. Although insulin consists of two peptide chains, 21 and 30 amino acids long, these are coded for by a single gene, which has a total of 330 base pairs between the initiator and stop codons. As you would expect for a secreted protein, there is a signal sequence coding for 24 amino acids at the 5' end of the gene.

TABLE 10.1 *Serum insulin by biological assay and radioimmunoassay*

	Fasting		One hour after glucose	
	Louis C	**Control subjects**	**Louis C**	**Control subjects**
Biological assay	0.8	6 ± 2	5	40 ± 11
Radioimmunoassay	10	6 ± 2	50	40 ± 11

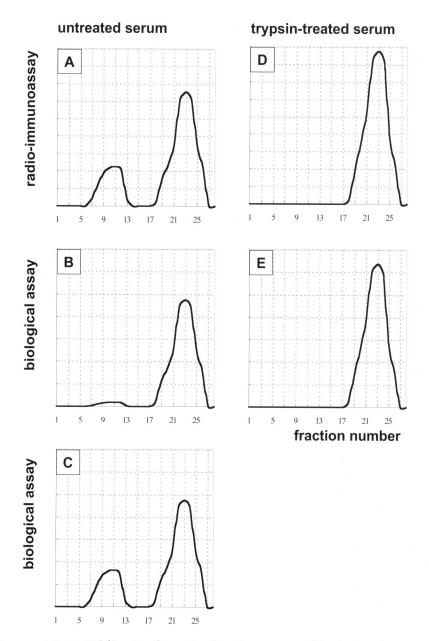

FIGURE 10.16 *Gel filtration of serum insulin and measurement of insulin by radioimmunoassay and biological assay. Graphs A and B show gel filtration of untreated serum. Graphs D and E show gel filtration of serum after brief treatment with trypsin. Graph C shows the effect of treatment of each fraction with trypsin after separation by gel filtration.*

What does this information suggest about the processes that occur in the synthesis of insulin?

What is likely to be the underlying biochemical basis of Louis' problem?

Problem 10.2: Lucinda K

Lucinda is the second child of unrelated parents. She was born at term after an uneventful pregnancy, weighing 3.4 kg, and was breast fed, with gradual introduction of solids from 3 months of age. Her mother reported that, although Lucinda liked cheese, meat and fish, she frequently became irritable and grizzly after meals, and became lethargic, drowsy and 'floppy' after eating relatively large amounts of protein-rich foods. Her urine had a curious odour, described by her mother as being 'cat-like', on such occasions.

At 9 months of age she was admitted to the Accident and Emergency Department of UCL Hospital in a coma and suffering convulsions. She had been unwell for the previous 3 days, with a slight fever, and for the previous 12 hours had been refusing all food and drink. At this time she weighed 8.8 kg, and her body length was 70.5 cm.

Emergency blood tests revealed moderate acidosis (pH 7.25) and severe hypoglycaemia (glucose < 1 mmol/L); a dipstick test for plasma ketone bodies was negative. A blood sample was taken for full clinical chemistry tests and she was given intravenous glucose. Within a short time she recovered consciousness. The results of the blood tests are shown in Table 10.2.

Lucinda remained in hospital for several weeks while further tests were performed. She was generally well through this time, but became drowsy and severely hypoglycaemic, and hyperventilated, if she was deprived of food for more than about 8–9 hours. Her muscle tone was poor and she was very weak, with considerably less strength (e.g. in pushing her arms or legs against the paediatrician's hand) than would be expected for a girl of her age.

TABLE 10.2 *Clinical chemistry results for a plasma sample from Lucinda K on admission and reference range for 24 hours fasting*

	Lucinda K	Reference range
Glucose (mmol/L)	0.22	4–5
pH	7.25	7.35–7.45
Bicarbonate (mmol/L)	11	21–29
Ammonium (μmol/L)	120	< 50
Ketone bodies (mmol/L)	Undetectable	2.5–3.5
Non-esterified fatty acids (mmol/L)	2	1.0–1.2
Insulin (mU/L)	5	5–35
Glucagon (ng/mL)	140	130–160

On one occasion her blood glucose was monitored at 30 minute intervals over 3 hours from waking, without being fed; it fell from 3.4 mmol/L on waking to 1.3 mmol/L 3 hours later. She was deprived of breakfast again the next day, and again blood glucose was measured at 30 minute intervals for 3 hours, during which time she received an intravenous infusion of β-hydroxybutyrate (50 μmol/min/kg body weight). During the infusion of β-hydroxybutyrate her plasma glucose remained between 3.3 and 3.5 mmol/L.

At no time were ketone bodies detected in her urine, and there was no evidence of any abnormal excretion of amino acids. However, a number of abnormal organic acids were detected in her urine, including relatively large amounts of 3-hydroxy-3-methylglutaric and 3-hydroxy-3-methylglutaconic acids. The excretion of these two acids increased considerably under two conditions:

- When she was fed a relatively high-protein meal (when she became grizzly, lethargic and irritable). A blood sample taken after such a meal showed significant hyperammonaemia (130 μmol/L) but normal glucose (5.5 mmol/L).
- When she was fasted for more than the normal overnight fast, with or without the infusion of β-hydroxybutyrate.

One obvious metabolic precursor of 3-hydroxy-3-methylglutaric acid is 3-hydroxy-3-methylglutaryl CoA (HMG CoA), which is normally cleaved to yield acetoacetate and acetyl CoA by the enzyme hydroxymethyglutaryl CoA lyase (see Figure 5.25). Therefore, the activity of this enzyme was determined in leucocytes from blood samples from Lucinda and her parents. The results are shown in Table 10.3.

Analysis of Lucinda's urine also revealed considerable excretion of carnitine, as shown in Table 10.4.

What is the likely biochemical basis of Lucinda's problem? To what extent can you account for her various metabolic problems from the information you are given?

TABLE 10.3 *Leucocyte HMG CoA lyase activity (nmol product formed per min per g protein)*

Lucinda K	1.7
Mother	10.2
Father	11.4
Control subjects	19.7 ± 2.0

TABLE 10.4 *Urinary excretion of carnitine (nmol per mg creatinine)*

	Lucinda K	**Reference range**
Total carnitine	680	125 ± 75
Free carnitine	31	51 ± 40
Acyl carnitine	649	74 ± 40

What dietary manipulation(s) would be likely to maintain her in good health and prevent further emergency hospital admissions?

Problem 10.4: Barry B

Barry is the second child of unrelated parents; his brother is 5 years old, fit and healthy. Barry was born at full term after an uneventful pregnancy, weighing 3.4 kg (the 50th centile), and developed normally until he was 6 months old, after which time he showed some retardation of development. He also developed a fine scaly skin rash about this time, and his hair, which had been normal, became thin and sparse.

At 9 months of age he was admitted to UCL Hospital in a coma; the results of clinical chemistry tests on a plasma sample are shown in Table 10.5.

The acidosis was treated by intravenous infusion of bicarbonate, and he recovered consciousness. Over the next few days he continued to show signs of acidosis (rapid respiration), and even after a meal he showed ketonuria. His plasma lactate, pyruvate and ketones remained high; plasma glucose was in the low normal range and his plasma insulin was normal both in the fasting state and after an oral glucose load.

Urine analysis revealed the presence of significant amounts of a number of organic acids that are not normally excreted in the urine, including:

- lactate, pyruvate and alanine;
- propionate, hydroxypropionate and propionylglycine;
- methyl citrate;
- tiglate and tiglylglycine;
- 3-methylcrotonate, 3-methylcrotonylglycine and 3-hydroxyisovalerate.

His skin rash and hair loss were reminiscent of the signs of biotin deficiency, as caused by excessive consumption of uncooked egg-white (section 11.12). However, his mother said that Barry did not eat raw or undercooked eggs at all, although he was fond of hard-boiled eggs and yeast extract (which are rich sources of biotin). His plasma biotin was 0.2 nmol/L (normal level > 0.8 nmol/L), and he excreted a

TABLE 10.5 *Clinical chemistry results for a plasma sample from Barry B on admission and reference range for 24 hours fasting*

	Barry B	**Reference range**
Glucose (mmol/L)	3.3	3.5–5.5
pH	6.9	7.35–7.45
Bicarbonate (mmol/L)	2.0	21–25
Ketone bodies (mmol/L)	21	1–2.5
Lactate (mmol/L)	7.3	0.5–2.2
Pyruvate (mmol/L)	0.31	< 0.15

significant amount of biotin in the form of biocytin and small biocytin-containing peptides (see Figure 11.25); these are not normally detectable in urine.

He was treated with 5 mg of biotin per day. After 3 days the various abnormal organic acids were no longer detectable in his urine, and his plasma lactate, pyruvate and ketones had returned to normal, although his excretion of biocytin and biocytin-containing peptides increased. At this stage he was discharged from hospital, with a supply of biotin tablets. After 3 weeks his skin rash began to clear and his hair loss ceased.

Three months later, at a regular out-patient visit, it was decided to cease the biotin supplements. Within a week the abnormal organic acids were detected in his urine again and he was treated with varying doses of biotin until the organicaciduria ceased. This was achieved at an intake of 150 µg/day (compared with the reference intake of 10–20 µg/day for an infant under 2 years old).

He has continued to take 150 µg of biotin daily, and has remained in good health for the last 4 years.

Can you account for the biochemical basis of Barry's problem?

Problem 10.5: Amelia Q

Amelia is the only child of non-consanguineous parents, born at term after an uneventful pregnancy. At 14 months of age she was admitted to hospital with a 1 day

TABLE 10.6 *Clinical chemistry results for plasma and urine samples from Amelia Q on admission and again 1 week later*

	Acute admission	One week later	Reference range
Plasma			
Glucose (mmol/L)	14	5.1	3.5–5.5
Sodium (mmol/L)	132	137	135–145
Chloride (mmol/L)	111	105	100–106
Bicarbonate, mmol/L	1.5	20	21–25
Urea (mmol/L)	4.1	4.9	2.9–8.9
Lactate (mmol/L)	7.3	5.5	0.5–2.2
Pyruvate (mmol/L)	0.31	0.25	< 0.15
Alanine (mmol/L)	–	852	99–313
Aspartate (mmol/L)	–	Undetectable	3–11
pH	6.89	7.36	7.35–7.45
Urine			
Lactate (mg per g creatinine)	–	1.48	< 0.1
Ketone bodies, using Ketostix	very high	negative	negative

TABLE 10.7 *Activities of mitochondrial enzymes from cultured skin fibroblasts (nmol product formed per min per mg protein)*

	Amelia Q	**Control subjects**
Citrate synthase	32.8	76.3 ± 15.1
Cytochrome c reduction by NADH	11.6	16.7 ± 4.6
Cytochrome c reduction by succinate	9.43	12.3 ± 3.2
Cytochrome oxidase	37.7	50.3 ± 11.6
NADH dehydrogenase	633	910 ± 169
Pyruvate carboxylase	0.03	1.62 ± 0.39
Pyruvate dehydrogenase	1.86	1.72 ± 0.35
Succinate oxidase	190	210 ± 30

history of persistent vomiting, rapid shallow respiration and dehydration. On admission her respiration rate was 60/min and her pulse 178/min. The first column in Table 10.6 shows the results of clinical chemistry tests at that time. She responded rapidly to intravenous bicarbonate and a single intramuscular injection of insulin.

The results of a glucose tolerance test 3 days after admission were normal, and her plasma insulin response to an oral glucose load was within the normal range. She was discharged from hospital 7 days after admission, apparently fit and well. The second column in Table 10.6 shows the results of clinical chemistry tests taken shortly before her discharge.

Amelia was readmitted to hospital at 16, 25, 31 and 48 months of age, suffering from restlessness, unsteady gait, rapid shallow respiration, persistent vomiting and dehydration. Each time the crisis was preceded by a common childhood illness and decreased appetite, and she responded well to intravenous fluids and bicarbonate. A number of milder episodes were treated at home by oral fluid and bicarbonate.

During her admission at age 25 months, a skin biopsy was taken, fibroblasts were cultured, and the mitochondrial enzyme activities shown in Table 10.7 were determined.

Can you explain the biochemical basis of Lucinda's condition?

Problem 10.6: David B

David is a 70 kg student; as part of a research project he performed exercise on a treadmill. Table 10.8 shows his oxygen consumption and carbon dioxide production at different speeds.

From these results and using information in Table 5.1, calculate:

- his energy expenditure at each speed of walking (in kJ/30 min);
- his PAR at each speed;

TABLE 10.8 *Oxygen consumption and carbon dioxide production during 30 minutes of exercise on a treadmill at different speeds*

	Litres O$_2$	kJ/30 min	PAR	Litres CO$_2$	RQ	Per cent fat metabolized
At rest (= BMR)	161		1.0	4.72		
1 km/h	158			5.66		
3.5 km/h	394			14.18		
4.5 km/h	525			19.95		
6.5 km/h	656			26.25		
6.5 km/h, incline + load	919			41.8		

TABLE 10.9 *Oxygen consumption and carbon dioxide production during 30 minutes exercise on a treadmill at 3.5 km/h before and after breakfast*

	Litres O$_2$	Litres CO$_2$	RQ	Per cent fat metabolized
Fasting	394	285		
Fed	394	390		

- his RQ (respiratory quotient, the ratio of CO$_2$ produced/O$_2$ consumed) at each speed;
- the percentage of fat and carbohydrate he is metabolizing at each speed (assuming that these are the only fuels he is utilizing).

Table 10.9 shows his oxygen consumption and carbon dioxide production walking on the treadmill at 3.5 km/h for 30 minutes early in the morning (after an overnight fast) and again 2 hours after eating breakfast.

What conclusions can you draw from these data?

CHAPTER **11**

Micronutrients – the vitamins and minerals

In addition to an adequate source of metabolic fuels (carbohydrates, fats and proteins, see Chapter 5) and protein (Chapter 9), there is a requirement for very much smaller amounts of other nutrients: the vitamins and minerals. Collectively these are referred to as micronutrients because of the small amounts that are required.

Vitamins are organic compounds which are required for the maintenance of normal health and metabolic integrity. They cannot be synthesized in the body, but must be provided in the diet. They are required in very small amounts, of the order of mg or μg/day, and thus can be distinguished from the essential fatty acids (section 4.3.1.1 and section 5.6.1.1) and the essential amino acids (section 9.1.3), which are required in amounts of grams/day.

The essential minerals are those inorganic elements which have a physiological function in the body. Obviously, since they are elements, they must be provided in the diet, because elements cannot be interconverted. The amounts required vary from grams/day for sodium and calcium, through mg/day (e.g. iron) to μg/day for the trace elements (so called because they are required in such small amounts).

Objectives

After reading this chapter you should be able to:

- Describe and explain the way in which micronutrient requirements are determined and how reference intakes are calculated; explain how it is that different national and international authorities have different reference intakes for some nutrients.

- Describe and explain the chemistry, metabolic functions and deficiency signs associated with each of the vitamins and the main minerals.

11.1 *The determination of requirements and reference intakes*

For any nutrient, there is a range of intakes between that which is clearly inadequate, leading to clinical deficiency disease, and that which is so much in excess of the body's metabolic capacity that there may be signs of toxicity. Between these two extremes is a level of intake that is adequate for normal health and the maintenance of metabolic integrity and a series of more precisely definable levels of intake that are adequate to meet specific criteria and may be used to determine requirements and appropriate levels of intake:

- Clinical deficiency disease, with clear anatomical and functional lesions, and severe metabolic disturbances, possibly proving fatal. Prevention of deficiency disease is a minimal goal in determining requirements.
- Covert deficiency, in which there are no signs of deficiency under normal conditions but any trauma or stress reveals the precarious state of the body reserves and may precipitate clinical signs. For example, as discussed in section 11.14.4, an intake of 10 mg of vitamin C per day is adequate to prevent clinical deficiency, but at least 20 mg/day is required for healing of wounds.
- Metabolic abnormalities under normal conditions, such as impaired carbohydrate metabolism in thiamin deficiency (section 11.6.3) or excretion of methylmalonic acid in vitamin B_{12} deficiency (section 11.10.5.2).
- Abnormal response to a metabolic load, such as the inability to metabolize a test dose of histidine in folate deficiency (section 11.11.6.1) or tryptophan in vitamin B_6 deficiency (section 11.9.5.1), although at normal levels of intake there may be no metabolic impairment.
- Inadequate saturation of enzymes with (vitamin-derived) coenzymes. This can be tested for three vitamins, using red blood cell enzymes: thiamin (section 11.6.4.1), riboflavin (section 11.7.4.1) and vitamin B_6 (section 11.9.5).
- Low plasma concentration of the nutrient, indicating that there is an inadequate amount in tissue reserves to permit normal transport between tissues. For some nutrients this may reflect failure to synthesize a transport protein rather than primary deficiency of the nutrient itself.
- Low urinary excretion of the nutrient, reflecting low intake and changes in metabolic turnover.
- Incomplete saturation of body reserves.
- Adequate body reserves and normal metabolic integrity. This is the (untestable) goal.
- Possibly beneficial effects of intakes more than adequate to meet requirements: the promotion of optimum health and life expectancy. There is evidence that relatively high intakes of vitamin E and possibly other antioxidant nutrients (section

7.4.3) may reduce the risk of developing cardiovascular disease and some forms of cancer. High intakes of folate during early pregnancy reduce the risk of neural tube defects in the fetus (section 11.11.5.1).

- Pharmacological (drug-like) actions at very high levels of intake.
- Abnormal accumulation in tissues and overloading of normal metabolic pathways, leading to signs of toxicity and possibly irreversible lesions. Iron (section 11.15.2.3), selenium (section 11.15.2.5), niacin (section 11.8.5.2) and vitamins A (section 11.2.5.2), D (section 11.3.5.1) and B$_6$ (section 11.9.6.1) are all known to be toxic in excess.

Having decided on an appropriate criterion of adequacy, requirements are determined by feeding volunteers a diet that is an otherwise adequate but lacks the nutrient under investigation until there is a detectable metabolic or other abnormality. The volunteers are then repleted with graded intakes of the nutrient until the abnormality is just corrected.

Problems arise in interpreting the results, and therefore defining requirements, when different markers of adequacy respond to different levels of intake. This explains the difference in the tables of reference intakes published by different national and international authorities (see Tables 11.1–11.3).

11.1.1 DIETARY REFERENCE VALUES

Individuals do not all have the same requirement for nutrients, even when calculated on the basis of body size or energy expenditure. There is a range of individual requirements of up to 25% around the average. Therefore, in order to set population goals, and assess the adequacy of diets, it is necessary to set a reference level of intake that is high enough to ensure that no-one will either suffer from deficiency or be at risk of toxicity.

As shown in the upper graph in Figure 11.1, if it is assumed that individual requirements are distributed in a statistically normal fashion around the observed mean requirement, then a range of $\pm$ 2 times the standard deviation (SD) around the mean will include the requirements of 95% of the population. This 95% range is conventionally used as the 'normal' or reference range (e.g. in clinical chemistry to assess the normality or otherwise of a test result) and is used to define three levels of nutrient intake:

- The estimated average requirement (EAR). This is the observed mean requirement to meet the chosen criterion of adequacy in experimental studies.
- The reference nutrient intake (RNI). This is $2 \times$ SD above the observed mean requirement, and is therefore **more than** adequate to meet the individual requirements of 97.5% of the population. This is the goal for planning diets, e.g. in institutional feeding, and the standard against which the intake of a population can be assessed. In the European Union tables (Table 11.2) this is called the

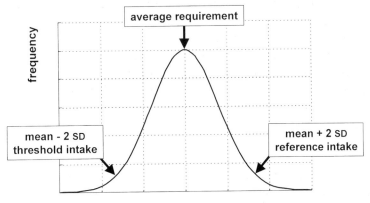

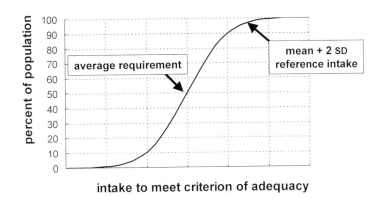

FIGURE 11.1 *The derivation of reference intakes of nutrients from the distribution around the observed mean requirement. The values are plotted below as a cumulative distribution curve, permitting estimation of the probability that a given level of intake is adequate to meet an individual's requirement.*

population reference intake (PRI); in the USA it is called the recommended dietary allowance (RDA; Table 11.3).

*   The lower reference nutrient intake (LNRI). This is $2 \times$ SD below the observed mean requirement, and is therefore adequate to meet the requirements of only 2.5% of the population. In the European Union tables this is called the lower threshold intake, to show that it is a level of intake at or below which it is extremely unlikely that normal metabolic integrity could be maintained.

The lower graph in Figure 11.1 shows the distribution of requirements plotted as the cumulative percentage of the population whose requirements have been met at each level of intake. This can therefore be used to estimate the probability that a given level of intake is adequate to meet an individual's requirements.

TABLE 11.1 *Reference nutrient intakes of vitamins and minerals, UK 1991*

Age	B_1 (mg)	B_2 (mg)	Niacin (mg)	B_6 (mg)	B_{12} (µg)	Folate (µg)	C (mg)	A (µg)	D (µg)	Ca (mg)	P (mg)	Mg (mg)	Fe (mg)	Zn (mg)	Cu (mg)	Se (µg)	I (µg)
										Mineral							
0–3 months	0.2	0.4	3	0.2	0.3	50	25	350	8.5	525	400	55	1.7	4.0	0.2	10	50
4–6 months	0.2	0.4	3	0.2	0.3	50	25	350	8.5	525	400	60	4.3	4.0	0.3	13	60
7–9 months	0.2	0.4	4	0.3	0.4	50	25	350	7	525	400	75	7.8	5.0	0.3	10	60
10–12 months	0.3	0.4	5	0.4	0.4	50	25	350	7	525	400	80	7.8	5.0	0.3	10	60
1–3 years	0.5	0.6	8	0.7	0.5	70	30	400	7	350	270	85	6.9	5.0	0.4	15	70
4–6 years	0.7	0.8	11	0.9	0.8	100	30	500	–	450	350	120	6.1	6.5	0.6	20	100
7–10 years	0.7	1.0	12	1.0	1.0	150	30	500	–	550	450	200	8.7	7.0	0.7	30	110
Males																	
11–14 years	0.9	1.2	15	1.2	1.2	200	35	600	–	1000	775	280	11.3	9.0	0.8	45	130
15–18 years	1.1	1.3	18	1.5	1.5	200	40	700	–	1000	775	300	11.3	9.5	1.0	70	140
19–50 years	1.0	1.3	17	1.4	1.5	200	40	700	–	700	550	300	8.7	9.5	1.2	75	140
50+ years	0.9	1.3	16	1.4	1.5	200	40	700	10	700	550	300	8.7	9.5	1.2	75	140
Females																	
11–14 years	0.7	1.1	12	1.0	1.2	200	35	600	–	800	625	280	14.8	9.0	0.8	45	130
15–18 years	0.8	1.1	14	1.2	1.5	200	40	600	–	800	625	300	14.8	7.0	1.0	60	140
19–50 y	0.8	1.1	13	1.2	1.5	200	40	600	–	700	550	270	14.8	7.0	1.2	60	140
50+ years	0.8	1.1	12	1.2	1.5	200	40	600	10	700	550	270	8.7	7.0	1.2	60	140
Pregnant	+0.1	+0.3	–	–	–	+100	+10	+100	10	–	–	–					
Lactating	+0.1	+0.5	–	–	+0.5	+60	+30	+350	10	+550	+440	+50		+6.0	+0.3	+15	

Source: Department of Health (1991) *Dietary Reference Values for Food Energy and Nutrients for the United Kingdom*. HMSO, London.

TABLE 11.2 *Population reference intakes of vitamins and minerals, European Union, 1993*

Age	Vitamin								Mineral						
	A (mg)	B_1 (mg)	B_2 (mg)	Niacin (mg)	B_6 (µg)	Folate (µg)	B_{12} (mg)	C (µg)	Ca (mg)	P (mg)	Fe (mg)	Zn (mg)	Cu (mg)	Se (µg)	I (µg)
6–12 months	350	0.3	0.4	5	0.4	50	0.5	20	400	300	6	4	0.3	8	50
1–3 years	400	0.5	0.8	9	0.7	100	0.7	25	400	300	4	4	0.4	10	70
4–6 years	400	0.7	1.0	11	0.9	130	0.9	25	450	350	4	6	0.6	15	90
7–10 years	500	0.8	1.2	13	1.1	150	1.0	30	550	450	6	7	0.7	25	100
Males															
11–14 years	600	1.0	1.4	15	1.3	180	1.3	35	1000	775	10	9	0.8	35	120
15–17 years	700	1.2	1.6	18	1.5	200	1.4	40	1000	775	13	9	1.0	45	130
18+ years	700	1.1	1.6	18	1.5	200	1.4	45	700	550	9	9.5	1.1	55	130
Females															
11–14 years	600	0.9	1.2	14	1.1	180	1.3	35	800	625	18	9	0.8	35	120
15–17 years	600	0.9	1.3	14	1.1	200	1.4	40	800	625	17	7	1.0	45	130
18+ years	600	0.9	1.3	14	1.1	200	1.4	45	700	550	16	7	1.1	55	130
Pregnant	700	1.0	1.6	14	1.3	400	1.6	55	700	550	16	7	1.1	55	130
Lactating	950	1.1	1.7	16	1.4	350	1.9	70	1200	950	16	12	1.4	70	160

Source: Scientific Committee for Food (1993) *Nutrient and energy intakes for the European Community*, Commission of the European Communities, Luxembourg.

TABLE 11.3 *Recommended dietary allowances and acceptable intakes for vitamins and minerals, USA and Canada, 1997–2001*

	Vitamin											Mineral						
Age	A (µg)	D (µg)	E (mg)	K (µg)	B_1 (mg)	B_2 (mg)	Niacin (mg)	B_6 (mg)	Folate (µg)	B_{12} (µg)	C (mg)	Ca (mg)	P (mg)	Fe (mg)	Zn (mg)	Cu (mg)	Se (µg)	I (µg)
0–6 months	400	5	4	2.0	0.2	0.3	2	0.1	65	0.4	40	210	100	–	2.0	200	15	110
7–12 months	500	5	5	2.5	0.3	0.4	4	0.3	80	0.5	50	270	275	11	3	220	20	130
1–3 years	300	5	6	30	0.5	0.5	6	0.5	150	0.9	15	500	460	7	3	340	20	90
4–8 years	400	5	7	55	0.5	0.6	8	0.6	200	1.2	25	800	500	10	5	440	30	90
Males																		
9–13 years	600	5	11	60	0.9	0.9	12	1.0	300	1.8	45	1300	1250	8	8	700	40	120
14–18 years	900	5	15	75	1.2	1.3	16	1.3	400	2.4	75	1300	1250	11	11	890	55	150
19–30 years	900	5	15	120	1.2	1.3	16	1.3	400	2.4	90	1000	700	8	11	900	55	150
31–50 years	900	5	15	120	1.2	1.3	16	1.3	400	2.4	90	1000	700	8	11	900	55	150
51–70 years	900	10	15	120	1.2	1.3	16	1.7	400	2.4	90	1200	700	8	11	900	55	150
>70 years	900	15	15	120	1.2	1.3	16	1.7	400	2.4	90	1200	700	8	11	900	55	150
Females																		
9–13 years	600	5	11	60	0.9	0.9	12	1.0	300	1.8	45	1300	1250	8	8	700	40	120
14–18 years	700	5	15	75	1.0	1.0	14	1.2	400	2.4	65	1300	1250	15	9	890	55	150
19–30 years	700	5	15	90	1.1	1.1	14	1.3	400	2.4	75	1000	700	18	8	900	55	150
31–50 years	700	5	15	90	1.1	1.1	14	1.3	400	2.4	75	1000	700	18	8	900	55	150
51–70 years	700	10	15	90	1.1	1.1	14	1.5	400	2.4	75	1200	700	8	8	900	55	150
> 70 years	700	15	15	90	1.1	1.1	14	1.5	400	2.4	75	1200	700	8	8	900	55	150
Pregnant	770	5	15	90	1.4	1.4	18	1.9	600	2.6	85	1000	700	27	11	1000	60	220
Lactating	900	5	16	90	1.4	1.6	17	2.0	500	2.8	120	1000	700	9	12	1300	70	290

Figures for infants under 12 months are adequate intakes, based on the observed mean intake of infants fed principally on breast milk; for nutrients other than vitamin K figures are RDA, based on estimated average requirement + 2 SD; figures for vitamin K are adequate intakes, based on observed average intakes.

Sources: Standing Committee on the Scientific Evaluation of Dietary Reference Intakes, Food and Nutrition Board, Institute of Medicine: Dietary Reference Intakes for calcium, phosphorus, magnesium, vitamin D and fluoride, 1997; Dietary reference intakes for thiamin, riboflavin, niacin, vitamin B_6, folate, vitamin B_{12}, pantothenic acid, biotin and choline, 1998; Dietary reference intakes for vitamin C, vitamin E, selenium and carotenoids, 2000; Dietary Reference Intakes for vitamin A, vitamin K, arsenc, boron, chromium, copper, iodine, iron, manganese, molybdenum, nickel, silicon, vanadium and zinc, 2001, National Academy Press: Washington, DC.

The reference intakes of vitamins and minerals published in the USA, UK and European Union are shown in Tables 11.1–11.3.

11.1.1.1 Safe and adequate levels of intake

For some nutrients, such as the vitamins biotin (section 11.12) and pantothenic acid (section 11.13), and a number of trace minerals, deficiency is unknown except under experimental conditions. For these nutrients there are no estimates of average requirements, and therefore no reference intakes. As deficiency does not occur, it is obvious that average levels of intake are more than adequate to meet requirements. For these nutrients there is a range of intakes that is defined as safe and adequate, based on the observed range of intakes.

11.1.1.2 Labelling reference values

Reference intakes depend on age and gender. For nutritional labelling of foods it is obviously essential to have a single labelling reference value that will permit the consumer to compare the nutrient yields of different foods. Apart from foods aimed at infants and small children, for which age-related reference intakes are used, there are two ways of determining labelling reference values:

- To use the highest value of reference intake of any group in the population. This is the basis of labelling in the USA and (at present) the European Union. The disadvantage of this is that the highest reference intakes are considerably higher than are appropriate for most groups in the population, and therefore perfectly adequate foods may appear to be poor sources of nutrients, and consumers may be encouraged to take inappropriate and unnecessary supplements.
- To use the average requirement for adult men, which in most cases equals the reference intake for women. This is the approach favoured by the Scientific Committee for Food of the European Union but has not yet been adopted in EU labelling legislation.

11.1.2 THE VITAMINS

A vitamin is defined as an organic compound that is required in small amounts for the maintenance of normal metabolic function. Deficiency causes a specific disease, which is cured or prevented only by restoring the vitamin to the diet. This is important – it is not enough just to show that the compound has effects when added to the diet, as these may be pharmacological actions unrelated to the maintenance of normal health and metabolic integrity. The metabolic functions of all the vitamins are now known. Therefore, before a new substance could be accepted as a possible vitamin, there must be not only evidence that deprivation causes a specific deficiency disease that can be cured only with that compound, but also definition of a clear metabolic function.

As can be seen from Table 11.4, the vitamins are named in a curious way. This is a historical accident, and results from the way in which they were discovered. Studies at the beginning of the twentieth century showed that there was something in milk that was essential, in very small amounts, for the growth of animals fed on a diet consisting of purified fat, carbohydrate, protein and mineral salts. Two factors were found to be essential: one was found in the cream and the other in the watery part of milk. Logically, they were called factor A (fat-soluble, in the cream) and factor B (water-soluble, in the watery part of the milk). Factor B was identified chemically as an amine, and in 1913 the name 'vitamin' was coined for these 'vital amines'.

Further studies showed that 'vitamin B' was a mixture of a number of compounds, with different actions in the body, and so they were given numbers as well: vitamin B_1, vitamin B_2, and so on. There are gaps in the numerical order of the B vitamins. When what might have been called vitamin B_3 was discovered, it was found to be a chemical compound that was already known, nicotinic acid. It was therefore not given a number. Other gaps resulted because compounds that were assumed to be vitamins, and were given numbers, such as B_4, B_5, etc., were later shown either not to be vitamins or to be vitamins that had already been described by other workers and given other names.

Vitamins C, D and E were named in the order of their discovery. The name 'vitamin F' was used at one time for what we now call the essential fatty acids (section 4.3.1.1); 'vitamin G' was later found to be what was already known as vitamin B_2. Biotin is still sometimes called vitamin H.

As the chemistry of the vitamins was elucidated, so they were given names as well, as shown in Table 11.4. Where only one chemical compound has the biological activity of the vitamin, this is quite easy. Thus, vitamin B_1 is thiamin, vitamin B_2 is riboflavin, etc. However, in the case of several of the vitamins, a number of chemically related compounds found in foods can be interconverted in the body, and all show the same biological activity. Such chemically related compounds are called *vitamers*, and a general name (a generic descriptor) is used to include all compounds that display the same biological activity. Thus, niacin is the generic descriptor for two compounds, nicotinic acid and nicotinamide, which have the same biological activity. Vitamin B_6 is used to describe the six compounds that have vitamin B_6 activity.

Correctly, for a compound to be classified as a vitamin, it should be a dietary essential that cannot be synthesized in the body. By this strict definition, two vitamins should not really be included, as they can be made in the body. However, both were discovered as a result of investigations of deficiency diseases, and they are usually considered as vitamins:

- Vitamin D is made in the skin after exposure to sunlight (section 11.3.2.1) and should really be regarded as a steroid hormone rather than a vitamin. It is only when sunlight exposure is inadequate that a dietary source is required.
- Niacin (section 11.8.2) can be formed from the essential amino acid tryptophan. Indeed, synthesis from tryptophan is probably more important than a dietary intake of preformed niacin.

TABLE 11.4 *The vitamins*

Vitamin		Functions	Deficiency disease
A	Retinol β-Carotene	Visual pigments in the retina; regulation of gene expression and cell differentiation (β-carotene is an antioxidant)	Night blindness, xerophthalmia; keratinization of skin
D	Calciferol	Maintenance of calcium balance; enhances intestinal absorption of Ca^{2+} and mobilizes bone mineral	Rickets = poor mineralization of bone; osteomalacia = bone demineralization
E	Tocopherols Tocotrienols	Antioxidant, especially in cell membranes	Extremely rare – serious neurological dysfunction
K	Phylloquinone Menaquinones	Coenzyme in formation of γ-carboxyglutamate in enzymes of blood clotting and bone matrix proteins	Impaired blood clotting, haemorrhagic disease
B_1	Thiamin	Coenzyme in pyruvate and α-ketoglutarate dehydrogenases, and transketolase; poorly defined function in nerve conduction	Peripheral nerve damage (beriberi) or central nervous system lesions (Wernicke–Korsakoff syndrome)
B_2	Riboflavin	Coenzyme in oxidation and reduction reactions; prosthetic group of flavoproteins	Lesions of corner of mouth, lips and tongue, seborrhoeic dermatitis
Niacin	Nicotinic acid Nicotinamide	Coenzyme in oxidation and reduction reactions, functional part of NAD and NADP	Pellagra – photosensitive dermatitis, depressive psychosis
B_6	Pyridoxine Pyridoxal Pyridoxamine	Coenzyme in transamination and decarboxylation of amino acids and glycogen phosphorylase; role in steroid hormone action	Disorders of amino acid metabolism, convulsions
	Folic acid	Coenzyme in transfer of one-carbon fragments	Megaloblastic anaemia
B_{12}	Cobalamin	Coenzyme in transfer of one-carbon fragments and metabolism of folic acid	Pernicious anaemia = megaloblastic anaemia with degeneration of the spinal cord
	Pantothenic acid	Functional part of CoA and acyl carrier protein: fatty acid synthesis and metabolism	Peripheral nerve damage (burning foot syndrome)
H	Biotin	Coenzyme in carboxylation reactions in gluconeogenesis and fatty acid synthesis	Impaired fat and carbohydrate metabolism, dermatitis
C	Ascorbic acid	Coenzyme in hydroxylation of proline and lysine in collagen synthesis; antioxidant; enhances absorption of iron	Scurvy – impaired wound healing, loss of dental cement, subcutaneous haemorrhage

11.2 *Vitamin A*

Vitamin A was the first vitamin to be discovered, initially as an essential dietary factor for growth. It has roles in vision (as the prosthetic group of the light-sensitive proteins in the retina) and the regulation of gene expression and tissue differentiation. Deficiency is a major problem of public health in large areas of the world.

11.2.1 VITAMIN A VITAMERS AND INTERNATIONAL UNITS

Two groups of compounds, shown in Figure 11.2, have vitamin A activity: retinol, retinaldehyde and retinoic acid (preformed vitamin A); and a variety of carotenes and related compounds (collectively known as carotenoids), which can be cleaved oxidatively to yield retinaldehyde, and hence retinol and retinoic acid. Those carotenoids that can be cleaved to yield retinaldehyde are known as are known as pro-vitamin A carotenoids.

Retinol is found only in foods of animal origin and a small number of bacteria, mainly as the ester retinyl palmitate. Retinoic acid is a metabolite of retinol and has important biological activities in its own right. The oxidation of retinaldehyde to retinoic acid is irreversible, and retinoic acid cannot be converted to retinol *in vivo*, and does not support either vision or fertility in deficient animals.

Some 50 or more dietary carotenoids are potential sources of vitamin A: α-, β- and γ-carotenes and cryptoxanthin are quantitatively the most important. Although it would appear from its structure that one molecule of β-carotene will yield two of retinol, this is not so in practice (section 11.2.2.1); 6 μg of β-carotene is equivalent to 1 μg of preformed retinol. For other carotenes with vitamin A activity, 12 μg is equivalent to 1 μg of preformed retinol.

The total amount of vitamin A in foods is expressed as μg retinol equivalents, calculated from the sum of μg preformed vitamin A + $\frac{1}{6}$ × μg β-carotene + $\frac{1}{12}$ × μg other pro-vitamin A carotenoids.

Before pure vitamin A was available for chemical analysis, the vitamin A content of foods was determined by biological assays, and the results expressed in standardized international units (iu): 1 iu = 0.3 μg retinol, or 1 μg of retinol = 3.33 iu. Although obsolete, international units are sometimes still used in food labelling.

11.2.2 METABOLISM OF VITAMIN A
AND PRO-VITAMIN A CAROTENOIDS

Retinol is absorbed from the small intestine dissolved in lipid. About 70–90% of dietary retinol is normally absorbed, and even at high levels of intake this falls only slightly. Some 5–60% of dietary carotene is absorbed, depending on the nature of the food and whether it is cooked or raw. In people whose diet provides less than about 10% of energy from fat, absorption of both retinol and carotene is impaired, and very low-fat diets are associated with vitamin A deficiency.

FᴵɢᴜʀE 11.2 *Vitamin A – retinoids and pro-vitamin A carotenoids.*

Retinyl esters formed in the intestinal mucosa enter the lymphatic circulation, in chylomicrons (section 5.6.2.1) together with dietary lipid and carotenoids. Tissues can take up retinyl esters from chylomicrons, but most remains in the chylomicron remnants that are taken up by the liver. Here the esters are hydrolysed, and the vitamin may be either secreted from the liver bound to retinol-binding protein or transferred to stellate cells in the liver, where it is stored as esters in intracellular lipid droplets.

At normal levels of intake, most retinol is catabolized by oxidation to retinoic acid and excreted in the bile as retinoyl glucuronide. As the liver concentration or retinol rises above 70 µmol/kg, there is microsomal cytochrome P_{450}-dependent oxidation, leading to a number of polar metabolites, which are excreted in the urine and bile. At high intakes this pathway becomes saturated, and excess retinol is toxic because there is no further capacity for its catabolism and excretion.

11.2.2.1 Carotene dioxygenase and the formation of retinol from carotenes

As shown in Figure 11.3, β-carotene and other pro-vitamin A carotenoids are cleaved in the intestinal mucosa by carotene dioxygenase, yielding retinaldehyde, which is reduced to retinol, esterified and secreted in chylomicrons together with esters formed from dietary retinol.

Only a proportion of carotene is oxidized in the intestinal mucosa, and a significant amount enters the circulation in chylomicrons. Carotene in the chylomicron remnants is cleared by the liver; some is cleaved by hepatic carotene dioxygenase, and the remainder is secreted in VLDL and may be taken up and cleaved by carotene dioxygenase in a variety of tissues.

Central oxidative cleavage of β-carotene, as shown in Figure 11.3, should give rise to two molecules of retinaldehyde, which can be reduced to retinol. However, the biological activity of β-carotene, on a molar basis, is considerably lower than that of retinol, not twofold higher as might be expected. In addition to the relatively poor absorption of carotene from the diet, three factors may account for this:

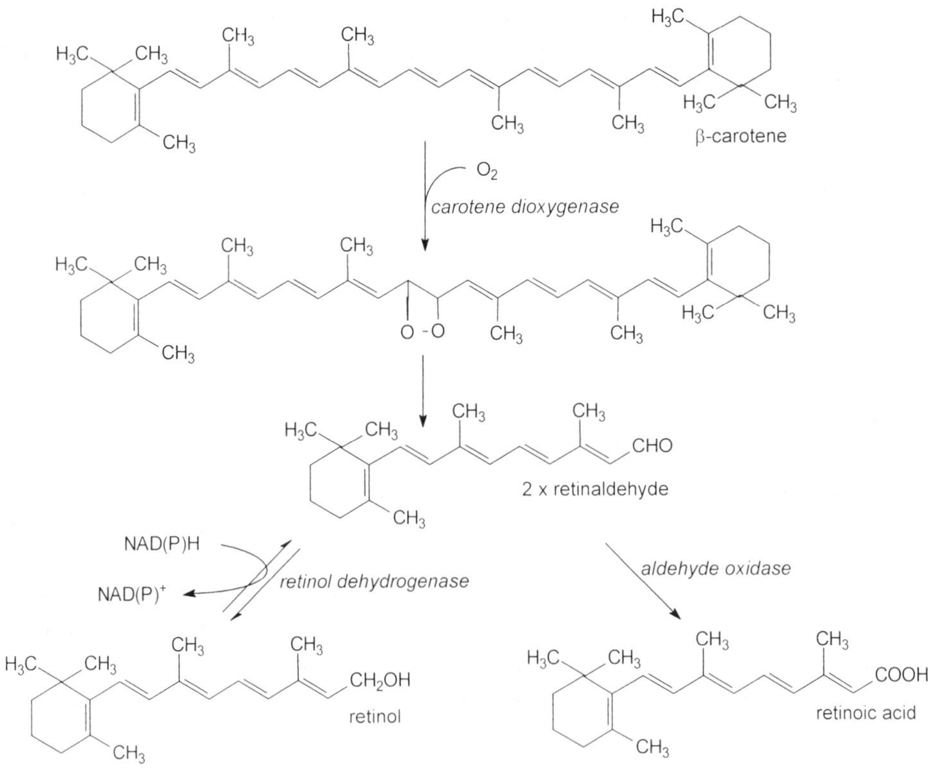

FIGURE 11.3 *The reaction of carotene dioxygenase.*

- The intestinal activity of carotene dioxygenase is relatively low, so that a relatively large proportion of ingested β-carotene may appear in the circulation unchanged. Although this has confounded attempts to prevent vitamin A deficiency by increasing intakes of dark-green leafy vegetables in developing countries, it also provides a measure of protection – although excessive intakes of preformed vitamin A are toxic, high intakes of carotene are not.
- Other carotenoids in the diet, which are not substrates, such as canthaxanthin and zeaxanthin, may inhibit carotene dioxygenase and reduce the proportion that is converted to retinol.
- While the principal site of carotene dioxygenase attack is the central bond of β-carotene, asymmetric cleavage may also occur, leading to the formation of 8′-, 10′- and 12′-apo-carotenals, which are oxidized to retinoic acid but cannot be used as sources of retinol or retinaldehyde.

11.2.2.2 Plasma retinol-binding protein (RBP)

Retinol is released from the liver bound to an α-globulin, retinol-binding protein (RBP); this serves to maintain the vitamin in aqueous solution, protects it against oxidation and also delivers the vitamin to target tissues. RBP is secreted from the liver as a 1:1 complex with the thyroxine-binding prealbumin, transthyretin. This is important to prevent urinary loss of retinol bound to the relatively small RBP, which would otherwise be filtered by the kidney, with a considerable loss of vitamin A from the body.

Cell-surface receptors on target tissues take up retinol from the RBP–transthyretin complex. The cell-surface receptors also remove the carboxy-terminal arginine residue from RBP, so inactivating it by reducing its affinity for both transthyretin and retinol. The apoprotein is not recycled; it is filtered at the glomerulus, reabsorbed in the proximal renal tubules and then hydrolysed.

11.2.3 METABOLIC FUNCTIONS OF VITAMIN A AND CAROTENES

The best-known function of vitamin A, and historically the first to be defined, is in vision. More recently, retinoic acid has also been shown to have a major function in regulation of gene expression and tissue differentiation.

At least *in vitro*, and under conditions of low oxygen availability, carotenes can act as radical-trapping antioxidants (section 7.4.3.4), and there is epidemiological evidence that associates high intakes of carotene with a low incidence of cardiovascular disease and some forms of cancer, although the results of intervention trials with β-carotene have been disappointing.

11.2.3.1 Vitamin A in vision

In the retina, retinaldehyde functions as the prosthetic group of the light-sensitive opsin proteins, forming rhodopsin (in rods) and iodopsin (in cones). Any one cone cell contains only one type of opsin and is sensitive to only one colour of light. Colour blindness results from loss or mutation of one or other of the cone opsins.

In the pigment epithelium of the retina, all-*trans*-retinol is isomerized to 11-*cis*-retinol and oxidized to 11-*cis*-retinaldehyde. This reacts with a lysine residue in opsin, forming the holoprotein rhodopsin. Opsins are cell type specific; they shift the absorption of 11-*cis*-retinaldehyde from the ultraviolet (UV) into what we call, in consequence, the visible range – either a relatively broad spectrum of sensitivity for vision in dim light (in the rods) or more defined spectral peaks for differentiation of colours in bright light (in the cones).

As shown in Figure 11.4, the absorption of light by rhodopsin causes isomerization of the retinaldehyde bound to opsin from 11-*cis* to all-*trans* and a conformational change in opsin. This results in the release of retinaldehyde from the protein and the initiation of a nerve impulse. The overall process is known as bleaching, as it results in the loss of the colour of rhodopsin.

The all-*trans*-retinaldehyde released from rhodopsin is reduced to all-*trans*-retinol and joins the pool of retinol in the pigment epithelium for isomerization to 11-*cis*-retinol and regeneration of rhodopsin. The key to initiation of the visual cycle is the availability of 11-*cis*-retinaldehyde, and hence vitamin A. In deficiency both the time taken to adapt to darkness and the ability to see in poor light are impaired.

The formation of the initial excited form of rhodopsin, bathorhodopsin, occurs within picoseconds of illumination and is the only light-dependent step in the visual cycle. Thereafter, there is a series of conformational changes leading to the formation of metarhodopsin II. The conversion of metarhodopsin II to metarhodopsin III is relatively slow, with a time-course of minutes. The final step is hydrolysis to release all-*trans*-retinaldehyde and opsin.

Metarhodopsin II is the excited form of rhodopsin, which initiates a guanine nucleotide amplification cascade (section 10.3.1) and then initiates a nerve impulse.

11.2.3.2 Retinoic acid and the regulation of gene expression

The most important function of vitamin A is in the control of cell differentiation and turnover. All-*trans*-retinoic acid and 9-*cis*-retinoic acid (Figure 11.3) act in the regulation of growth, development and tissue differentiation; they have different actions in different tissues. Like the steroid hormones (section 10.4) and vitamin D (section 11.3.3), retinoic acid binds to nuclear receptors that bind to response elements (control regions) of DNA and regulate the transcription of specific genes.

As shown in Figure 11.5, there are two families of nuclear retinoid receptors: the retinoic acid receptors (RAR) bind all-*trans*-retinoic acid or 9-*cis*-retinoic acid and the retinoid X receptors (RXR) bind 9-*cis*-retinoic acid. Retinoic acid is involved in the regulation of a wide variety of genes; there are three types of activated retinoid receptor dimers, which bind to different response elements on DNA:

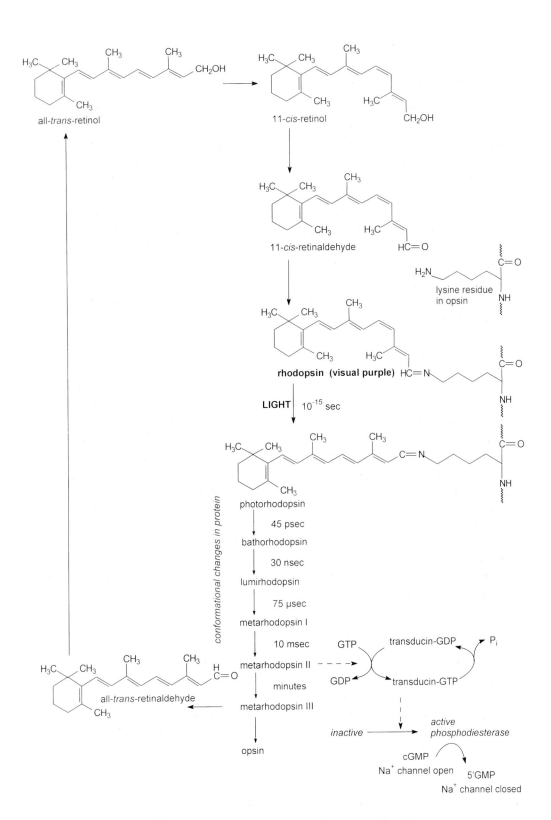

FIGURE 11.4 *The role of retinaldehyde in the visual cycle.*

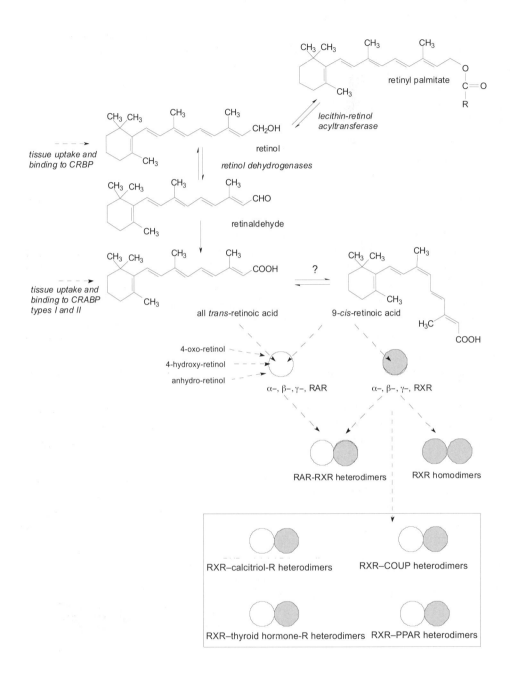

retinyl palmitate

*lecithin-retinol
acyltransferase*

CH₂OH

retinol

*tissue uptake and
binding to CRBP*

retinol dehydrogenases

CHO

retinaldehyde

COOH

?

*tissue uptake and
binding to CRABP
types I and II*

all *trans*-retinoic acid

9-*cis*-retinoic acid

4-oxo-retinol
4-hydroxy-retinol
anhydro-retinol

α–, β–, γ–, RAR

α–, β–, γ–, RXR

RAR-RXR heterodimers

RXR homodimers

RXR–calcitriol-R heterodimers

RXR–COUP heterodimers

RXR–thyroid hormone-R heterodimers

RXR–PPAR heterodimers

FIGURE 11.5 *Retinoic acid and retinoid receptors.*

- RXR can form homodimers (i.e. RXR–RXR dimers).
- They can form RAR–RXR heterodimers.
- RXR can form heterodimers with a wide variety of other nuclear-acting receptors, including those for vitamin D (section 11.3.3), thyroid hormone (section 11.15.3.3), long-chain polyunsaturated fatty acids derivatives (the so-called PPAR receptor) and one for which the physiological ligand has not yet been identified (the COUP receptor).

11.2.4 VITAMIN A DEFICIENCY –
NIGHT BLINDNESS AND XEROPHTHALMIA

World-wide, vitamin A deficiency is a major public health problem and the most important preventable cause of blindness. Table 11.5 shows the numbers of pre-school children at risk of, or suffering from, deficiency.

The earliest signs of deficiency are connected with vision. Initially, there is a loss of sensitivity to green light; this is followed by impairment of the ability to adapt to dim light, followed by inability to see at all in dim light: night blindness. More prolonged or severe deficiency leads to the condition called xerophthalmia: keratinization of the cornea, followed by ulceration – irreversible damage to the eye that causes blindness. At the same time there are changes in the skin, again with excessive formation of keratinized tissue.

Vitamin A also has an important role in the differentiation of immune system cells, and mild deficiency, not severe enough to cause any disturbance of vision, leads to increased susceptibility to a variety of infectious diseases. At the same time, the synthesis of RBP is reduced in response to infection (it is a negative acute-phase protein), so that there is a reduction in the circulating concentration of the vitamin, and hence further impairment of immune responses.

Signs of vitamin A deficiency also occur in protein–energy malnutrition (section 8.2), regardless of whether or not the intake of vitamin A is adequate. This is due to impairment of the synthesis of RBP. Hence, functional vitamin A deficiency can occur secondary to protein–energy malnutrition. In this case, there is severely impaired immunity to infection, as a result of both the functional vitamin A deficiency and also the impairment of immune responses associated with undernutrition.

TABLE 11.5 *Millions of children at risk of, or suffering from, vitamin A deficiency*

	At risk	**Children with xerophthalmia**
South-East Asia	138	10.0
Western Pacific	19	1.4
Africa	18	1.3
Eastern Mediterranean	13	1.0
Americas	2	0.1
Europe	–	–

Source: World Health Organization data, 1995.

11.2.5 VITAMIN A REQUIREMENTS AND REFERENCE INTAKES

There have been relatively few studies of vitamin A requirements in which subjects have been depleted of the vitamin for long enough to permit the development of clear deficiency signs. Current estimates of requirements are based on the intakes required to maintain a concentration of 70 µmol retinol per kg in the liver, as determined by measurement of the rate of metabolism of isotopically labelled vitamin A. This is adequate to maintain normal plasma concentrations of the vitamin, and people with this level of liver reserves can be maintained on a vitamin A-free diet for many months before they develop any detectable signs of deficiency.

The average requirement to maintain a concentration of 70 µmol per kg of liver is 6.7 µg retinol equivalents per kg body weight, and this is the basis for calculation of reference intakes.

11.2.5.1 Assessment of vitamin A status

In field surveys, clinical signs of vitamin A deficiency can be used to identify those suffering from vitamin A deficiency. The earliest signs of corneal damage are detected by conjunctival impression cytology; abnormalities develop only when liver reserves are seriously depleted.

The ability to adapt to dim light is impaired early in deficiency, and dark adaptation time is sometimes used to assess vitamin A status. The test is not suitable for use on children (the group most at risk of deficiency) and the apparatus is not suited to use in the field.

The plasma concentration of vitamin A falls only when the liver reserves are nearly depleted. In deficiency there is accumulation of apo-RBP in the liver, which can only be secreted when vitamin A is available. This provides the basis for the relative dose–response test for vitamin A status – the ability of a dose of retinol to raise the plasma concentration several hours later, after chylomicrons have been cleared from the circulation.

11.2.5.3 Toxicity of vitamin A

Although there is an increase in the rate of metabolism and excretion of retinol as the concentration in the liver rises above 70 µmol/kg, there is only a limited capacity to metabolize the vitamin. Excessively high intakes led to accumulation in the liver and other tissues, beyond the capacity of normal binding proteins, so that free, unbound, vitamin A is present, leading to tissue damage.

Single doses of 60 mg of retinol are given to children in developing countries as prophylaxis against vitamin A deficiency – an amount adequate to meet the child's needs for 4–6 months. About 1% of children so treated show transient signs of toxicity, but this is considered an acceptable risk in view of the high prevalence and devastating effects of deficiency.

The chronic toxicity of vitamin A is a more general cause for concern; prolonged and regular intake of more than about 7.5–9 mg/day by adults (and significantly less for children) causes signs and symptoms of toxicity affecting:

- the central nervous system: headache, nausea, ataxia and anorexia, all associated with increased cerebrospinal fluid pressure;
- the liver: hepatomegaly with histological changes in the liver, increased collagen formation and hyperlipidaemia;
- bones: joint pains, thickening of the long bones, hypercalcaemia and calcification of soft tissues;
- the skin: excessive dryness, scaling and chapping of the skin, desquamation and alopecia.

The recommended upper limits of habitual intake of retinol, compared with reference intakes, are shown in Table 11.6.

The synthetic retinoids 13-*cis*-retinoic acid and etretinate are highly teratogenic in experimental animals and human beings. After women have been treated with them for dermatological problems, it is generally recommended that contraceptive precautions be continued for 12 months, because of the retention of retinoids in the body. By extrapolation, it has been assumed that retinol is also teratogenic, although there is little evidence; pregnant women are advised not to consume more than 3300 μg of preformed vitamin A per day.

High intakes of carotene are not known to have any adverse effects, apart from giving an orange–yellow colour to the skin. However, in two intervention studies in the 1990s with supplements of β-carotene, there was increased mortality from lung cancer in those receiving the supplements. It is likely that under conditions of high oxygen availability β-carotene (and presumably also other carotenoids) has a more marked pro-oxidant action than an antioxidant action (section 7.4.3.4).

TABLE 11.6 *Recommended upper limits of habitual intakes of preformed retinol*

	Upper limit of intake (μg/day)	RNI (μg/day)
Infants	900	350
1–3 years	1800	400
4–6 years	3000	500
6–12 years	4500	500
13–20 years	6000	600–700
Adult men	9000	700
Adult women	7500	600
Pregnant women	3300	700

11.3 *Vitamin D*

Vitamin D is not strictly a vitamin, as it can be synthesized in the skin, and indeed under most conditions endogenous synthesis is the major source of the vitamin – it is only when sunlight exposure is inadequate that a dietary source is required. Its main function is in the regulation of calcium absorption and homeostasis; most of its actions are mediated by way of nuclear receptors that regulate gene expression. Deficiency, leading to rickets in children and osteomalacia in adults, continues to be a problem in northern latitudes, where sunlight exposure is poor.

11.3.1 VITAMERS AND INTERNATIONAL UNITS

The normal dietary form of vitamin D is cholecalciferol (also known as calciol). This is also the compound that is formed in the skin by UV irradiation of 7-dehydrocholesterol. Some foods are enriched or fortified with the synthetic compound ergocalciferol, which is synthesized by UV irradiation of the steroid ergosterol. Ergocalciferol undergoes the same metabolism as cholecalciferol, and has the same biological activity. Early studies assigned the name vitamin D_1 to an impure mixture of products derived from the irradiation of ergosterol; when ergocalciferol was identified it was called vitamin D_2, and when the physiological compound was identified as cholecalciferol it was called vitamin D_3.

Like vitamin A, vitamin D was originally measured in international units of biological activity before the pure compound was isolated: 1 iu = 25 ng of cholecalciferol; 1 μg of cholecalciferol = 40 iu.

There are relatively few sources of vitamin D, mainly oily fish, with eggs, liver and butter providing modest amounts. As a result, strict vegetarians are at risk of deficiency, especially in northern latitudes with little sunlight exposure.

Although meat provides apparently negligible quantities of vitamin D, it may be an important source, as what is present is largely the final active metabolite, calcitriol, which is many-fold more potent on a molar basis than is cholecalciferol.

11.3.2 ABSORPTION AND METABOLISM OF VITAMIN D

Like vitamin A, dietary vitamin D is absorbed in lipid micelles and incorporated into chylomicrons; therefore people consuming a low-fat diet will absorb little of such dietary vitamin D as is available.

11.3.2.1 Synthesis of vitamin D in the skin

As shown in Figure 11.6, the steroid 7-dehydrocholesterol (an intermediate in the synthesis of cholesterol that accumulates in the skin but not other tissues), undergoes a non-enzymic reaction on exposure to UV light, yielding previtamin D. This undergoes

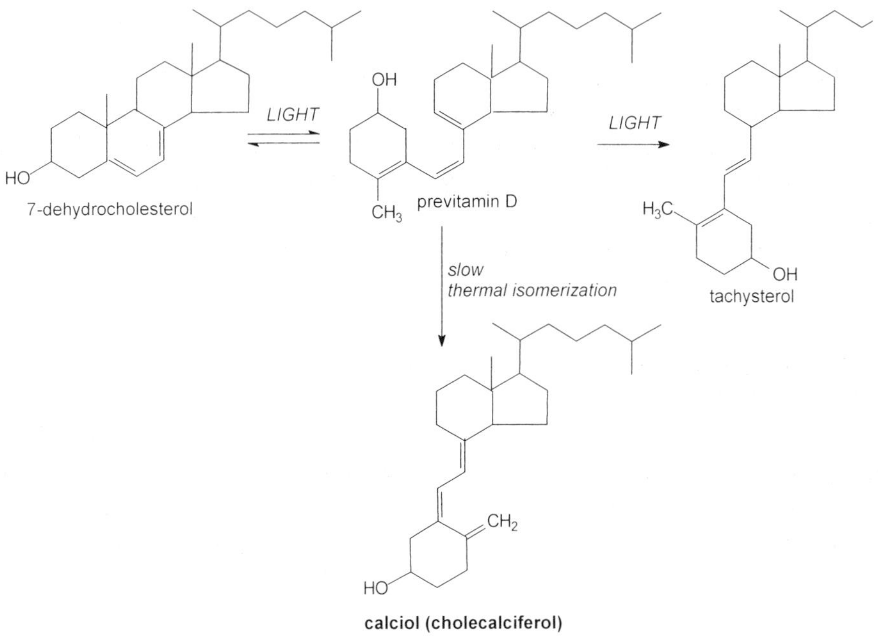

FIGURE 11.6 *The synthesis of vitamin D in the skin.*

a further reaction over a period of hours to form cholecalciferol, which is absorbed into the bloodstream. The photolytic reaction occurs with radiation in the UV-B range, between 290 and 310 nm, with a relatively sharp peak at 296.5 nm.

In temperate climates there is a marked seasonal variation in the plasma concentration of vitamin D; it is highest at the end of summer and lowest at the end of winter. Although there may be bright sunlight in winter, beyond about 40°N or 40°S there is very little UV radiation of the appropriate wavelength for cholecalciferol synthesis when the sun is low in the sky. By contrast, in summer, when the sun is more or less overhead, there is a considerable amount of UV light even on a moderately cloudy day, and enough can penetrate thin clothes to result in significant formation of vitamin D.

In northerly climates, and especially in polluted industrial cities with little sunlight, people may not be exposed to enough UV light to meet their vitamin D needs and will be reliant on the few dietary sources of the vitamin.

11.3.2.2 Metabolism to the active metabolite, calcitriol

Cholecalciferol, either synthesized in the skin or taken in from foods, undergoes two hydroxylations to yield the active metabolite, 1,25-dihydroxyvitamin D or calcitriol, as shown in Figure 11.7. Ergocalciferol from fortified foods undergoes similar hydroxylation to yield ercalcitriol. The nomenclature of the vitamin D metabolites is shown in Table 11.7.

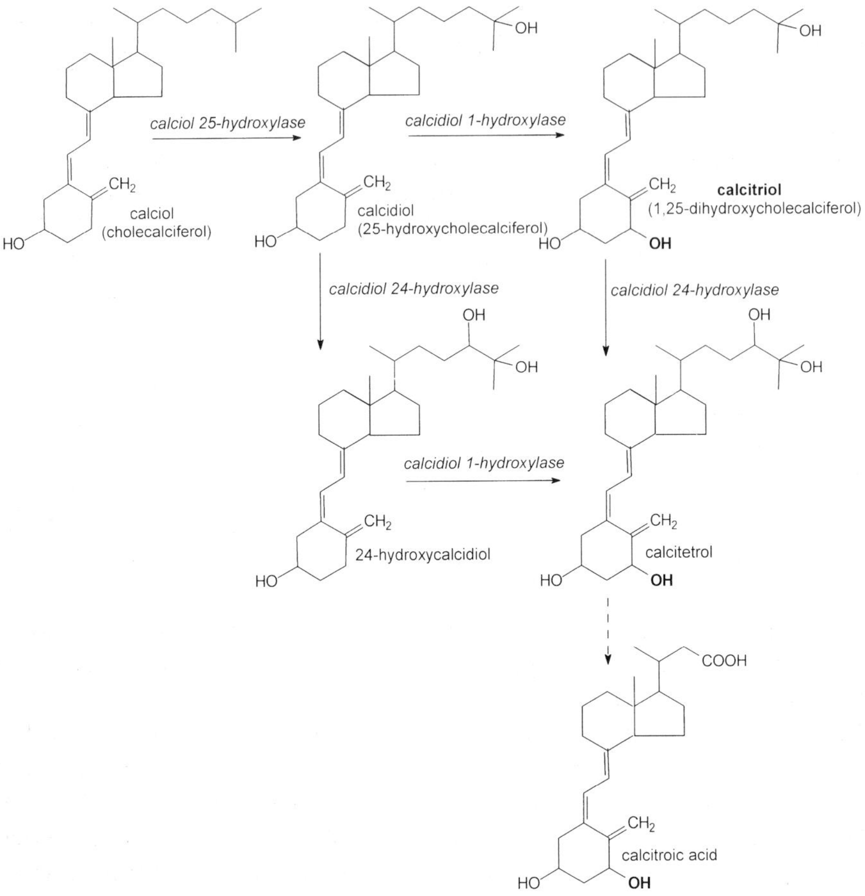

FIGURE 11.7 *Metabolism of vitamin D.*

The first stage in vitamin D metabolism occurs in the liver, where it is hydroxylated to form the 25-hydroxy derivative, calcidiol. This is released into the circulation bound to a vitamin D-binding globulin. There is no tissue storage of vitamin D; plasma calcidiol is the main storage form of the vitamin, and it is plasma calcidiol that shows the most significant seasonal variation in temperate climates.

The second stage of vitamin D metabolism occurs in the kidney, where calcidiol undergoes either 1-hydroxylation to yield the active metabolite 1,25-dihydroxyvitamin D (calcitriol) or 24-hydroxylation to yield an apparently inactive metabolite, 24,25-dihydroxyvitamin D (24-hydroxycalcidiol).

The main function of vitamin D is in the control of calcium homeostasis (section 11.15.1) and, in turn, vitamin D metabolism is regulated, at the level of 1- or 24-hydroxylation, by factors that respond to plasma concentrations of calcium and phosphate:

TABLE 11.7 *Nomenclature of vitamin D metabolites*

Trivial name	Recommended name	Abbreviation
Vitamin D$_3$		
Cholecalciferol	Calciol	–
25-Hydroxycholecalciferol	calcidiol	$25(OH)D_3$
1α-Hydroxycholecalciferol	1(S)-Hydroxycalciol	$1α(OH)D_3$
24,25-Dihydroxycholecalciferol	24(R)-Hydroxycalcidiol	$24,25(OH)_2D_3$
1,25-Dihydroxycholecalciferol	Calcitriol	$1,25(OH)_2D_3$
1,24,25-Trihydroxycholecalciferol	Calcitetrol	$1,24,25(OH)_3D_3$
Vitamin D$_2$		
Ergocalciferol	Ercalciol	–
25-Hydroxyergocalciferol	Ercalcidiol	$25(OH)D_2$
24,25-Dihydroxyergocalciferol	24(R)-Hydroxyercalcidiol	$24,25(OH)_2D_2$
1,25-Dihydroxyergocalciferol	Ercalcitriol	$1,25(OH)_2 D_2$
1,24,25-Trihydroxyergocalciferol	Ercalcitetrol	$1,24,25(OH)_3D_2$

The abbreviations shown in column 3 are not recommended but are frequently used in the literature.

- Calcitriol acts to reduce its own synthesis. It induces the 24-hydroxylase and represses the synthesis of 1-hydroxylase in the kidney, acting on gene expression by way of calcitriol receptors.
- Parathyroid hormone is secreted in response to a fall in plasma calcium. In the kidney it acts to increase the activity of calcidiol 1-hydroxylase and decrease that of the 24-hydroxylase. This is not an effect on protein synthesis, but the result of changes in the activity of existing enzyme protein, mediated by cAMP (section 10.3.2). In turn, both calcitriol and high concentrations of calcium repress the synthesis of parathyroid hormone.
- Calcium exerts its main effect on the synthesis and secretion of parathyroid hormone. However, calcium ions also have a direct effect on the kidney, reducing the activity of calcidiol 1-hydroxylase (but with no effect on the activity of 24-hydroxylase).

11.3.3 METABOLIC FUNCTIONS OF VITAMIN D

Calcitriol acts like a steroid hormone, binding to a nuclear receptor protein (section 10.4). The calcitriol–receptor complex then binds to the enhancer site of the gene coding for a calcium-binding protein, increasing its transcription and so increasing the amount of calcium-binding protein in the cell.

The principal function of vitamin D is to maintain the plasma concentration of calcium. Calcitriol achieves this in three ways:

- increased intestinal absorption of calcium;
- reduced excretion of calcium (by stimulating resorption in the distal renal tubules);
- mobilization of bone mineral.

In addition, calcitriol has a variety of permissive or modulatory effects. It is a necessary, but not sufficient, factor, in:

- insulin secretion;
- synthesis and secretion of parathyroid and thyroid hormones;
- inhibition of production of interleukin by activated T-lymphocytes and of immunoglobulin by activated B-lymphocytes;
- differentiation of monocyte precursor cells.
- modulation of cell proliferation.

In all of these actions, the role of calcitriol seems to be the induction or maintenance of synthesis of calcium-binding proteins, and the effects are secondary to increased calcium uptake into the target cells. Several of these actions are also modulated by vitamin A; as discussed in section 11.2.3.2, vitamin A (RXR) receptors form heterodimers with calcitriol receptors, so that both vitamins are required together for some actions.

The best-studied actions of vitamin D are in the intestinal mucosa, where the intracellular calcium-binding protein is essential for the absorption of calcium from the diet. Here the vitamin has another action as well: to increase the transport of calcium across the mucosal membrane. The increase in transport of calcium is seen immediately after feeding vitamin D, whereas the increase in absorption is a slower response, as it depends on new synthesis of the binding protein. The rapid response to vitamin D does not involve new protein synthesis, but presumably reflects an effect on preformed calcium transport proteins in the cell membrane.

11.3.3.1 The role of calcitriol in bone metabolism

The maintenance of bone structure is due to balanced activity of osteoclasts, which erode existing bone mineral and organic matrix, and osteoblasts, which synthesize and secrete the proteins of bone matrix. Mineralization of the organic matrix is largely controlled by the availability of calcium and phosphate.

Calcitriol raises plasma calcium by activating osteoclasts to stimulate the mobilization of calcium from bone. It acts later to stimulate the laying down of new bone to replace the loss, by stimulating the differentiation and recruitment of osteoblast cells.

11.3.4 VITAMIN D DEFICIENCY: RICKETS AND OSTEOMALACIA

Historically, rickets is a disease of toddlers, especially in northern industrial cities. Their bones are undermineralized, as a result of poor absorption of calcium in the absence of adequate amounts of calcitriol. When the child begins to walk, the long bones of the legs are deformed, leading to bow-legs or knock knees. More seriously, rickets can also lead to collapse of the rib-cage and deformities of the bones of the pelvis. Similar problems may also occur in adolescents who are deficient in vitamin D during the adolescent growth spurt, when there is again a high demand for calcium for new bone formation.

Osteomalacia is the adult equivalent of rickets. It results from the demineralization of bone, rather than the failure to mineralize it in the first place, as is the case with rickets. Women who have little exposure to sunlight are especially at risk from osteomalacia after several pregnancies because of the strain that pregnancy places on their marginal reserve of calcium.

Osteomalacia also occurs in the elderly. Here again the problem may be inadequate exposure to sunlight, but there is also evidence that the capacity to form 7-dehydrocholesterol in the skin decreases with advancing age, so that the elderly are more reliant on the few dietary sources of vitamin D.

Although vitamin D is essential for prevention and treatment of osteomalacia in the elderly, there is little evidence that it is beneficial in treating or preventing the other common degenerative bone disease of advancing age, osteoporosis (section 11.15.1.1).

11.3.5 VITAMIN D REQUIREMENTS AND REFERENCE INTAKES

It is difficult to determine requirements for dietary vitamin D, as the major source is synthesis in the skin. The main criterion of adequacy is the plasma concentration of calcidiol. In elderly subjects with little sunlight exposure, a dietary intake of 10 μg of vitamin D per day results in a plasma calcidiol concentration of 20 nmol/L, the lower end of the reference range for younger adults at the end of winter. Therefore, the reference intake for the elderly is 10 μg/day. Average intakes of vitamin D are less than 4 μg/day, so to achieve an intake of 10 μg/day will almost certainly require either fortification of foods or the use of vitamin D supplements.

11.3.5.1 Vitamin D toxicity

During the 1950s, rickets was more or less totally eradicated in Britain and other temperate countries. This was due to enrichment of a large number of infant foods with vitamin D. However, a small number of infants suffered from vitamin D poisoning, the most serious effect of which is an elevated plasma concentration of calcium. This can lead to contraction of blood vessels, and hence dangerously high blood pressure, and calcinosis – the calcification of soft tissues, including the kidney, heart, lungs and blood vessel walls.

Some infants are sensitive to intakes of vitamin D as low as 50 μg/day. In order to avoid the serious problem of vitamin D poisoning in these susceptible infants, the fortification of infant foods with vitamin D was reduced considerably. Unfortunately, this means that a small proportion of infants who have relatively high requirements are at risk of developing rickets. The problem is to identify those who have high requirements and provide them with supplements.

The toxic threshold in adults is not known, but patients suffering from vitamin D intoxication who have been investigated were taking more than 250 μg of vitamin D per day.

Although excess dietary vitamin D is toxic, excessive exposure to sunlight does not lead to vitamin D poisoning. There is a limited capacity to form the precursor, 7-dehydrocholesterol, in the skin, and a limited capacity to take up cholecalciferol from the skin. Furthermore, prolonged exposure of previtamin D to UV light results in further reactions to yield biologically inactive compounds.

11.4   *Vitamin E*

Although vitamin E was identified as a dietary essential for animals in the 1920s, it was not until 1983 that it was clearly demonstrated to be a dietary essential for human beings. Unlike other vitamins, no unequivocal physiological function for vitamin E has been defined; it acts as a lipid-soluble antioxidant in cell membranes, but many of its functions can be replaced by synthetic antioxidants. As discussed in section 7.4.3.3, there is epidemiological evidence that high intakes of vitamin E are associated with a lower incidence of cardiovascular disease.

11.4.1 VITAMERS AND UNITS OF ACTIVITY

Vitamin E is the generic descriptor for two families of compounds, the tocopherols and the tocotrienols (Figure 11.8). The different vitamers have different biological potency, as shown in Table 11.8. The most active is α-tocopherol, and it is usual to express vitamin E intake in terms of milligrams of α-tocopherol equivalents. This is the sum of mg α-tocopherol + 0.5 × mg β-tocopherol + 0.1 × mg γ-tocopherol + 0.3 × mg α-tocotrienol. The other vitamers either occur in negligible amounts in foods or have negligible vitamin activity.

The obsolete international unit of vitamin E activity is still sometimes used: 1 iu = 0.67 mg α-tocopherol equivalent; 1 mg α-tocopherol = 1.49 iu.

Synthetic α-tocopherol does not have the same biological potency as the naturally occurring compound, because the side-chain of tocopherol has three centres of asymmetry (Figure 11.9), and when it is synthesized chemically the result is a mixture of the various isomers. In the naturally occurring compound all three centres of asymmetry have the *R*-configuration, and naturally occurring α-tocopherol is called all-*R*- or *RRR*-α-tocopherol.

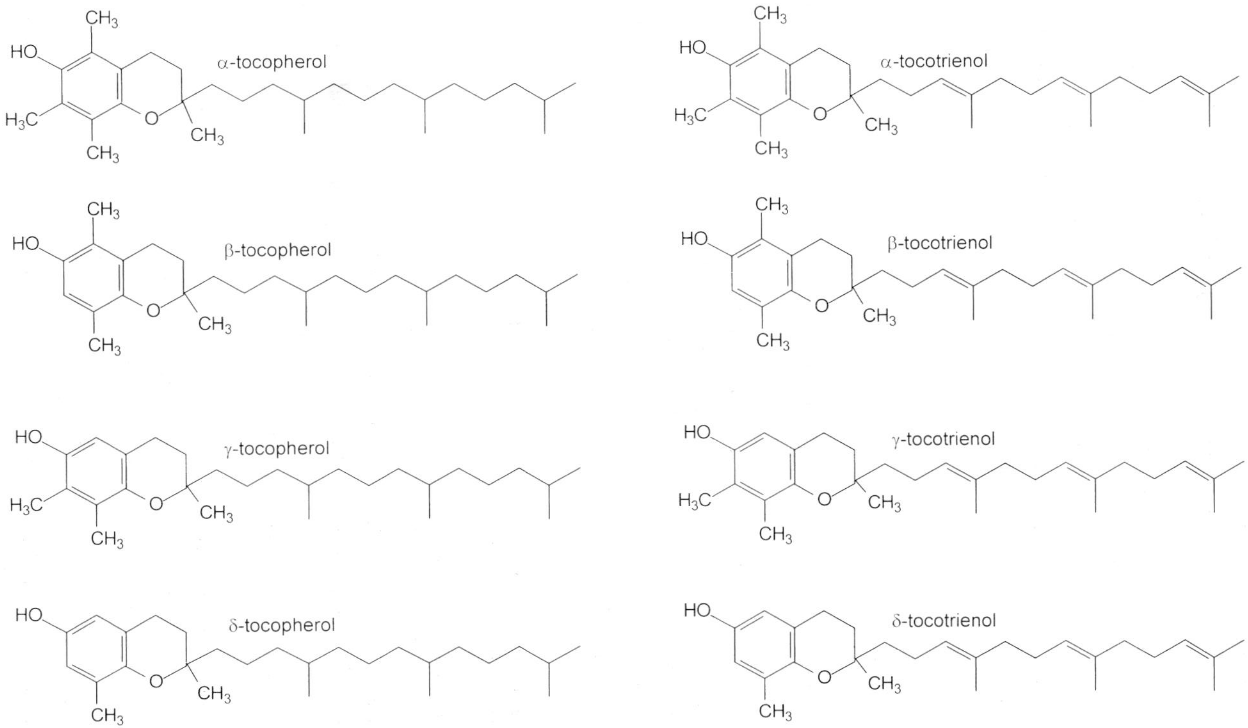

FIGURE 11.8 *Vitamin E vitamers.*

TABLE 11.8 *Relative biological activity of the vitamin E vitamers*

	iu/mg	Relative activity
D-α-Tocopherol (*RRR*)	1.49	1.00
D-β-Tocopherol (*RRR*)	0.75	0.49
D-γ-Tocopherol (*RRR*)	0.15	0.10
D-δ-Tocopherol (*RRR*)	0.05	0.03
D-α-Tocotrienol	0.45	0.29
D-β-Tocotrienol	0.08	0.05
D-γ-Tocotrienol	–	–
D-δ-Tocotrienol	–	–
L-α-Tocopherol (SRR)	0.46	0.31
RRS-α-Tocopherol	1.34	0.90
SRS-α-Tocopherol	0.55	0.37
RSS-α-Tocopherol	1.09	0.73
SSR-α-Tocopherol	0.31	0.21
RSR-α-Tocopherol	0.85	0.57
SSS-α-Tocopherol	1.10	0.74

11.4.2 ABSORPTION AND METABOLISM OF VITAMIN E

Tocopherols and tocotrienols are absorbed unchanged from the small intestine, in micelles with other dietary lipids. They are incorporated into chylomicrons (section 5.6.2.1), then secreted by the liver in VLDL. The major route of excretion is in the bile, largely as unidentified metabolites, including glucuronides and other conjugates. There may also be significant excretion of the vitamin by the skin.

There are two mechanisms for tissue uptake of vitamin E. Lipoprotein lipase releases the vitamin by hydrolysing the triacylglycerols in chylomicrons and VLDL, while separately there is uptake of LDL-bound vitamin E by means of LDL receptors. Retention within tissues depends on binding proteins, and it is likely that the differences in biological activity of the vitamers are due to differential protein binding. γ-Tocopherol and α-tocotrienol bind relatively poorly, whereas *SRR*-α-tocopherol and *RRR*-α-tocopherol acetate do not bind to liver tocopherol-binding protein to any significant extent.

11.4.3 METABOLIC FUNCTIONS OF VITAMIN E

The main function of vitamin E is as a radical-trapping antioxidant in cell membranes and plasma lipoproteins. It is especially important in limiting radical damage resulting from oxidation of polyunsaturated fatty acids, by reacting with the lipid peroxide radicals before they can establish a chain reaction. The radical formed from vitamin E is relatively unreactive and persists long enough to undergo reaction to yield non-radical products. Commonly, the vitamin E radical in a membrane or lipoprotein is

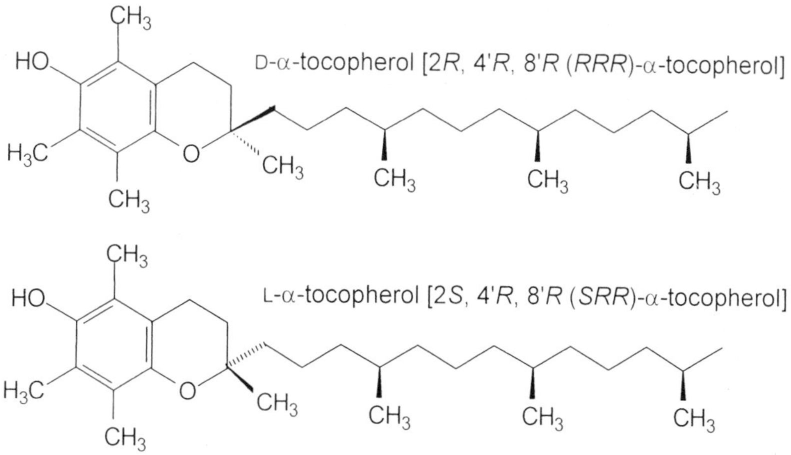

FIGURE 11.9 *Asymmetric centres in α-tocopherol.*

reduced back to tocopherol by reaction with vitamin C in plasma, as shown in Figure 7.17. The resultant monodehydroascorbate radical then undergoes enzymic or non-enzymic reaction to yield ascorbate and dehydroascorbate (see Figure 7.18), neither of which is a radical.

The antioxidant function of vitamin E is dependent on the stability of the tocopheroxyl radical, which means that it survives long enough to undergo reaction to yield non-radical products. However, this stability also means that the tocopheroxyl radical can penetrate further into cells, or deeper into plasma lipoproteins, and potentially propagate a chain reaction. Therefore, although it is regarded as an antioxidant, vitamin E may, like other antioxidants, also have pro-oxidant actions, especially at high concentrations. This may explain why, although epidemiological studies have shown a clear association between high blood concentrations of vitamin E and lower incidence of atherosclerosis, the results of intervention studies with relatively high doses of vitamin E have generally been disappointing (section 7.4.3.3).

There is a considerable overlap between the functions of vitamin E and selenium (section 11.15.2.5). As shown in Figure 7.17, vitamin E reduces lipid peroxide radicals to yield unreactive fatty acids; the selenium-dependent enzyme glutathione peroxidase reduces hydrogen peroxide to water (see Figure 5.15), thus lowering the intracellular concentration of potentially lipid-damaging peroxide. Glutathione peroxidase will also reduce the tocopheroxyl radical back to tocopherol. Thus, vitamin E acts to remove the products of lipid peroxidation, whereas selenium acts both to remove the cause of lipid peroxidation and also to recycle vitamin E. In vitamin E-deficient animals, selenium will prevent testicular atrophy, necrotizing myopathy and exudative diathesis but not central nervous system necrosis (section 11.4.4).

11.4.3.1 Hypocholesterolaemic actions of tocotrienols

Tocotrienols have lower biological activity that tocopherols, and indeed it is conventional to consider only γ-tocotrienol as a significant part of vitamin E intake. However, the tocotrienols have a hypocholesterolaemic action not shared by the tocopherols. In plants, tocotrienols are synthesized from hydroxymethylglutaryl CoA (HMG CoA), which is also the precursor for cholesterol synthesis (see Figure 7.21). High levels of tocotrienols reduce the activity of HMG CoA reductase, which is the rate-limiting enzyme in the pathway for synthesis of both cholesterol and tocotrienols, by repressing synthesis of the enzyme.

11.4.4 VITAMIN E DEFICIENCY

In experimental animals, vitamin E deficiency results in a number of different conditions:

- Deficient female animals suffer the death and resorption of the fetuses. This provided the basis of the original biological assay of vitamin E.
- In male animals, deficiency results in testicular atrophy and degeneration of the germinal epithelium of the seminiferous tubules.
- Both skeletal and cardiac muscle are affected in deficient animals. This is sometimes called nutritional muscular dystrophy. This is an unfortunate term as there is no evidence that human muscular dystrophy is related to vitamin E deficiency, and it is better called necrotizing myopathy.
- The integrity of blood vessel walls is affected, with leakage of blood plasma into subcutaneous tissues and accumulation under the skin of a green-coloured fluid – exudative diathesis.
- The nervous system is affected, with the development of central nervous system necrosis and axonal dystrophy. This is exacerbated by feeding diets rich in polyunsaturated fatty acids.

Dietary deficiency of vitamin E in human beings is unknown, although patients with severe fat malabsorption, cystic fibrosis, some forms of chronic liver disease or (very rare) congenital lack of plasma β-lipoprotein suffer deficiency because they are unable to absorb the vitamin or transport it around the body. They suffer from severe damage to nerve and muscle membranes.

Premature infants are at risk of vitamin E deficiency because they are often born with inadequate reserves of the vitamin. The red blood cell membranes of deficient infants are abnormally fragile as a result of unchecked oxidative radical attack. This may lead to haemolytic anaemia if they are not given supplements of the vitamin.

Experimental animals which are depleted of vitamin E become sterile. However, there is no evidence that vitamin E nutritional status is in any way associated with human fertility, and there is certainly no evidence that vitamin E supplements increase sexual potency, prowess or vigour.

11.4.5 VITAMIN E REQUIREMENTS

It is difficult to establish vitamin E requirements, partly because deficiency is more or less unknown but also because the requirement depends on the intake of polyunsaturated fatty acids. It is generally accepted, albeit with little experimental evidence, that an acceptable intake of vitamin E is 0.4 mg α-tocopherol equivalent per gram of dietary polyunsaturated fatty acid. This does not present any problem as the plant oils that are rich sources of polyunsaturated fatty acids are also rich sources of vitamin E.

11.4.5.1 Indices of vitamin E status

Erythrocytes are incapable of *de novo* lipid synthesis, so peroxidative damage resulting from oxygen stress has a serious effect, shortening red cell life and possibly precipitating haemolytic anaemia in vitamin E deficiency. This can be used as a method of assessing status (although unrelated factors affect the results) by measuring the haemolysis of red cells induced by dilute hydrogen peroxide.

An alternative method of assessing functional antioxidant status, again one that is affected by both vitamin E and other antioxidants, is by measuring the exhalation of pentane arising from the metabolism of the peroxides of ω-6 polyunsaturated fatty acids or ethane from peroxides of ω-3 polyunsaturated fatty acids.

11.5 *Vitamin K*

Vitamin K was discovered as a result of investigations into the cause of a bleeding disorder (haemorrhagic disease) of cattle fed on silage made from sweet clover and of chickens fed on a fat-free diet. The missing factor in the diet of the chickens was identified as vitamin K, while the problem in the cattle was that the feed contained dicoumarol, an antagonist of the vitamin. Because of its importance in blood coagulation, it was called the *koagulations-vitamine* (vitamin K) when the original results were reported (in German).

As the effect of an excessive intake of dicoumarol was severely impaired blood clotting, it was isolated and tested in low doses as an anticoagulant, for use in patients at risk of thrombosis. Although it was effective, it had unwanted side-effects, and synthetic vitamin K antagonists were developed for clinical use as anticoagulants. The most commonly used of these is warfarin, which is also used, in larger amounts, to kill rodents (see also Problem 9.2).

11.5.1 VITAMERS OF VITAMIN K

Three compounds have the biological activity of vitamin K (Figure 11.10):

*   phylloquinone, the normal dietary source, found in green leafy vegetables;
*   menaquinones, a family of related compounds synthesized by intestinal bacteria, with differing lengths of side-chain;
*   menadione and menadiol diacetate, synthetic compounds that can be metabolized to phylloquinone.

Phylloquinone is found in all green leafy vegetables, the richest sources being spring (collard) greens, spinach and Brussels sprouts. In addition, soybean, rapeseed, cottonseed and olive oils are relatively rich in vitamin K, although other oils are not.

About 80% of dietary phylloquinone is normally absorbed into the lymphatic system in chylomicrons, and is then taken up by the liver from chylomicron remnants and released into the circulation in VLDL.

Intestinal bacteria synthesize a variety of menaquinones, which are absorbed to a limited extent from the large intestine, again into the lymphatic system, cleared by the liver and released in VLDL. It is often suggested that about half the requirement for vitamin K is met by intestinal bacterial synthesis, but there is little evidence for this, other than the fact that about half the vitamin K in liver is phylloquinone and the remainder a variety of menaquinones. It is not clear to what extent the menaquinones are biologically active – it is possible to induce signs of vitamin K deficiency simply be feeding a phylloquinone-deficient diet without inhibiting intestinal bacterial action.

11.5.2 METABOLIC FUNCTIONS OF VITAMIN K

Although it had been known since the 1920s that vitamin K was required for blood clotting, it was not until the 1970s that its function was established. It is the cofactor for the carboxylation of glutamate residues in the post-synthetic modification of proteins to form the unusual amino acid γ-carboxyglutamate, abbreviated to Gla (Figure 11.11, and see also Problem 9.2).

The first step in the reaction is oxidation of vitamin K hydroquinone to the epoxide. This epoxide then activates a glutamate residue in the protein substrate to a carbanion that reacts non-enzymically with carbon dioxide to form γ-carboxyglutamate. Vitamin K epoxide is then reduced to the quinone by a warfarin-sensitive reductase, and the quinone is reduced to the active hydroquinone by either the same warfarin-sensitive reductase or a warfarin-insensitive quinone reductase.

In the presence of warfarin, vitamin K epoxide cannot be reduced back to the active hydroquinone, but accumulates, and is excreted as a variety of conjugates. If enough vitamin K is provided in the diet, the quinone can be reduced to the active

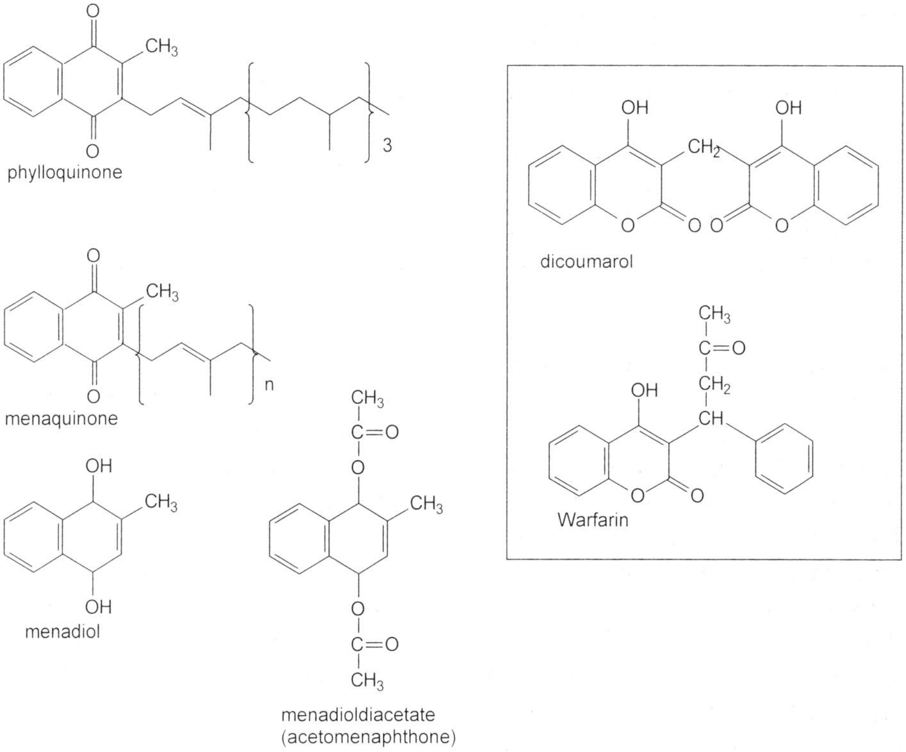

FIGURE 11.10 *Vitamin K vitamers; the vitamin K antagonists dicoumarol and warfarin are shown in the box. Menadione and menadiol diacetate are synthetic compounds that are converted to menaquinone in the liver and have vitamin activity..*

hydroquinone by the warfarin-insensitive enzyme, and carboxylation can continue, with stoichiometric utilization of vitamin K and excretion of the epoxide. High doses of vitamin K are used to treat patients who have received an overdose of warfarin, and at least part of the resistance of some populations of rats to the action of warfarin is due to a high consumption of vitamin K from maram grass, although there are also genetically resistant populations of rodents.

Prothrombin and several other proteins of the blood clotting system (factors VII, IX and X, and proteins C and S) each contain 4–6 γ-carboxyglutamate residues per mol. γ-Carboxyglutamate chelates calcium ions, and so permits the binding of the blood clotting proteins to membranes. In vitamin K deficiency, or in the presence of an antagonist such as warfarin, an abnormal precursor of prothrombin (preprothrombin) containing little or no γ-carboxyglutamate is released into the circulation. Preprothrombin cannot chelate calcium or bind to phospholipid membranes, and so is unable to initiate blood clotting. Preprothrombin is sometimes known as PIVKA – the protein induced by vitamin K absence.

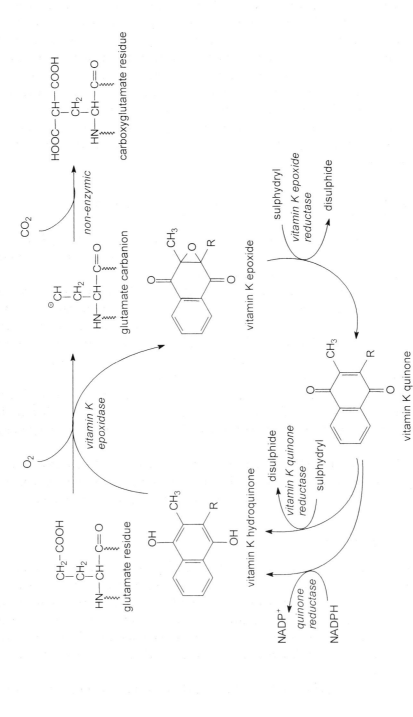

FIGURE 11.11 *The role of vitamin K in γ-carboxyglutamate synthesis.*

11.5.2.1 Bone vitamin K-dependent proteins

It has long been known that treatment of pregnant women with warfarin or other anticoagulants can lead to bone abnormalities in the child – the fetal warfarin syndrome. There are two proteins in bone matrix that contain γ-carboxyglutamate: osteocalcin and a less well-characterized protein known simply as bone matrix Gla protein. Osteocalcin is interesting in that, as well as γ-carboxyglutamate, it also contains hydroxyproline, so its synthesis is dependent on both vitamins K and C (section 11.14.2.2). In addition, its synthesis is induced by vitamin D, and the release into the circulation of osteocalcin provides a sensitive index of vitamin D action (section 11.3.3). Osteocalcin constitutes some 1–2% of total bone protein and, although it obviously functions as a calcium-binding protein and modifies the crystallization of bone mineral, its precise function remains unclear.

11.5.3 VITAMIN K DEFICIENCY AND REQUIREMENTS

Apart from deliberate experimental manipulation, vitamin K deficiency is unknown, and determination of requirements is complicated by a lack of data on the importance of menaquinones synthesized by intestinal bacteria.

The main way of determining vitamin K status, and monitoring the efficacy of anticoagulant therapy, is by measuring the time required for the formation of a fibrin clot in citrated blood plasma after the addition of calcium ions and thromboplastin – the prothrombin time. A more sensitive index is provided by direct measurement of preprothrombin in plasma, most commonly by immunoassay using antisera against preprothrombin that do not react with prothrombin.

Based on determination of clotting time, and direct measurement of prothrombin and preprothrombin, an intake of 1 μg per kg body weight per day is considered adequate; this forms the basis of reference intakes of between 65 and 80 μg/day for adults.

A small number of newborn infants have very low reserves of vitamin K and are at risk of potentially fatal haemorrhagic disease. It is therefore generally recommended that all neonates should be given a single prophylactic dose of vitamin K.

11.5.3.1 Toxicity of vitamin K

There is no evidence that phylloquinone has any significant toxicity. However, the synthetic analogue menadione can undergo non-enzymic redox cycling, and injection of menadione in newborn infants has been implicated in the later development of leukaemia. For this reason it is generally advised that prophylactic vitamin K given at birth should be as phylloquinone by mouth rather than menadione by injection. Menadione may also cause haemolytic anaemia, hyperbilirubinaemia and kernicterus in the newborn.

It was noted above (section 11.5.2) that high intakes of vitamin K can overcome the effects of warfarin and other anticoagulants, by permitting stoichiometric utilization of vitamin K for carboxylation of glutamate, with excretion of vitamin K epoxide. This means that patients who are being treated with warfarin could overcome the beneficial effects of their medication if they took supplements of vitamin K. The danger is that, if their dose of warfarin is increased to counteract the effects of the vitamin supplements and they then stop taking the supplements, they would be receiving considerably too much warfarin and would be at risk of haemorrhage. It is relatively unlikely that a normal diet could provide a sufficient excess of vitamin K to lead to problems.

11.6 *Vitamin B$_1$ (thiamin)*

Historically, thiamin deficiency affecting the peripheral nervous system (beriberi) was a major public health problem in South-East Asia following the introduction of the steam-powered mill that made highly polished (thiamin-depleted) rice widely available. There are still sporadic outbreaks of deficiency among people whose diet is rich in carbohydrate and poor in thiamin. More commonly, thiamin deficiency affecting the heart and central nervous system is a problem in people with an excessive consumption of alcohol – to the extent that there was it was seriously suggested in Australia at one time that thiamin should be added to beer.

The structures of thiamin and the coenzyme thiamin diphosphate are shown in Figure 11.12.

Like other water-soluble vitamins, thiamin is readily lost by leaching into cooking water. Furthermore, it is unstable to light and, although bread and flour contain significant amounts of thiamin, much or all of this can be lost when baked goods are exposed to sunlight in a shop window.

Thiamin is also destroyed by sulphites, and in potato products that have been blanched by immersion in sulphite solution there is little or no thiamin remaining. Polyphenols, including tannic acid in tea and betel nuts, also destroy thiamin and have been associated with thiamin deficiency.

11.6.1 ABSORPTION AND METABOLISM OF THIAMIN

Most dietary thiamin is present as phosphates, which are readily hydrolysed by intestinal phosphatases, and free thiamin is readily absorbed in the duodenum and proximal jejunum and then transferred to the portal circulation as free thiamin or thiamin monophosphate. This is an active transport process, and is inhibited by alcohol, which may explain why alcoholics are especially susceptible to thiamin deficiency.

Tissues take up both free thiamin and thiamin monophosphate, then phosphorylate them further to yield thiamin diphosphate (the active coenzyme) and thiamin

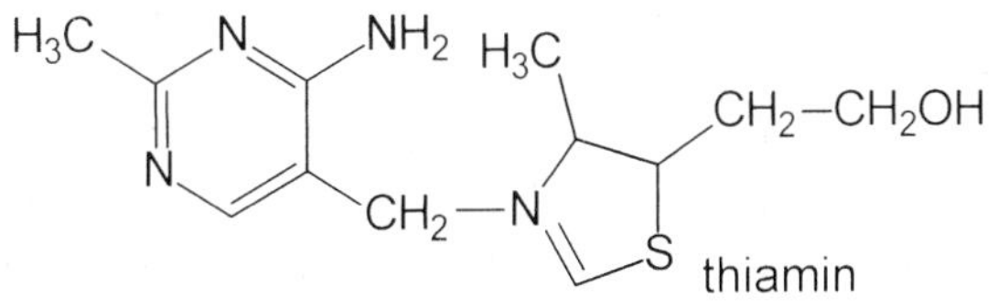

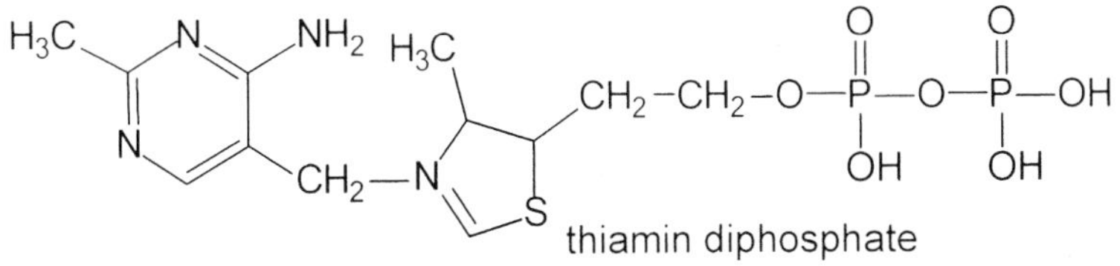

Figure 11.12 *Thiamin (vitamin B₁) and the coenzyme thiamin diphosphate.*

triphosphate. Some free thiamin is excreted in the urine, increasing with diuresis, and a significant amount may also be lost in sweat. Most urinary excretion is as thiochrome, the result of non-enzymic cyclization, as well as a variety of products of side-chain oxidation and ring cleavage.

There is little storage of thiamin in the body, and biochemical signs of deficiency can be observed within a few days of initiating a thiamin-free diet.

11.6.2 METABOLIC FUNCTIONS OF THIAMIN

Thiamin has a central role in energy-yielding metabolism, and especially the metabolism of carbohydrates. Thiamin diphosphate (also known as thiamin pyrophosphate; see Figure 11.12) is the coenzyme for three multienzyme complexes that catalyse oxidative decarboxylation of the substrate linked to reduction of enzyme-bound lipoamide, and eventually reduction of NAD^+ to NADH:

*   pyruvate dehydrogenase in carbohydrate metabolism (section 5.4.3.1 and Figure 5.16);
* α-ketoglutarate dehydrogenase in the citric acid cycle (section 5.4.4);
*   the branched-chain ketoacid dehydrogenase involved in the metabolism of leucine, isoleucine and valine.

Thiamin diphosphate is also the coenzyme for transketolase, in the pentose phosphate pathway of carbohydrate metabolism (section 5.4.2).

Thiamin triphosphate has a function in nerve conduction. Electrical stimulation of nerve leads to a fall in membrane thiamin triphosphate and release of free thiamin. It is likely that thiamin triphosphate acts as a phosphate donor for phosphorylation of the nerve membrane sodium transport channel.

11.6.3 THIAMIN DEFICIENCY

Thiamin deficiency can result in three distinct syndromes:

- a chronic peripheral neuritis, beriberi, which may or may not be associated with heart failure and oedema;
- acute pernicious (fulminating) beriberi (shoshin beriberi), in which heart failure and metabolic abnormalities predominate, with little evidence of peripheral neuritis;
- Wernicke's encephalopathy with Korsakoff's psychosis, a thiamin-responsive condition associated especially with alcohol and narcotic abuse.

In general, a relatively acute deficiency is involved in the central nervous system lesions of the Wernicke–Korsakoff syndrome, and a high energy intake, as in alcoholics, is also a predisposing factor. Dry beriberi is associated with a more prolonged, and presumably less severe, deficiency, with a generally low food intake, whereas higher carbohydrate intake and physical activity predispose to wet beriberi.

The role of thiamin diphosphate in pyruvate dehydrogenase means that in deficiency there is impaired conversion of pyruvate to acetyl CoA, and hence impaired entry of pyruvate into the citric acid cycle (section 5.4.3.1). Especially in subjects on a relatively high-carbohydrate diet, this results in increased plasma concentrations of lactate and pyruvate, which may lead to life-threatening lactic acidosis (see also Problem 5.2).

11.6.3.1 Dry beriberi

Chronic deficiency of thiamin, especially associated with a high-carbohydrate diet, results in beriberi, which is a symmetrical ascending peripheral neuritis. Initially the patient complains of weakness, stiffness and cramps in the legs and is unable to walk more than a short distance. There may be numbness of the dorsum of the feet and ankles, and vibration sense may be diminished. As the disease progresses, the ankle jerk reflex is lost, and the muscular weakness spreads upwards, involving first the extensor muscles of the foot, then the muscles of the calf, and finally the extensors and flexors of the thigh. At this stage there is pronounced toe and foot drop – the patient is unable to keep either the toe or the whole foot extended off the ground. When the arms are affected there is a similar inability to keep the hand extended – wrist drop.

The affected muscles become tender, numb and hyperaesthetic. The hyperaesthesia extends in the form of a band around the limb, the so-called stocking and glove distribution, and is followed by anaesthesia. There is deep muscle pain and, in the terminal stages, when the patient is bed-ridden, even slight pressure, as from bed clothes, causes considerable pain.

11.6.3.2 Wet beriberi

The heart may also be affected in beriberi, with dilatation of arterioles, rapid blood flow, increased pulse rate and pressure and increased jugular venous pressure leading to right-sided heart failure and oedema – so-called wet beriberi. The signs of chronic heart failure may be seen without peripheral neuritis. The arteriolar dilatation, and possibly also the oedema, probably result from high circulating concentrations of lactate and pyruvate as a result of impaired activity of pyruvate dehydrogenase.

11.6.3.3 Acute pernicious (fulminating) beriberi – shoshin beriberi

Heart failure without increased cardiac output, and no peripheral oedema, may also occur acutely, associated with severe lactic acidosis. This was a common presentation of deficiency in Japan, where it was called shoshin (= acute) beriberi; in the 1920s some 26,000 deaths a year were recorded.

With improved knowledge of the cause, and improved nutritional status, the disease had become more or less unknown, although in the 1980s it reappeared among Japanese adolescents consuming a diet based largely on such high-carbohydrate, low-nutrient foods as sweet carbonated drinks, 'instant' noodles and polished rice. It also occurs among alcoholics, when the lactic acidosis may be life-threatening, without clear signs of heart failure. Acute beriberi has also been reported when previously starved subjects are given intravenous glucose.

11.6.3.4 The Wernicke–Korsakoff syndrome

While peripheral neuritis and acute cardiac beriberi with lactic acidosis occur in thiamin deficiency associated with alcohol abuse, the more usual presentation is as the Wernicke–Korsakoff syndrome, due to central nervous system lesions. Initially there is a confused state, Korsakoff's psychosis, which is characterized by confabulation and loss of recent memory, although memory for past events may be unimpaired. Later, clear neurological signs develop – Wernicke's encephalopathy. This is characterized by nystagmus and extraocular palsy. Post-mortem examination shows characteristic brain lesions.

Like shoshin beriberi, Wernicke's encephalopathy can develop acutely, without the more gradual development of Korsakoff's psychosis, among previously starved patients given intravenous glucose and seriously ill patients given parenteral hyperalimentation.

11.6.4 THIAMIN REQUIREMENTS

Because thiamin has a central role in energy-yielding, and especially carbohydrate, metabolism, requirements depend mainly on carbohydrate intake, and have been related to 'non-fat' energy. In practice, requirements and reference intakes are calculated on the basis of total energy intake, assuming that the average diet provides 40% of energy from fat. For diets that are lower in fat content, and hence higher in carbohydrate and protein, thiamin requirements may be somewhat higher.

From depletion/repletion studies, an intake of at least 0.2 mg of thiamin per 1000 kcal is required to prevent the development of deficiency signs and maintain normal urinary excretion, but an intake of 0.23 mg/1000 kcal is required for a normal transketolase activation coefficient (section 11.6.4.1).

Reference intakes are calculated on the basis of 0.5 mg/1000 kcal (100 µg/MJ), with a minimum requirement for people with a low energy intake of 0.8–1.0 mg/day to allow for metabolism of endogenous substrates.

11.6.4.1 Assessment of thiamin status

The impairment of pyruvate dehydrogenase in thiamin deficiency results in a considerable increase in the plasma concentrations of lactate and pyruvate. This was formerly used as a means of assessing thiamin status, by measuring changes in the plasma concentrations of lactate and pyruvate after an oral dose of glucose and mild exercise, but is now little used.

For enzymes that have a tightly bound cofactor, such as thiamin diphosphate (and also riboflavin derivatives; see section 11.7 and vitamin B_6, section 11.9), the extent to which red blood cells can compete with other tissues for the vitamin-derived coenzyme provides a sensitive means of assessing nutritional status. Tissue contains:

- Enzyme protein with coenzyme bound (the holoenzyme) – this is catalytically active.
- Enzyme protein without coenzyme (the apoenzyme) – this is catalytically inactive.

Incubation of a red blood cell lysate without added coenzyme permits measurement of what was initially present as holoenzyme, whereas incubation after addition of coenzyme permits activation (and hence measurement) of the apoenzyme as well. The increase in catalytic activity after addition of coenzyme is the activation coefficient.

The activation of apo-transketolase in erythrocyte lysate by thiamin diphosphate added *in vitro* has become the most widely used and accepted index of thiamin nutritional status. An activation coefficient > 1.25 is indicative of deficiency, and < 1.15 is considered to reflect adequate thiamin nutrition.

11.7 *Vitamin B₂ (riboflavin)*

Riboflavin deficiency is a significant public health problem in many areas of the world. The vitamin has a central role as a coenzyme in energy-yielding metabolism, yet deficiency is rarely, if ever, fatal – there is very efficient conservation and recycling of riboflavin in deficiency. The structures of riboflavin and the riboflavin-derived coenzymes (also known as flavin coenzymes) are shown in Figures 2.14 and 2.15.

The main dietary sources of riboflavin are milk and dairy products, which provide 25% or more of the total intake in most diets, and it is noteworthy that average riboflavin status in different countries reflects milk consumption to a considerable extent. In addition, because of its intense yellow colour, riboflavin is widely used as a food colour.

Photolysis of riboflavin leads to the formation of lumiflavin (in alkaline solution) and lumichrome (in acidic or neutral solution), both of which are biologically inactive. Exposure of milk in clear-glass bottles to sunlight or fluorescent light (with a peak wavelength of 400–550 nm) can result in the loss of nutritionally important amounts of riboflavin. Lumiflavin and lumichrome catalyse oxidation of lipids (to peroxides) and methionine (to methional), resulting in the development of an unpleasant flavour – the so-called 'sunlight' flavour. Light of 400–550 nm can penetrate both clear-glass bottles and cardboard cartons; cartons for milk include a protective lining that is opaque at this wavelength.

11.7.1 ABSORPTION AND METABOLISM OF RIBOFLAVIN

Apart from milk and eggs, which contain relatively large amounts of free riboflavin, most of the vitamin in foods is present as flavin coenzymes bound to enzymes, which are released when the protein is hydrolysed. Intestinal phosphatases then hydrolyse the coenzymes to riboflavin, which is absorbed in the upper small intestine. Much of the absorbed riboflavin is phosphorylated in the intestinal mucosa by flavokinase and enters the bloodstream as riboflavin phosphate.

Most tissues contain very little free riboflavin; most is present as FAD and riboflavin phosphate bound to enzymes. Uptake into tissues is by passive carrier-mediated transport of free riboflavin, followed by metabolic trapping (section 3.2.2.2) by phosphorylation to riboflavin phosphate, then onward metabolism to FAD.

FAD that is not protein bound is rapidly hydrolysed to riboflavin phosphate by nucleotide pyrophosphatase; unbound riboflavin phosphate is hydrolysed to riboflavin by non-specific phosphatases, and free riboflavin will diffuse out of tissues into the bloodstream.

Riboflavin and riboflavin phosphate that are not bound to plasma proteins are filtered at the glomerulus. Renal tubular resorption of riboflavin is saturated at normal plasma concentrations. There is also active tubular secretion of the vitamin; urinary excretion of riboflavin after high doses can be two- to threefold greater than the glomerular filtration rate.

There is no significant storage of riboflavin; any surplus intake is excreted rapidly, so that once metabolic requirements have been met urinary excretion of riboflavin and its metabolites reflects intake until intestinal absorption is saturated. In depleted animals, the maximum growth response is achieved with intakes that give about

75% saturation of tissues, and the intake to achieve tissue saturation is that at which there is quantitative excretion of the vitamin.

There is very efficient conservation of tissue riboflavin in deficiency, with only a fourfold difference between the minimum concentration of flavins in the liver in deficiency and the level at which saturation occurs. In deficiency, almost the only loss of riboflavin from tissues will be the small amount that is covalently bound to enzymes; the 8-α linkage is not cleaved by mammalian enzymes and 8-α derivatives of riboflavin are not substrates for flavokinase and cannot be reutilized.

11.7.2 METABOLIC FUNCTIONS OF THE FLAVIN COENZYMES

The metabolic function of the flavin coenzymes is as electron carriers in a wide variety of oxidation and reduction reactions central to all metabolic processes (see Figure 2.15), including the mitochondrial electron transport chain (section 3.3.12), and key enzymes in fatty acid (section 5.5.2) and amino acid (section 9.3.1.1) oxidation and the citric acid cycle (section 5.4.4). The flavin coenzymes remain bound to the enzyme throughout the catalytic cycle. The majority of flavoproteins have FAD as the prosthetic group; some have both flavin coenzymes, and some have other prosthetic groups as well.

Reoxidation of the reduced flavin in oxygenases and mixed-function oxidases proceeds by way of formation of the flavin radical and flavin hydroperoxide, with the intermediate generation of superoxide and perhydroxyl radicals and hydrogen peroxide. Because of this, flavin oxidases make a significant contribution to the total oxidant stress of the body (section 7.4.2.1).

11.7.3 RIBOFLAVIN DEFICIENCY

Although riboflavin is involved in all areas of metabolism, and deficiency is widespread on a global scale, deficiency is not fatal. There seem to be two reasons for this:

*   Although deficiency is common, the vitamin is widespread in foods, and most diets will provide minimally adequate amounts to permit maintenance of central metabolic pathways.
*   In deficiency there is extremely efficient reutilization of the riboflavin that is released by the turnover of flavoproteins, so that only a very small amount is metabolized or excreted.

Riboflavin deficiency is characterized by lesions of the margin of the lips (cheilosis) and corners of the mouth (angular stomatitis), a painful desquamation of the tongue, so that it is red, dry and atrophic (magenta tongue), and a seborrhoeic dermatitis, with filiform excrescences.

The main metabolic effect of riboflavin deficiency is on lipid metabolism. Riboflavin-deficient animals have a lower metabolic rate than controls, and require a 15–20% higher food intake to maintain body weight. Feeding a high-fat diet leads to more marked impairment of growth and a higher requirement for riboflavin to restore growth.

11.7.3.1 Resistance to malaria in riboflavin deficiency

A number of studies have noted that in areas where malaria is endemic riboflavin-deficient subjects are relatively resistant and have a lower parasite burden than adequately nourished subjects. The biochemical basis of this resistance to malaria in riboflavin deficiency is not known, but two possible mechanisms have been proposed:

- The malarial parasites may have a particularly high requirement for riboflavin. A number of flavin analogues have antimalarial action.
- As a result of impaired antioxidant activity in erythrocytes, there may be increased fragility of erythrocyte membranes. As in sickle cell trait, which also protects against malaria, this may result in exposure of the parasites to the host's immune system at a vulnerable stage in their development, resulting in the production of protective antibodies.

11.7.4 RIBOFLAVIN REQUIREMENTS

Estimates of riboflavin requirements are based on depletion/repletion studies to determine the minimum intake at which there is significant excretion of the vitamin. In deficiency there is virtually no excretion of the vitamin; as requirements are met, so any excess is excreted in the urine. On this basis the minimum adult requirement for riboflavin is 0.5–0.8 mg/day. At intakes between 1.1 and 1.6 mg/day urinary excretion rises sharply because tissue reserves are saturated.

A more generous estimate of requirements, and the basis of reference intakes, is the intake at which there is normalization of the activity of the red cell enzyme glutathione reductase, a flavoprotein whose activity is especially sensitive to riboflavin nutritional status. Normal values of the activation coefficient (section 11.7.4.1) are seen in subjects whose habitual intake of riboflavin is between 1.2 and 1.5 mg/day.

11.7.4.1 Assessment of riboflavin nutritional status

Although urinary excretion of riboflavin and its metabolites can be used as an index of status, excretion is correlated with intake only in subjects who are maintaining nitrogen balance (section 9.1). In subjects in negative nitrogen balance urinary excretion may be higher than expected, largely as a result of the catabolism of tissue flavoproteins and failure of replacement synthesis, leading to loss of their prosthetic groups. Higher intakes of protein than are required to maintain nitrogen balance do not affect the requirement for riboflavin.

Glutathione reductase is especially sensitive to riboflavin depletion, and the usual way of assessing riboflavin status is by measurement of the activation of red blood cell glutathione reductase by FAD added *in vitro* (section 11.6.4.1). An activation coefficient > 1.7 indicates deficiency.

11.8 *Niacin*

Niacin is not strictly a vitamin, as it can be synthesized in the body from the essential amino acid tryptophan. Indeed, it is only when tryptophan metabolism is deranged that dietary preformed niacin becomes important. Nevertheless, niacin was discovered as a nutrient during studies of the deficiency disease pellagra, which was a major public health problem in the southern USA throughout the first half of the twentieth century, and continued to be a problem in parts of India and sub-Saharan Africa until the 1990s.

Two compounds, nicotinic acid and nicotinamide, have the biological activity of niacin. When nicotinic acid was discovered to be a curative and preventive factor for pellagra, it was already known as a chemical compound, and was therefore never assigned a number among the B vitamins. The name niacin was coined in the USA when it was decided to enrich maize meal with the vitamin to prevent pellagra – it was considered that the name nicotinic acid was not desirable because of the similarity to nicotine. In USA, the term niacin is commonly used to mean specifically nicotinic acid, and nicotinamide is known as niacinamide; elsewhere 'niacin' is used as a generic descriptor for both vitamers. Figure 2.16 shows the structures of nicotinic acid, niacin and the nicotinamide nucleotide coenzymes, NAD and NADP.

11.8.1 METABOLISM OF NIACIN

The nicotinamide ring of NAD can be synthesized in the body from the essential amino acid tryptophan, as shown in Figure 11.13. In adults, almost all of the dietary intake of tryptophan is metabolized by this pathway and hence is potentially available for NAD synthesis.

A number of studies have investigated the equivalence of dietary tryptophan and preformed niacin as precursors of the nicotinamide nucleotides, generally by determining the excretion of niacin metabolites in response to test doses of the precursors in subjects maintained on deficient diets. There is a considerable variation between subjects in the response to tryptophan and niacin, and in order to allow for this it is generally assumed that 60 mg of tryptophan is equivalent to 1 mg of preformed niacin.

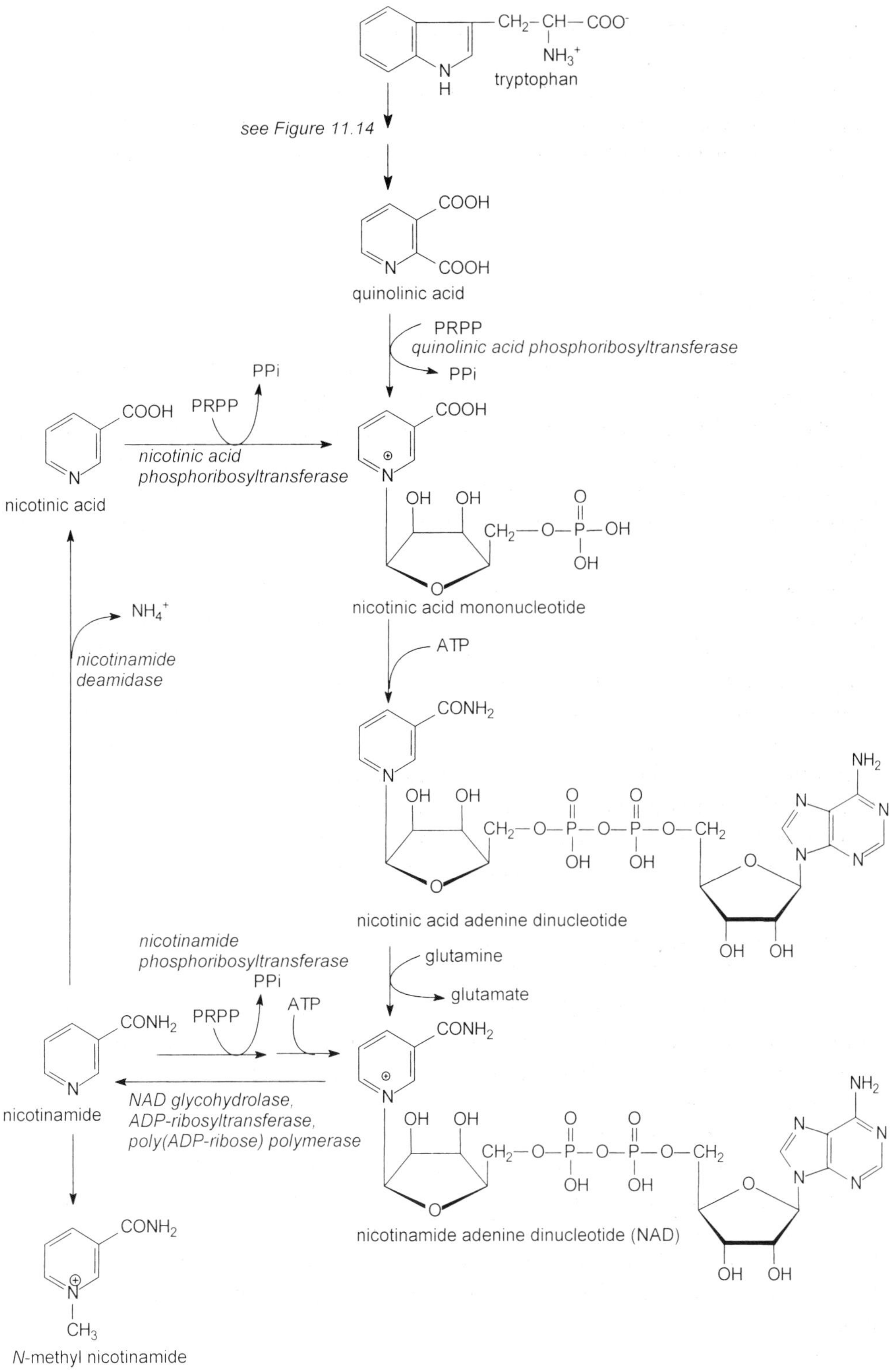

FIGURE 11.13 *The metabolism of the nicotinamide nucleotide coenzymes.*

Changes in hormonal status may result in considerable changes in this ratio, with between 7 and 30 mg of dietary tryptophan equivalent to 1 mg of preformed niacin in late pregnancy. The intake of tryptophan also affects the ratio, and at low intakes 1 mg of tryptophan may be equivalent to only 1/125 mg preformed niacin.

The niacin content of foods is generally expressed as mg niacin equivalents; 1 mg niacin equivalent = mg preformed niacin + 1/60 × mg tryptophan. Because most of the niacin in cereals is biologically unavailable (section 11.8.1.1), it is conventional to ignore preformed niacin in cereal products.

11.8.1.1 Unavailable niacin in cereals

Chemical analysis reveals niacin in cereals (largely in the bran), but this is biologically unavailable, as it is bound as niacytin – nicotinoyl esters to polysaccharides, polypeptides and glycopeptides.

Treatment of cereals with alkali (for example soaking overnight in calcium hydroxide solution, as is the traditional method for the preparation of tortillas in Mexico) releases much of the nicotinic acid. This may explain why pellagra has always been rare in Mexico, despite the fact that maize is the dietary staple. Up to 10% of the niacin in niacytin may be biologically available as a result of hydrolysis by gastric acid.

11.8.1.2 Absorption and metabolism of niacin

Niacin is present in tissues, and therefore in foods, largely as the nicotinamide nucleotides. The post-mortem hydrolysis of NAD(P) is extremely rapid in animal tissues, so it is likely that much of the niacin of meat (a major dietary source of the vitamin) is free nicotinamide. Both nicotinic acid and nicotinamide are absorbed from the small intestine by a sodium-dependent saturable process.

11.8.1.3 Metabolism of the nicotinamide nucleotide coenzymes.

As shown in Figure 11.13, the nicotinamide nucleotide coenzymes can be synthesized from either of the niacin vitamers, and from quinolinic acid, an intermediate in the metabolism of tryptophan. In the liver, the oxidation of tryptophan results in a considerably greater synthesis of NAD than is required, and this is catabolized to release nicotinic acid and nicotinamide, which are taken up and used by other tissues for synthesis of the coenzymes.

The catabolism of NAD^+ is catalysed by four enzymes:

- NAD glycohydrolase, which releases nicotinamide and ADP–ribose.
- NAD pyrophosphatase, which releases nicotinamide mononucleotide. This can either be hydrolysed by NAD glycohydrolase to release nicotinamide, or can be a reutilized to form NAD;

- ADP–ribosyltransferases.
- Poly(ADP–ribose) polymerase.

The activation of ADP–ribosyltransferase and poly(ADP–ribose) polymerase by toxins or DNA damage (section 11.8.3.1) may result in considerable depletion of intracellular NAD(P), and may indeed provide a suicide mechanism to ensure that cells that have suffered very severe damage die, as a result of NAD(P) depletion. The administration of DNA-breaking carcinogens to experimental animals results in the excretion of large amounts of nicotinamide metabolites and depletion of tissue NAD(P). Chronic exposure to such carcinogens and mycotoxins may be a contributory factor in the aetiology of pellagra when dietary intakes of tryptophan and niacin are marginal.

Under normal conditions there is little or no urinary excretion of either nicotinamide or nicotinic acid. This is because both vitamers are actively resorbed from the glomerular filtrate. It is only when the concentration is so high that the resorption mechanism is saturated that there is any significant excretion. The main urinary metabolites of niacin are N^1-methyl nicotinamide and onward metabolic products, methyl pyridone-2-carboxamide and methyl pyridone-4-carboxamide.

11.8.2 The synthesis of nicotinamide nucleotides from tryptophan

The oxidative pathway of tryptophan metabolism is shown in Figure 11.14. Under normal conditions almost all of the dietary intake of tryptophan, apart from the small amounts that are used for net new protein synthesis and synthesis of 5-hydroxytryptophan, is metabolized by this pathway, and hence is potentially available for NAD synthesis.

The synthesis of NAD from tryptophan involves the non-enzymic cyclization of aminocarboxymuconic semialdehyde to quinolinic acid. The alternative metabolic fate of aminocarboxymuconic semialdehyde is decarboxylation, catalysed by picolinate carboxylase, leading to acetyl CoA and total oxidation. There is thus competition between an enzyme-catalysed reaction, which has hyperbolic, saturable kinetics, and a non-enzymic reaction, which has linear kinetics. At low rates of flux through the pathway, most metabolism will be by way of the enzyme-catalysed pathway, leading to oxidation. As the rate of formation of aminocarboxymuconic semialdehyde increases, and picolinate carboxylase becomes more or less saturated, so an increasing proportion will be available to undergo cyclization to quinolinic acid and onward metabolism to NAD. There is thus not a simple stoichiometric relationship between tryptophan and niacin, and the equivalence of the two coenzyme precursors will vary as the amount of tryptophan to be metabolized and the rate of metabolism vary.

The activities of three enzymes, tryptophan dioxygenase, kynurenine hydroxylase and kynureninase, affect the rate of formation of aminocarboxymuconic semialdehyde, as may the rate of uptake of tryptophan into the liver.

Tryptophan dioxygenase is the enzyme that controls the entry of tryptophan into the oxidative pathway. It has a short half-life (of the order of 2 hours) and is subject to regulation by three mechanisms:

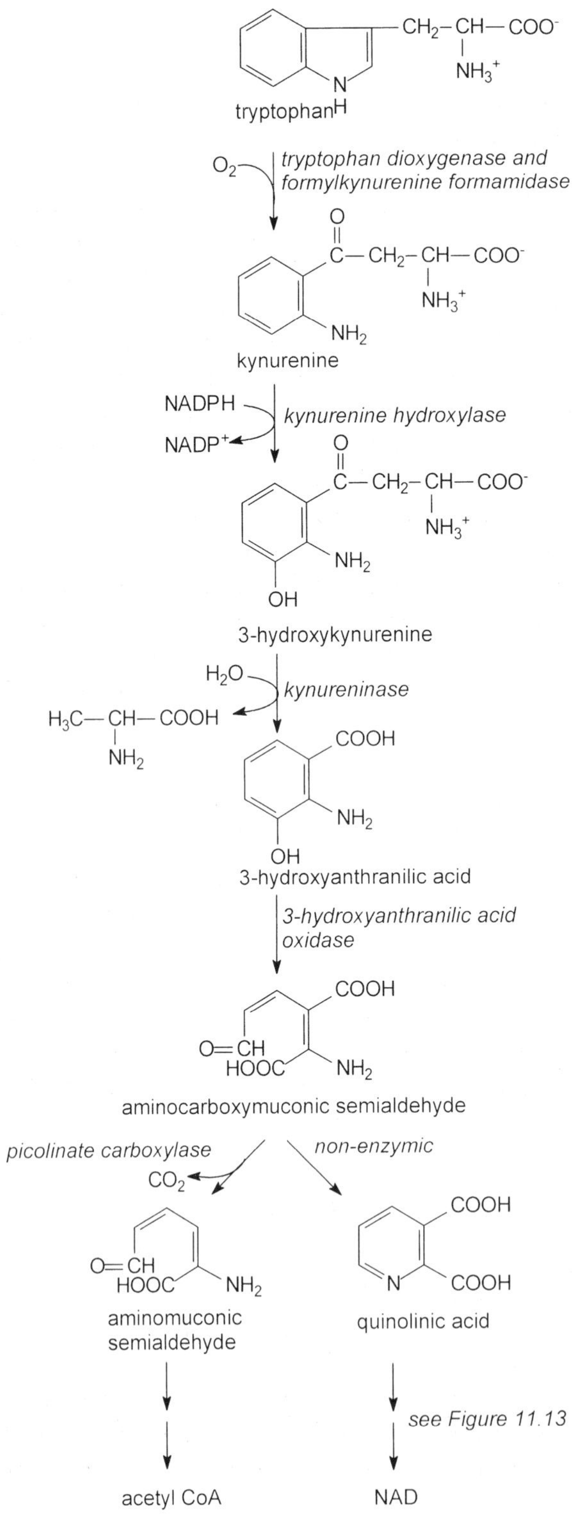

FIGURE 11.14 *The oxidative pathway of tryptophan metabolism.*

- stabilization by its haem cofactor;
- hormonal induction by glucocorticoid hormones and glucagon (section 9.1.2.2);
- feedback inhibition and repression by NAD(P).

The activities of both kynurenine hydroxylase and kynureninase are only slightly higher than that of tryptophan dioxygenase under basal conditions, and increased tryptophan dioxygenase activity in response to glucocorticoid action is accompanied by increased accumulation and excretion of kynurenine, hydroxykynurenine and their transamination products, kynurenic and xanthurenic acids. Impairment of the activity of either enzyme may impair the onward metabolism of kynurenine and so reduce the accumulation of aminocarboxymuconic semialdehyde, and hence the synthesis of NAD.

Kynurenine hydroxylase is FAD dependent, and the activity of kynurenine hydroxylase in the liver of riboflavin deficient rats is only 30–50% of that in control animals. Riboflavin deficiency (section 11.7.3) may thus be a contributory factor in the aetiology of pellagra when intakes of tryptophan and niacin are marginal.

Kynureninase is a pyridoxal phosphate (vitamin B_6)-dependent enzyme, and its activity is extremely sensitive to vitamin B_6 depletion. Indeed, the ability to metabolize a test dose of tryptophan has been used to assess vitamin B_6 nutritional status (section 11.9.5.1). Deficiency of vitamin B_6 will lead to severe impairment of NAD synthesis from tryptophan. Kynureninase is also inhibited by oestrogen metabolites.

11.8.3 METABOLIC FUNCTIONS OF NIACIN

The best-defined role of niacin is in oxidation and reduction reactions, as the functional nicotinamide part of the coenzymes NAD and NADP (section 2.4.1.3). In general, NAD^+ is involved as an electron acceptor in energy-yielding metabolism, being oxidized by the mitochondrial electron transport chain (section 3.3.1.2), whereas the major coenzyme for reductive synthetic reactions is NADPH. An exception to this general rule is the pentose phosphate pathway of glucose metabolism (section 5.4.2), which results in the reduction of $NADP^+$ to NADPH and is a major metabolic source of reductant for fatty acid synthesis (section 5.6.1).

11.8.3.1 The role of NAD in ADP–ribosylation

In addition to its coenzyme role, NAD is the source of ADP–ribose for the ADP–ribosylation of proteins and poly(ADP–ribosylation) of nucleoproteins involved in the DNA repair mechanism. Only NAD^+ is a substrate for these enzymes, not NADP, and not the reduced coenzyme.

ADP–ribosyltransferases modify the activity of target enzymes by catalysing the transfer of ADP–ribose onto arginine, lysine or asparagine residues. ADP–ribosylation is a reversible modification of proteins, and there are specific hydrolases which cleave the *N*-glycoside linkage.

Poly(ADP–ribose) polymerase is primarily a nuclear enzyme. The acceptor for the initial ADP–ribose moiety is a glutamate or the carboxyl group of a terminal lysine in the acceptor enzyme, forming an O-glycoside. This is followed by successive ADP–ribosyl transfer to form poly(ADP–ribose), which may be a linear or branched polymer.

In the nucleus, poly(ADP–ribose) polymerase is activated by binding to breakage points in DNA fragments and is involved in activation of the DNA repair mechanism in response to strand breakage. In the immediate vicinity of a double-strand break several hundred ADP–ribose molecules may be polymerized per minute. The acceptor protein may be DNA ligase II, which is activated by poly(ADP–ribosylation) or a histone, resulting in reduced histone inhibition of DNA ligase II.

11.8.4 Pellagra – a disease of tryptophan and niacin deficiency

Pellagra became common in Europe when maize was introduced from the New World as a convenient high-yielding dietary staple, and by the late nineteenth century it was widespread throughout southern Europe, North and South Africa and the southern USA. The proteins of maize are particularly lacking in tryptophan, and as with other cereals little or none of the preformed niacin is biologically available (see section 11.8.1.1).

Pellagra is characterized by a photosensitive dermatitis, like severe sunburn, affecting all parts of the skin that are exposed to sunlight. Similar skin lesions may also occur in areas not exposed to sunlight but subject to pressure, such as the knees, elbows, wrists and ankles. Advanced pellagra is also accompanied by dementia (more correctly a depressive psychosis), and there may be diarrhoea. Untreated pellagra is fatal.

The depressive psychosis is superficially similar to schizophrenia and the organic psychoses, but clinically distinguishable by the sudden lucid phases that alternate with the most florid psychiatric signs. It is probable that these mental symptoms can be explained by a relative deficit of the essential amino acid tryptophan, and hence reduced synthesis of the neurotransmitter serotonin, and not to a deficiency of niacin *per se*.

Although the nutritional aetiology of pellagra is well established, and tryptophan or niacin will prevent or cure the disease, additional factors, including deficiency of riboflavin (and hence impaired activity of kynurenine hydroxylase) or vitamin B_6 (and hence impaired activity of kynureninase), may be important when intakes of tryptophan and niacin are only marginally adequate.

Among the 87,000 people who died from pellagra in the United States during the first half of the twentieth century, there were twice as many women as men. Reports of individual outbreaks of pellagra, both in USA and more recently elsewhere, show a similar sex ratio. This may well be the result of inhibition of kynureninase, and impairment of the activity of kynurenine hydroxylase, by oestrogen metabolites, and hence reduced synthesis of NAD from tryptophan.

11.8.4.1 Non-nutritional pellagra

A number of genetic diseases are associated with the development of pellagra despite an apparently adequate intake of both tryptophan and niacin; all are defects of tryptophan metabolism, suggesting that endogenous synthesis from tryptophan is the more important source of NAD. In most cases, the pellagra-like signs resolve with (relatively high) niacin supplements.

Hartnup disease (see Problem 4.3) is a rare genetic condition in which there is a defect of the membrane transport mechanism for tryptophan and other large neutral amino acids. As a result, the intestinal absorption of free tryptophan is impaired, although dipeptide absorption is normal. There is a considerable urinary loss of tryptophan (and other amino acids) as a result of failure of the normal resorption mechanism in the renal tubules – renal aminoaciduria. In addition to neurological signs, which can be attributed to a deficit of tryptophan for the synthesis of 5-hydroxytryptamine in the central nervous system, the patients show clinical signs of pellagra, which respond to the administration of niacin.

Carcinoid is a tumour of the enterochromaffin cells, which synthesize 5-hydroxytryptophan and 5-hydroxytryptamine. The carcinoid syndrome is seen when there are significant metastases of the primary tumour, normally in the liver. It is characterized by much increased gastrointestinal motility and diarrhoea, as well as by regular periodic flushing. These symptoms can be attributed to systemic release of large amounts of 5-hydroxtryptamine. The synthesis of 5-hydroxytryptamine in advanced carcinoid syndrome may be so great that as much as 60% of the body's tryptophan metabolism proceeds by this pathway, compared with about 1% under normal conditions. A significant number of patients with advanced carcinoid syndrome develop clinical signs of pellagra because of this diversion of tryptophan away from the oxidative pathway.

11.8.5 NIACIN REQUIREMENTS

On the basis of depletion/repletion studies in which the urinary excretion of niacin metabolites was measured after feeding tryptophan or preformed niacin, the average requirement for niacin is 1.3 mg niacin equivalents per MJ energy expenditure, and reference intakes are based on 1.6 mg/MJ.

Average intakes of tryptophan in Western diets will more than meet requirements without the need for a dietary source of preformed niacin.

11.8.5.1 Assessment of niacin status

Although the nicotinamide nucleotide coenzymes function in a large number of oxidation and reduction reactions, this cannot be exploited as a means of assessing the state of the body's niacin reserves, because the coenzymes are not firmly attached to their apoenzymes, as are thiamin pyrophosphate, riboflavin and pyridoxal phosphate, but act as co-substrates of the reactions, binding to and leaving the enzyme as the reaction proceeds. No specific metabolic lesions associated with NAD(P) depletion have been identified.

The two methods of assessing niacin nutritional status are measurement of the ratio of NAD to NADP in red blood cells and the urinary excretion of niacin metabolites, neither of which is wholly satisfactory.

11.8.5.2 Niacin toxicity

Nicotinic acid has been used to lower blood triacylglycerol and cholesterol in patients with hyperlipidaemia. However, relatively large amounts are required (of the order of 1–6 g/day, compared with reference intakes of 18–20 mg/day). At this level of intake, nicotinic acid causes dilatation of blood vessels and flushing, with skin irritation, itching and a burning sensation. This effect wears off after a few days.

High intakes of both nicotinic acid and nicotinamide, in excess of 500 mg/day, also cause liver damage, and prolonged use can result in liver failure. This is especially a problem with sustained release preparations of niacin, which permit a high blood level to be maintained for a relatively long time.

11.9 *Vitamin B$_6$*

Apart from a single outbreak in the 1950s, due to overheated infant milk formula, vitamin B$_6$ deficiency is unknown except under experimental conditions. Nevertheless, there is a considerable body of evidence that marginal status, and biochemical deficiency, may be relatively widespread.

The generic descriptor vitamin B$_6$ includes six vitamers (see Figure 11.15): the alcohol pyridoxine, the aldehyde pyridoxal, the amine pyridoxamine and their 5'-phosphates. There is some confusion in the literature, because at one time 'pyridoxine' was used as a generic descriptor, with 'pyridoxol' as the specific name for the alcohol. The vitamers are metabolically interconvertible and have equal biological activity; they are all converted in the body to the metabolically active form, pyridoxal phosphate. 4-Pyridoxic acid is a biologically inactive end-product of vitamin B$_6$ metabolism.

When foods are heated, pyridoxal and pyridoxal phosphate, can react with the ε-amino groups of lysine to form a Schiff base (aldimine). This renders both the vitamin B$_6$ and the lysine biologically unavailable; more importantly, the pyridoxyl-lysine released during digestion is absorbed and has anti-vitamin B$_6$ antimetabolite activity.

11.9.1 ABSORPTION AND METABOLISM OF VITAMIN B$_6$

The phosphorylated vitamers are dephosphorylated by alkaline phosphatase in the intestinal mucosa; pyridoxal, pyridoxamine and pyridoxine are all absorbed rapidly

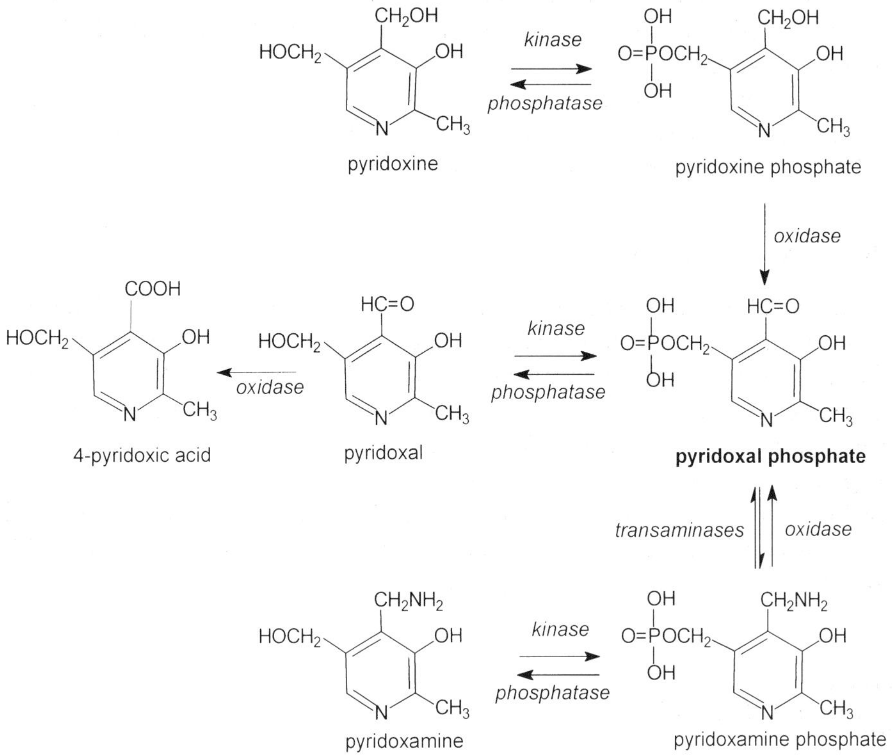

FIGURE 11.15 *Interconversion of the vitamin B$_6$ vitamers.*

by diffusion, then phosphorylated and oxidized. Much of the ingested vitamin is released into the portal circulation as pyridoxal, after dephosphorylation at the serosal surface.

Most of the absorbed vitamin is taken up by the liver by diffusion, followed by metabolic trapping as the phosphate. Pyridoxal phosphate and some pyridoxal are exported from the liver bound to albumin. Free pyridoxal remaining in the liver is rapidly oxidized to 4-pyridoxic acid, which is the main excretory product.

Extrahepatic tissues take up both pyridoxal and pyridoxal phosphate from the plasma. The phosphate is hydrolysed to pyridoxal, which can cross cell membranes, by extracellular alkaline phosphatase, then trapped intracellularly by phosphorylation.

Some 80% of the body's total vitamin B$_6$ is pyridoxal phosphate in muscle, mostly associated with glycogen phosphorylase (section 5.6.3.1). This does not function as a reserve of the vitamin and is not released from muscle in times of deficiency; it is released into the circulation (as pyridoxal) in starvation, when glycogen reserves are exhausted and there is less requirement for phosphorylase activity. Under these conditions it is available for redistribution to other tissues, and especially liver and kidney, to meet the increased requirement for gluconeogenesis (section 5.7) from amino acids.

11.9.2 METABOLIC FUNCTIONS OF VITAMIN B$_6$

Pyridoxal phosphate is a coenzyme in three main areas of metabolism:

- In a wide variety of reactions of amino acids, especially transamination, in which it functions as the intermediate carrier of the amino group (section 9.3.1.2), and decarboxylation to form amines.
- As the cofactor of glycogen phosphorylase (section 5.6.3.1) in muscle and liver, in which case it is the phosphate group that is catalytically important.
- In the regulation of the action of steroid hormones (section 10.4). Pyridoxal phosphate acts to remove the hormone–receptor complex from DNA binding and so terminate the action of the hormones. In vitamin B$_6$ deficiency there is increased sensitivity of target tissues to the actions of low concentrations of such hormones as the oestrogens, androgens, cortisol and vitamin D.

11.9.3 VITAMIN B$_6$ DEFICIENCY

Deficiency of vitamin B$_6$ severe enough to lead to clinical signs is extremely rare, and clear deficiency has been reported in only one outbreak, during the 1950s, when babies were fed on a milk preparation which had been severely overheated during manufacture. Many of the affected infants suffered convulsions, which ceased rapidly following the administration of vitamin B$_6$.

The cause of the convulsions was severe impairment of the activity of the enzyme glutamate decarboxylase, which is a pyridoxal phosphate-dependent enzyme. The product of glutamate decarboxylase is GABA (γ-aminobutyric acid), a regulatory neurotransmitter in the central nervous system (see Figure 5.19).

Moderate vitamin B$_6$ deficiency results in a number of abnormalities of amino acid metabolism, and especially of tryptophan (section 11.9.5.1) and methionine (section 11.9.5.2). In experimental animals, a moderate degree of deficiency leads to increased sensitivity of target tissues to steroid hormone action. This may be important in the development of hormone-dependent cancer of the breast, uterus and prostate, and may therefore affect the prognosis. Vitamin B$_6$ supplementation may be a useful adjunct to other therapy in these common cancers; certainly, there is evidence that poor vitamin B$_6$ nutritional status is associated with a poor prognosis in women with breast cancer.

11.9.4 VITAMIN B$_6$ REQUIREMENTS

Most studies of vitamin B$_6$ requirements have followed the development of abnormalities of tryptophan and methionine metabolism during depletion and normalization during repletion with graded intakes of the vitamin. Adults maintained on vitamin B$_6$-deficient diets develop abnormalities of tryptophan and methionine metabolism faster, and their blood vitamin B$_6$ falls more rapidly, when their protein intake is relatively high (80–160 g/day in various studies) than on low protein intakes (30–50 g/day). Similarly, during repletion of deficient subjects, tryptophan and methionine metabolism and blood vitamin B_6 are normalized faster at low than at high levels of protein intake.

From such studies the mean requirement for vitamin B_6 is estimated to be 13 μg per gram dietary protein, and reference intakes are based on 15–16 μg/g.

11.9.5 ASSESSMENT OF VITAMIN B_6 STATUS

Fasting plasma total vitamin B_6, or more specifically pyridoxal phosphate, is widely used as an index of vitamin B_6 nutritional status. Urinary excretion of 4-pyridoxic acid is also used, but it reflects recent intake of the vitamin rather than underlying nutritional status.

The most widely used method of assessing vitamin B_6 status is by the activation of erythrocyte transaminases by pyridoxal phosphate added *in vitro*, expressed as the activation coefficient (section 11.6.4.1). The ability to metabolize a test dose of tryptophan (section 11.9.5.1) or methionine (section 11.9.5.2) has also been used.

11.9.5.1 The tryptophan load test

The tryptophan load test for vitamin B_6 nutritional status (the ability to metabolize a test dose of tryptophan) is one of the oldest metabolic tests for functional vitamin nutritional status. It was developed as a result of observation of the excretion of an abnormal coloured compound, later identified as the tryptophan metabolite xanthurenic acid, in the urine of deficient animals.

Kynureninase (Figure 11.16) is a pyridoxal phosphate-dependent enzyme, and its activity falls markedly in vitamin B_6 deficiency, at least partly because it undergoes a slow mechanism-dependent inactivation that leaves catalytically inactive pyridoxamine phosphate at the active site of the enzyme. The enzyme can only be reactivated if there is an adequate supply of pyridoxal phosphate. This means that in vitamin B_6 deficiency there is a considerable accumulation of both hydroxykynurenine and kynurenine, sufficient to permit greater metabolic flux than usual through kynurenine transaminase, resulting in increased formation of kynurenic and xanthurenic acids.

Xanthurenic and kynurenic acids, and kynurenine and hydroxykynurenine, are easy to measure in urine, so the tryptophan load test (the ability to metabolize a test dose of 2–5 g of tryptophan) has been widely adopted as a convenient and very sensitive index of vitamin B_6 nutritional status. However, because glucocorticoid hormones increase tryptophan dioxygenase activity, abnormal results of the tryptophan load test must be regarded with caution, and cannot necessarily be interpreted as indicating vitamin B_6 deficiency. Increased entry of tryptophan into the pathway will overwhelm the capacity of kynureninase, leading to increased formation of xanthurenic and kynurenic acids. Similarly, oestrogen metabolites inhibit kynureninase, leading to results that have been misinterpreted as vitamin B_6 deficiency.

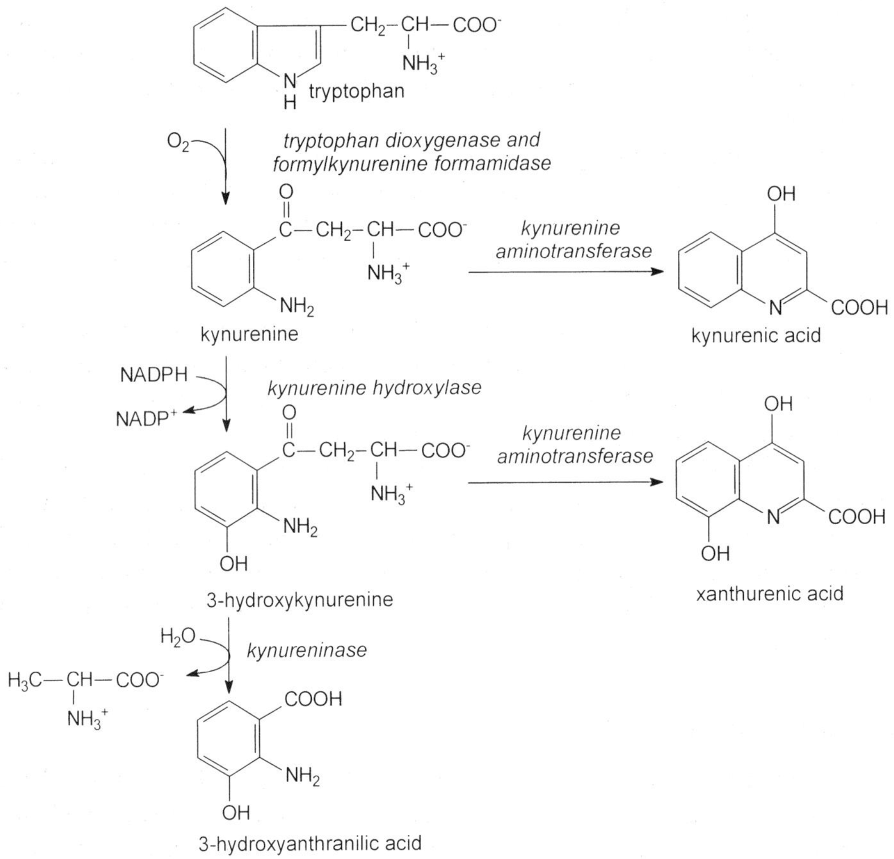

FIGURE 11.16 *The tryptophan load test for vitamin B$_6$ status.*

11.9.5.2 The methionine load test

The metabolism of methionine, shown in Figure 11.22, includes two pyridoxal phosphate-dependent steps: cystathionine synthetase and cystathionase. Cystathionase activity falls markedly in vitamin B$_6$ deficiency, and as a result there is an increase in the urinary excretion of homocysteine and cystathionine, both after a loading dose of methionine and under basal conditions. However, as discussed below, homocysteine metabolism is affected more by folate status than by vitamin B$_6$ status, and, like the tryptophan load test, the methionine load test is probably not reliable as an index of vitamin B$_6$ status in field studies.

11.9.6 NON-NUTRITIONAL USES OF VITAMIN B$_6$

A number of studies have suggested that oral contraceptives cause vitamin B$_6$ deficiency. As a result of this, supplements of vitamin B$_6$ of between 50 and 100 mg/day, and sometimes higher, have been used to overcome the side-effects of oral contraceptives. Similar supplements have also been recommended for the treatment of the premenstrual syndrome, although there is little evidence of efficacy from placebo-controlled trials.

All of the studies that suggested that oral contraceptives cause vitamin B_6 deficiency used the tryptophan load test (section 11.9.5.1). When other biochemical markers of status were also assessed, they were not affected by oral contraceptive use. Furthermore, most of these studies were performed using the now obsolete high-dose contraceptive pills.

Oral contraceptives do not cause vitamin B_6 deficiency. The problem is that oestrogen metabolites inhibit kynureninase and reduce the activity of kynurenine hydroxylase. This results in the excretion of abnormal amounts of tryptophan metabolites, similar to what is seen in vitamin B_6 deficiency, but for quite a different reason.

Doses of 50–200 mg of vitamin B_6 per day have an antiemetic effect, and the vitamin is widely used, alone or in conjunction with other antiemetics, to minimize the nausea associated with radiotherapy and to treat pregnancy sickness. There is no evidence that vitamin B_6 has any beneficial effect in pregnancy sickness, or that women who suffer from morning sickness have lower vitamin B_6 nutritional status than other pregnant women.

11.9.6.1 Vitamin B_6 toxicity

In experimental animals, doses of vitamin B_6 of 50 mg per kg body weight cause histological damage to dorsal nerve roots, and doses of 200 mg per kg body weight lead to the development of signs of peripheral neuropathy, with ataxia, muscle weakness and loss of balance. The clinical signs of vitamin B_6 toxicity in animals regress within 3 months after withdrawal of these massive doses, but sensory nerve conduction velocity, which decreases during the development of the neuropathy, does not recover fully.

The development of sensory neuropathy has been reported in seven patients taking 2–7 g of pyridoxine per day. Although there was some residual damage, withdrawal of these extremely high doses resulted in a considerable recovery of sensory nerve function. Other reports have suggested that intakes as low as 50 mg/day are associated with neurological damage, although these have been based on patients reporting symptoms rather than detailed neurological examination.

11.10 *Vitamin B_{12}*

Dietary deficiency of vitamin B_{12} occurs only in strict vegans, as the vitamin is found almost exclusively in animal foods. However, functional deficiency (pernicious anaemia, with spinal cord degeneration), as a result of impaired absorption, is relatively common, especially in elderly people with atrophic gastritis.

The structure of vitamin B$_{12}$ is shown in Figure 11.17. The term corrinoid is used as a generic descriptor for cobalt-containing compounds of this general structure, which, depending on the substituents in the pyrrole rings, may or may not have vitamin activity. The term 'vitamin B$_{12}$' is used as a generic descriptor for the cobalamins – those corrinoids having the biological activity of the vitamin. Some of the corrinoids that are growth factors for micro-organisms not only have no vitamin B$_{12}$ activity but may be antimetabolites of the vitamin.

Vitamin B$_{12}$ is found only in foods of animal origin, although it is also formed by some yeasts and bacteria. There are no plant sources of this vitamin. This means that strict vegetarians (vegans), who eat no foods of animal origin, are at risk of developing dietary vitamin B$_{12}$ deficiency. The small amounts of vitamin B$_{12}$ formed by bacteria on the surface of fruits may be adequate to meet requirements. Preparations of vitamin B$_{12}$ made by bacterial fermentation, which are ethically acceptable to vegans, are readily available.

There are claims that yeast and some plants (especially algae) contain vitamin B$_{12}$. This seems to be incorrect. The problem is that the officially recognized, and legally required, method of determining vitamin B$_{12}$ in food analysis depends on the growth of micro-organisms for which vitamin B$_{12}$ is an essential growth factor. However, these organisms can also use some corrinoids that have no vitamin activity. Therefore,

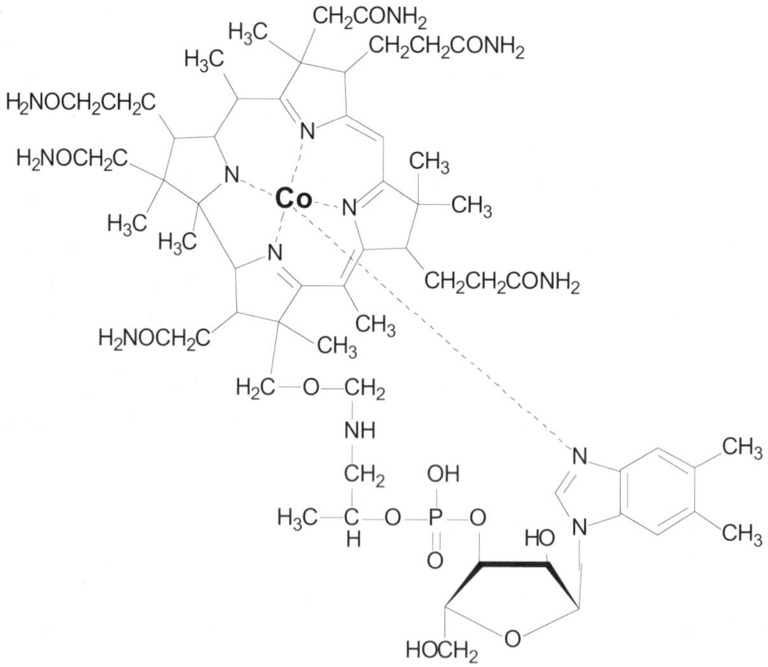

FIGURE 11.17 *Vitamin B$_{12}$. Four coordination sites on the central cobalt atom are chelated by the nitrogen atoms of the corrin ring, and one by the nitrogen of the dimethylbenzimidazole nucleotide. The sixth coordination site may be occupied by: CN$^-$ (cyanocobalamin), OH$^-$ (hydroxocobalamin), H$_2$O (aquocobalamin, –CH$_3$ (methylcobalamin) or 5′-deoxyadenosine (adenosylcobalamin).*

analysis reveals the presence of something that appears to be vitamin B_{12} but in fact is not the active vitamin and is useless in human nutrition. Where biologically active vitamin B_{12} has been identified in algae, it is almost certainly the result of bacterial contamination of the lakes from which the algae were harvested.

11.10.1 ABSORPTION AND METABOLISM OF VITAMIN B_{12}

Very small amounts of vitamin B_{12} can be absorbed by passive diffusion across the intestinal mucosa, but under normal conditions this is insignificant, accounting for less than 1% of large oral doses; the major route of vitamin B_{12} absorption is by way of attachment to a specific binding protein in the intestinal lumen.

This binding protein is 'intrinsic factor', so called because in the early studies of pernicious anaemia (section 11.10.3) it was found that two curative factors were involved – an extrinsic or dietary factor, which we now know to be vitamin B_{12}, and an intrinsic or endogenously produced factor. Intrinsic factor is a small glycoprotein secreted by the parietal cells of the gastric mucosa, which also secrete hydrochloric acid.

Gastric acid and pepsin have a role in vitamin B_{12} nutrition, serving to release the vitamin from protein binding and so make it available. Atrophic gastritis is a relatively common problem of advancing age; in the early stages there is failure of acid secretion but more or less normal secretion of intrinsic factor. This can result in vitamin B_{12} depletion as a result of failure to release the vitamin from dietary proteins, but the absorption of a test dose of free vitamin B_{12} is normal. In the stomach, vitamin B_{12} binds to cobalophilin, a binding protein secreted in the saliva.

In the duodenum cobalophilin is hydrolysed, releasing the vitamin B_{12} for binding to intrinsic factor. Pancreatic insufficiency can therefore be a factor in the development of vitamin B_{12} deficiency, as failure to hydrolyse cobalophilin will result in the excretion of cobalophilin-bound vitamin B_{12} rather than transfer to intrinsic factor. Intrinsic factor binds the various vitamin B_{12} vitamers, but not other corrinoids. Considerably more intrinsic factor is normally secreted than is needed for the binding and absorption of dietary vitamin B_{12}, which requires only about 1% of the total intrinsic factor available.

Vitamin B_{12} is absorbed from the distal third of the ileum. There are intrinsic factor–vitamin B_{12} binding sites on the brush border of the mucosal cells in this region; neither free intrinsic factor nor free vitamin B_{12} interacts with these receptors.

In plasma, vitamin B_{12} circulates bound to transcobalamin I, which is required for tissue uptake of the vitamin, and transcobalamin II, which seems to be a storage form of the vitamin.

There is a considerable enterohepatic circulation of vitamin B_{12}. Vitamin B_{12} and its metabolites (some of which are biologically inactive) are transferred from peripheral tissues to the liver bound to transcobalamin III. They are then secreted into the bile, bound to cobalophilins; 3–8 μg (2.25–6 nmol) of vitamin B_{12} may be secreted in the bile each day, about the same as the dietary intake. Like dietary vitamin B_{12} bound to salivary cobalophilin, the biliary cobalophilins are hydrolysed in the duodenum, and the vitamin binds to intrinsic factor, so permitting reabsorption in the ileum. Whereas cobalophilins and transcorrin III have low specificity, and will bind a variety of corrinoids, intrinsic factor binds only cobalamins, and so only the biologically active vitamin will be reabsorbed to any significant extent.

11.10.2 METABOLIC FUNCTIONS OF VITAMIN B_{12}

There are three vitamin B_{12}-dependent enzymes in human tissues: methylmalonyl CoA mutase, leucine aminomutase and methionine synthetase. Methionine synthetase is discussed in section 11.11.3.2.

Methylmalonyl CoA is formed as an intermediate in the catabolism of valine and by the carboxylation of propionyl CoA arising in the catabolism of isoleucine, cholesterol and (rare) fatty acids with an odd number of carbon atoms. As shown in Figure 11.18, it normally undergoes vitamin B_{12}-dependent rearrangement to succinyl CoA, catalysed by methylmalonyl CoA mutase. The activity of this enzyme is greatly reduced in vitamin B_{12} deficiency, leading to an accumulation of methylmalonyl CoA, some of which is hydrolysed to yield methylmalonic acid, which is excreted in the urine; urinary

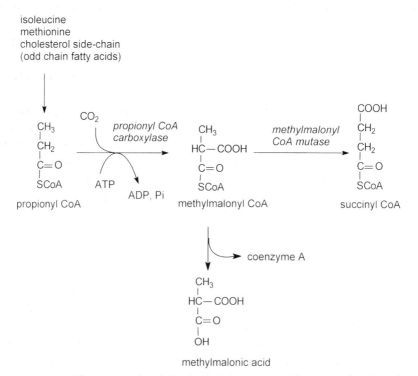

FIGURE 11.18 *The reaction of methylmalonyl CoA mutase and formation of methylmalonic acid in vitamin B_{12} deficiency.*

excretion of methylmalonic acid provides a means of assessing vitamin B$_{12}$ nutritional status and monitoring therapy in patients with pernicious anaemia (section 11.10.3).

11.10.3 VITAMIN B$_{12}$ DEFICIENCY: PERNICIOUS ANAEMIA

Vitamin B$_{12}$ deficiency causes pernicious anaemia – the release into the bloodstream of immature precursors of red blood cells (megaloblastic anaemia). As discussed in section 11.11.3.2, vitamin B$_{12}$ deficiency impairs the metabolism of folic acid, leading to the development of functional folate deficiency; this is what disturbs the rapid multiplication of red blood cells, causing immature precursors to be released into the circulation.

The other clinical feature of vitamin B$_{12}$ deficiency, which is very rarely seen in folic acid deficiency, is degeneration of the spinal cord – hence the name 'pernicious' for the anaemia of vitamin B$_{12}$ deficiency. The spinal cord degeneration is due to a failure of the methylation of one arginine residue on myelin basic protein and occurs in about one-third of patients with megaloblastic anaemia due to vitamin B$_{12}$ deficiency and in about one-third of patients who do not show signs of anaemia.

Dietary deficiency of vitamin B$_{12}$ does occur, rarely, in strict vegetarians. However, the commonest cause of pernicious anaemia is failure of the absorption of vitamin B$_{12}$, rather than dietary deficiency.

Failure of intrinsic factor secretion is commonly due to autoimmune disease; 90% of patients with pernicious anaemia have antibodies to the gastric parietal cells. Similar autoantibodies are found in 30% of the relatives of pernicious anaemia patients, suggesting that there is a genetic basis for the condition.

About 70% of patients also have anti-intrinsic factor antibodies in plasma, saliva and gastric juice. Although the oral administration of partially purified preparations of intrinsic factor will restore the absorption of vitamin B$_{12}$ in many patients with pernicious anaemia, this can result eventually in the production of anti-intrinsic factor antibodies, so parenteral administration of vitamin B$_{12}$ is the preferred means of treatment. For patients who secrete anti-intrinsic factor antibodies in the saliva or gastric juice, oral intrinsic factor will be useless.

11.10.4 VITAMIN B$_{12}$ REQUIREMENTS

Most estimates of vitamin B$_{12}$ requirements are based on the amounts given parenterally to maintain normal health in patients with pernicious anaemia due to a failure of vitamin B$_{12}$ absorption. This overestimates normal requirements because of the enterohepatic circulation of vitamin B$_{12}$ (section 11.10.1); in people with defective absorption, the vitamin that is excreted in the bile will be lost in the faeces, whereas normally it is almost completely reabsorbed.

The total body pool of vitamin B_{12} is of the order of 2.5 mg (1.8 μmol), with a minimum desirable body pool of about 1 mg (0.3 μmol). The daily loss is about 0.1% of the body pool in subjects with normal enterohepatic circulation of the vitamin; on this basis requirements are about 1–2.5 μg/day, and reference intakes for adults range between 1.4 and 2.0 μg.

11.10.5 ASSESSMENT OF VITAMIN B_{12} STATUS

Measurement of plasma concentrations of vitamin B_{12} is the method of choice, and a number of simple and reliable radioligand binding assays have been developed. Radioligand binding assays may give falsely high values if the binding protein is cobalophilin, which binds a number of metabolically inactive corrinoids as well as cobalamins; more precise determination of true vitamin B_{12} comes from assays in which the binding protein is purified intrinsic factor.

A serum concentration of vitamin B_{12} below 110 pmol/L is associated with megaloblastic bone marrow, incipient anaemia and myelin damage. Below 150 pmol/L there are early bone marrow changes, abnormalities of the dUMP suppression test (section 11.11.6.2) and methylmalonic aciduria after a valine load (section 11.10.2).

11.10.5.1 The Schilling test for vitamin B_{12} absorption

The absorption of vitamin B_{12} can be determined by the Schilling test. An oral dose of ^{57}Co- or ^{58}Co-labelled vitamin B_{12} is given with a parenteral flushing dose of 1 mg of non-radioactive vitamin to saturate body reserves, and the urinary excretion of radioactivity is followed as an index of absorption of the oral material. Normal subjects excrete 16–45% of the radioactivity over 24 hours, whereas patients lacking intrinsic factor excrete less than 5%.

The test can be repeated, giving intrinsic factor orally together with the radioactive vitamin B_{12}; if the impaired absorption was due to a simple lack of intrinsic factor, and not to anti-intrinsic factor antibodies in saliva or gastric juice, then a normal amount of the radioactive material should be absorbed and excreted.

11.11 *Folic acid*

Folic acid functions in the transfer of one-carbon fragments in a wide variety of biosynthetic and catabolic reactions; it is therefore metabolically closely related to vitamin B_{12}. Deficiency of either vitamin has similar clinical effects, and the main effects of vitamin B_{12} deficiency are exerted by effects on folate metabolism.

Although folate is widely distributed in foods, dietary deficiency is not uncommon, and a number of commonly used drugs can cause folate depletion. More importantly, there is good evidence that intakes of folate considerably higher than normal dietary levels reduce the risk of neural tube defects, and pregnant women are recommended to take supplements. There is also some evidence that high intakes of folate may also be effective in reducing plasma homocysteine in subjects genetically at risk of hyperhomocystinaemia (some 10–20% of the population), and hence reducing the risk of ischaemic heart disease and stroke.

11.11.1 FOLATE VITAMERS AND DIETARY EQUIVALENCE

The structure of folic acid (pteroyl glutamate) is shown in Figure 11.19. The folate coenzymes may have up to seven additional glutamate residues linked by γ-peptide bonds, forming pteroyldiglutamate ($PteGlu_2$), pteroyltriglutamate ($PteGlu_3$), etc., collectively known as folate or pteroyl polyglutamate conjugates ($PteGlu_n$).

'Folate' is the preferred trivial name for pteroylglutamate, although both 'folate' and 'folic acid' may also be used as generic descriptors to include various polyglutamates. $PteGlu_2$ is sometimes referred to as folic acid diglutamate, $PteGlu_3$ as folic acid triglutamate, etc.

As shown in Figure 11.19, tetrahydrofolate can carry one-carbon fragments attached to N-5 (formyl, formimino or methyl groups), N-10 (formyl) or bridging N-5–N-10 (methylene or methenyl groups). 5-Formyl-tetrahydrofolate is more stable to atmospheric oxidation than folate itself, and is therefore commonly used in pharmaceutical preparations; it is also known as folinic acid, and the synthetic (racemic) compound as leucovorin.

The extent to which the different forms of folate can be absorbed varies; in order to permit calculation of folate intakes, the dietary folate equivalent has been defined as 1 μg mixed food folates or 0.6 μg free folic acid. On this basis, total dietary folate equivalents = μg food folate + 1.7 × synthetic (free) folic acid.

11.11.2 ABSORPTION AND METABOLISM OF FOLATE

About 80% of dietary folate is in the form of polyglutamates; a variable amount may be replaced by various one-carbon fragments or be present as dihydrofolate derivatives. Folate conjugates are hydrolysed in the small intestine by conjugase (pteroyl-polyglutamate hydrolase), a zinc-dependent enzyme of the pancreatic juice, bile and mucosal brush border; zinc deficiency can impair folate absorption. Free folate, released by conjugase action, is absorbed by active transport in the jejunum.

The folate in milk is mainly bound to a specific binding protein; the protein–tetrahydrofolate complex is absorbed intact, mainly in the ileum, by a mechanism that is distinct from the active transport system for the absorption of free folate. The biological availability of folate from milk, or of folate from diets to which milk has been added, is considerably greater than that of unbound folate.

Much of the dietary folate undergoes methylation and reduction within the intestinal

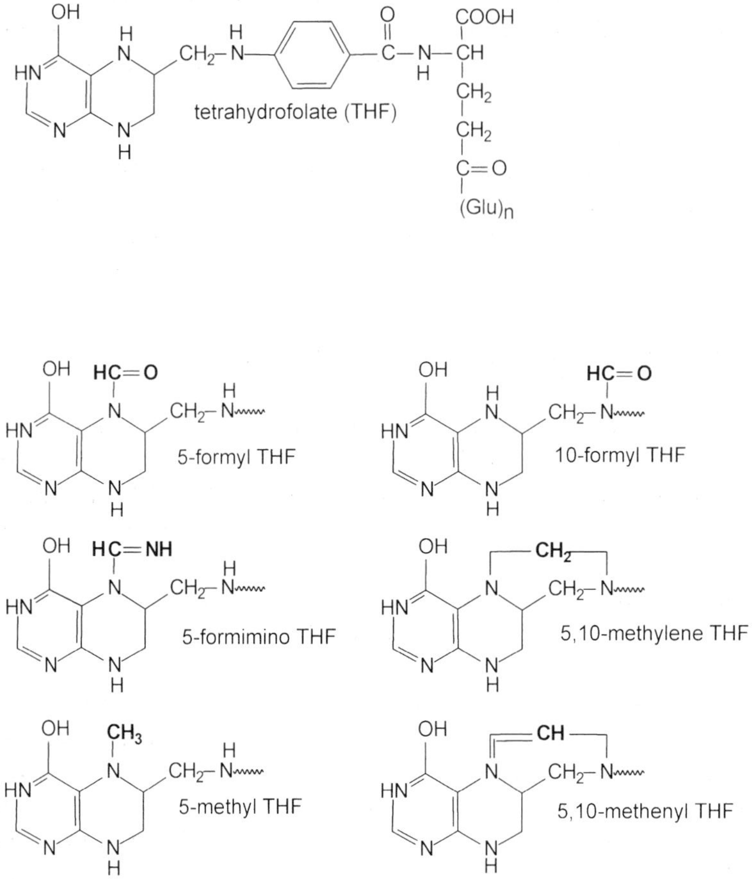

FIGURE 11.19 *Folic acid and the various one-carbon substituted folates.*

mucosa, so that what enters the portal bloodstream is largely 5-methyl-tetrahydrofolate (see Figure 11.19). Other substituted and unsubstituted folate monoglutamates and dihydrofolate are also absorbed; they are reduced and methylated in the liver, then secreted in the bile. The liver also takes up various folates released by tissues; again these are reduced, methylated and secreted in the bile.

The total daily enterohepatic circulation of folate is equivalent to about one-third of the dietary intake. Despite this, there is very little faecal loss of folate; jejunal absorption of methyl-tetrahydrofolate is a very efficient process, and the faecal excretion of some 200 μg (450 nmol) of folates per day represents synthesis by intestinal flora and does not reflect intake to any significant extent.

Methyl-tetrahydrofolate circulates bound to albumin, and is available for uptake by extrahepatic tissues. Small amounts of other one-carbon substituted folates also circulate, and will also enter cells by the same carrier-mediated process, where they are trapped by formation of polyglutamates, which do not cross cell membranes.

The main circulating folate is methyl-tetrahydrofolate, which is a poor substrate for polyglutamylation; demethylation by the action of methionine synthetase (section 11.11.3.2) is required for effective metabolic trapping of folate. In vitamin B_{12} deficiency, when methionine synthetase activity is impaired, there will therefore be impairment of the retention of folate in tissues.

The catabolism of folate is largely by cleavage of the C-9–N-10 bond, catalysed by carboxypeptidase G. The *p*-aminobenzoic acid moiety is amidated and excreted in the urine as *p*-acetamidobenzoate and *p*-acetamidobenzoyl-glutamate; pterin is excreted either unchanged or as isoxanthopterin and other biologically inactive metabolites.

11.11.3 METABOLIC FUNCTIONS OF FOLATE

The metabolic role of folate is as a carrier of one-carbon fragments, both in catabolism and in biosynthetic reactions. As shown in Figure 11.19, these may be carried as formyl, formimino, methyl, methylene or methylene residues. The major sources of these one-carbon fragments and their major uses, as well as the interconversions of the substituted folates, are shown in Figure 11.20.

The major point of entry for one-carbon fragments into substituted folates is methylene-tetrahydrofolate, which is formed by the catabolism of glycine, serine and choline.

Serine hydroxymethyltransferase is a pyridoxal phosphate-dependent enzyme that catalyses the cleavage of serine to glycine and methylene-tetrahydrofolate. Whereas folate is required for the catabolism of variety of compounds, serine is the most important source of substituted folates for biosynthetic reactions, and the activity of serine hydroxymethyltransferase is regulated by the state of folate substitution and the availability of folate. The reaction is freely reversible, and under appropriate conditions in liver it functions to form serine from glycine, as a substrate for gluconeogenesis (section 5.7).

The catabolism of histidine leads to the formation of formiminoglutamate (section 11.11.6). The formimino group is transferred onto tetrahydrofolate to form formimino-tetrahydrofolate, which is subsequently deaminated to form methenyl-tetrahydrofolate.

Methylene-, methenyl- and 10-formyl-tetrahydrofolates are freely interconvertible. This means that when one-carbon folates are not required for synthetic reactions, the oxidation of formyl-tetrahydrofolate to carbon dioxide and folate provides a means of maintaining an adequate tissue pool of free folate.

By contrast, the reduction of methylene-tetrahydrofolate to methyl-tetrahydrofolate is irreversible, and the only way in which free folate can be formed from methyl-tetrahydrofolate is by the reaction of methionine synthetase (section 11.11.3.2).

As shown in Figure 11.21, 10-formyl- and methylene-tetrahydrofolate are donors of one-carbon fragments in a number of biosynthetic reactions, including especially the synthesis of purines, pyrimidines and porphyrins. In most cases the reaction is a simple transfer of the one-carbon group from substituted folate onto the acceptor

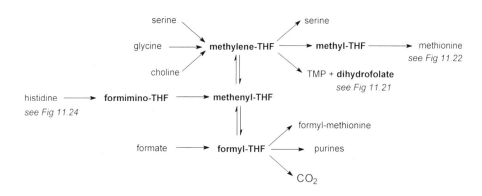

FIGURE 11.20 *Sources and utilization of folate derivatives carrying one-carbon fragments and interconversion of the one-carbon substituted folates.*

substrate. Two reactions are of especial interest: thymidylate synthetase and methionine synthetase.

11.11.3.1 Thymidylate synthetase and dihydrofolate reductase

The methylation of deoxyuridine monophosphate (dUMP) to thymidine monophosphate (TMP), catalysed by thymidylate synthetase (see Figure 11.21), is essential for the synthesis of DNA, although preformed TMP can be reutilized by salvage from the catabolism of DNA.

The methyl donor is methylene-tetrahydrofolate; the reaction involves reduction of the one-carbon fragment to a methyl group at the expense of the folate, which is oxidized to dihydrofolate. Dihydrofolate is then reduced to tetrahydrofolate by dihydrofolate reductase.

Thymidylate synthetase and dihydrofolate reductase are especially active in tissues with a high rate of cell division, and hence a high rate of DNA replication and a high requirement for thymidylate. Because of this, inhibitors of dihydrofolate reductase have been exploited as anti-cancer drugs. The most successful of these is methotrexate, an analogue of 10-methyl-tetrahydrofolate. Chemotherapy consists of alternating periods of administration of methotrexate and folate (normally as 5-formyl-tetrahydrofolate, leucovorin) in order to replete the normal tissues and avoid induction of folate deficiency – so-called 'leucovorin rescue'.

The dihydrofolate reductase of some bacteria and parasites differs significantly from the human enzyme, so that inhibitors of the enzyme can be used as antibacterial drugs (e.g. trimethoprim) and antimalarial drugs (e.g. pyrimethamine).

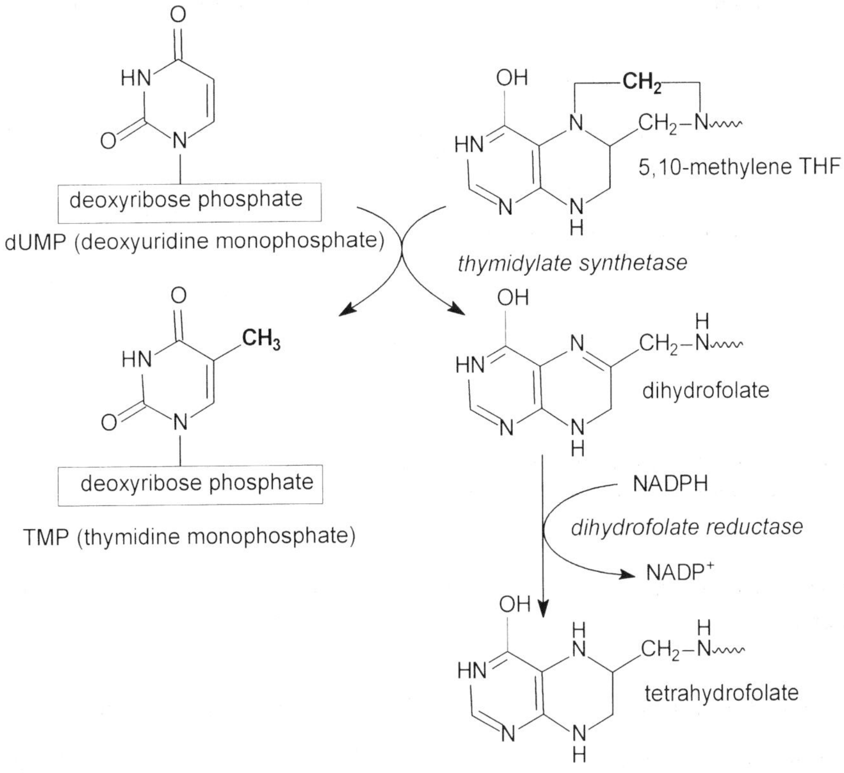

FIGURE 11.21 *The reaction of thymidylate synthetase and dihydrofolate reductase.*

11.11.3.2 Methionine synthetase and the methyl-folate trap

In addition to its role in the synthesis of proteins, methionine, as the *S*-adenosyl derivative, acts as a methyl donor in a wide variety of biosynthetic reactions. As shown in Figure 11.22, the resultant homocysteine may either be metabolized to yield cysteine or may be remethylated to yield methionine.

Two enzymes catalyse the methylation of homocysteine to methionine:

- methionine synthetase is a vitamin B$_{12}$-dependent enzyme, for which the methyl donor is methyl-tetrahydrofolate;
- homocysteine methyltransferase utilizes betaine (an intermediate in the catabolism of choline) as the methyl donor and is not vitamin B$_{12}$ dependent.

Both enzymes are found in most tissues, but only the vitamin B$_{12}$-dependent methionine synthetase is found in the central nervous system.

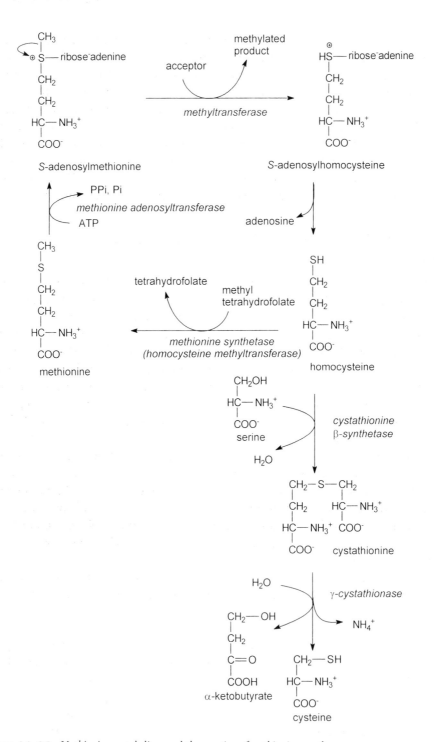

FIGURE 11.22 *Methionine metabolism and the reaction of methionine synthetase.*

The reduction of methylene-tetrahydrofolate to methyl-tetrahydrofolate is irreversible, and the major source of folate for tissues is methyl-tetrahydrofolate. The only metabolic role of methyl-tetrahydrofolate is the methylation of homocysteine to methionine, and this is the only way in which methyl-tetrahydrofolate can be demethylated to yield free folate in tissues. Methionine synthetase thus provides the link between the physiological functions of folate and vitamin B_{12}. Impairment of methionine synthetase activity in vitamin B_{12} deficiency will result in the accumulation of methyl-tetrahydrofolate, which can neither be utilized for any other one-carbon transfer reactions nor be demethylated to provide free folate. There is therefore functional deficiency of folate, secondary to the deficiency of vitamin B_{12}.

11.11.3.3 Methylene-tetrahydrofolate reductase and hyperhomocysteinaemia

Elevated blood homocysteine is a significant risk factor for atherosclerosis, thrombosis and hypertension, independent of factors such as dietary lipids and plasma lipoproteins (section 7.3.2). About 10–15% of the population, and almost 30% of people with ischaemic heart disease, have an abnormal variant of methylene-tetrahydrofolate reductase (Figure 11.23) that is unstable and loses activity faster than normal.

The result of this is that people with the abnormal form of the enzyme have an impaired ability to form methyl-tetrahydrofolate (the main form in which folate is taken up by tissues), and suffer from functional folate deficiency. Therefore, they are unable to remethylate homocysteine to methionine adequately and develop hyperhomocysteinaemia.

People with the abnormal variant of methylene-tetrahydrofolate reductase do not develop hyperhomocysteinaemia if they have a relatively high intake of folate. This seems to be due to the methylation of folate in the intestinal mucosa during absorption; intestinal mucosal cells have a rapid turnover (section 4.1), and therefore it is not important that methylene-tetrahydrofolate reductase is less stable than normal – there is still an adequate activity of the enzyme in the intestinal mucosa to maintain absorption of methyl-tetrahydrofolate.

This has led to the suggestion that supplements of folate will reduce the incidence of cardiovascular disease; to date there is no evidence from intervention studies that

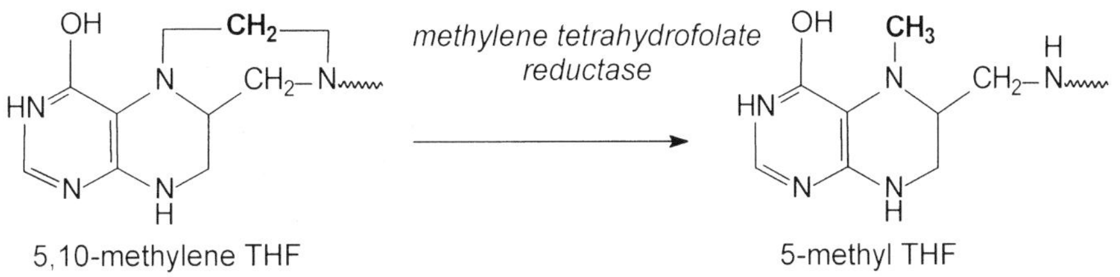

FIGURE 11.23 *The reaction of methylene tetrahydrofolate reductase.*

the lowering of plasma homocysteine by folate supplements does reduce the risk, but mandatory enrichment of foods with folate has been introduced in some countries.

11.11.4 FOLATE DEFICIENCY: MEGALOBLASTIC ANAEMIA

Dietary deficiency of folic acid is not uncommon, and, as noted above, deficiency of vitamin B_{12} also leads to functional folic acid deficiency. In either case, it is cells which are dividing rapidly, and which therefore have a large requirement for thymidine for DNA synthesis, which are most severely affected. These are the cells of the bone marrow which form red blood cells, the cells of the intestinal mucosa and the hair follicles. Clinically, folic acid deficiency leads to megaloblastic anaemia, the release into the circulation of immature precursors of red blood cells.

Megaloblastic anaemia is also seen in vitamin B_{12} deficiency, when it is due to functional folate deficiency as a result of trapping folate as methyl-tetrahydrofolate (section 11.11.3.2). However, the neurological degeneration of pernicious anaemia (section 11.10.3) is rarely seen in folate deficiency, and indeed a high intake of folate can mask the development of megaloblastic anaemia in vitamin B_{12} deficiency, so that the presenting sign is irreversible nerve damage.

11.11.5 FOLATE REQUIREMENTS

Depletion/repletion studies to determine folate requirements using folic acid monoglutamate suggest a requirement of the order of 80–100 µg (170–220 nmol)/ day. The total body pool of folate in adults is some 17 µmol (7.5 mg), with a biological half-life of 101 days. This suggests a minimum requirement for replacement of 85 nmol (37 µg)/day. Studies of the urinary excretion of folate metabolites in subjects maintained on folate-free diets suggest that there is catabolism of some 80 µg of folate per day.

Because of the problems of determining the biological availability of the various folate polyglutamate conjugates found in foods, reference intakes allow a wide margin of safety, and are based on an allowance of 3 µg (6.8 nmol) per kg body weight.

11.11.5.1 Folate in pregnancy

During the 1980s a considerable body of evidence accumulated that spina bifida and other neural tube defects (which occur in about 0.75–1% of pregnancies) were associated with low intakes of folate and that increased intake during pregnancy might be protective. It is now established that supplements of folate begun periconceptually result in a significant reduction in the incidence of neural tube defects, and it is recommended that intakes be increased by 400 µg/day before conception. The studies were conducted using folate monoglutamate, and it is unlikely that an equivalent increase in intake could be achieved from unfortified foods; supplements are recommended. Closure of the neural tube occurs by day 28 of pregnancy, which is before the woman knows she is pregnant. The advice therefore is that all women who are, or may be about to become, pregnant should take folate supplements.

11.11.5.2 Higher levels of folate intake

Folate supplements of 400 μg/day reduce the incidence of spina bifida and neural tube defect; about 1% of pregnant women are at risk. Similar supplements lower plasma homocysteine in people with the abnormal variant of methylene tetrahydrofolate reductase (section 11.3.3); between 10% and 20% of the population are homozygous for the abnormal gene.

There is some evidence that folate supplements in excess of 350 μg/day may impair zinc absorption. In addition, there are two potential problems that have to be considered when advocating either widespread use of folate supplements or enrichment of foods with folate for protection against heart disease and neural tube defect:

- Folate supplements will mask the megaloblastic anaemia of vitamin B_{12} deficiency (section 11.10.3), and may hasten the development of the (irreversible) nerve damage. This is especially a problem of the elderly, who may suffer impaired absorption of vitamin B_{12} as a result of gastric atrophy with increasing age. It has been suggested that the addition of relatively large amounts of vitamin B_{12} to foods, as well as folate, would permit passive absorption of adequate amounts of vitamin B_{12} to prevent deficiency developing.
- Antagonism between folic acid and the anticonvulsants used in the treatment of epilepsy is part of their mechanism of action; about 2% of the population have (drug-controlled) epilepsy. Relatively large supplements of folic acid (in excess of 1000 μg/day) may antagonize the beneficial effects of the anticonvulsants and lead to an increase in the frequency of epileptic attacks. If enrichment of a food such as bread with folate is to provide 400 μg/day to those who eat little bread, those who eat a relatively large amount may well have an intake in excess of 1000 μg/day.

11.11.6 ASSESSMENT OF FOLATE STATUS

Measurement of the serum or red blood cell concentration of folate is the method of choice, and a number of simple and reliable radioligand-binding assays have been developed. There are a number of problems involved in radioligand-binding assays for folate, and in some centres microbiological determination of plasma or whole-blood folates is the preferred technique.

11.11.6.1 Histidine metabolism – the FIGLU test

The ability to metabolize a test dose of histidine provides a sensitive functional test of

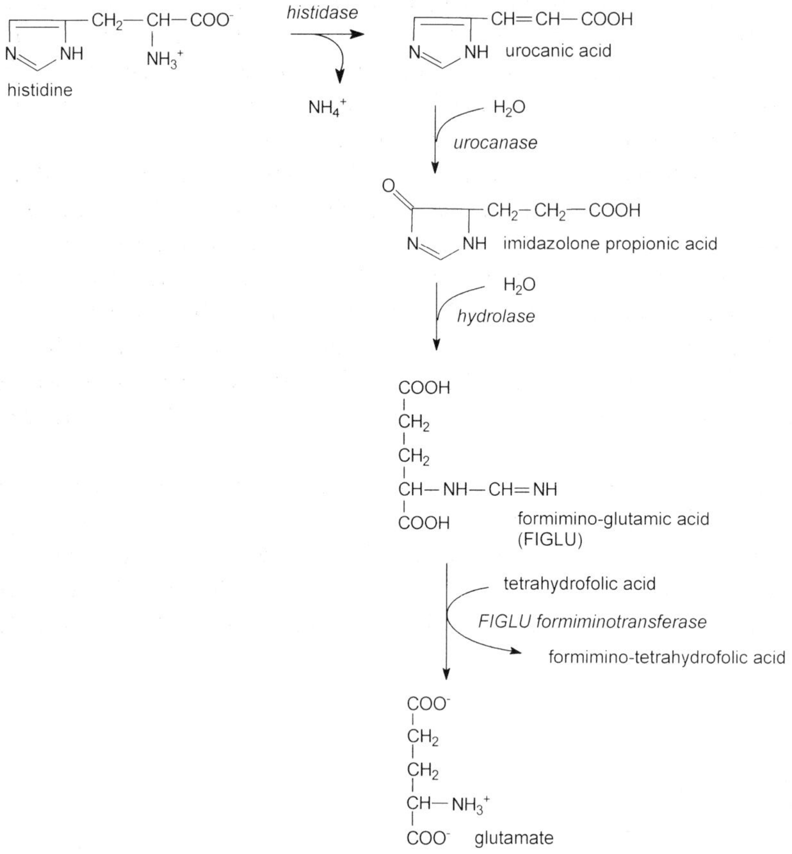

FIGURE 11.24 *Metabolism of histidine – the FIGLU test for folate status.*

folate nutritional status; formiminoglutamate (FIGLU) is an intermediate in histidine catabolism (Figure 11.24) and is metabolized by the folate-dependent enzyme formiminoglutamate formiminotransferase. In folate deficiency the activity of this enzyme is impaired and formiminoglutamate accumulates and is excreted in the urine, especially after a test dose of histidine – the so-called FIGLU test.

Although the FIGLU test depends on folate nutritional status, the metabolism of histidine will also be impaired, and hence a positive result obtained, in vitamin B_{12} deficiency because of the secondary deficiency of free folate. About 60% of vitamin B_{12}-deficient subjects show increased FIGLU excretion after a histidine load.

11.11.6.2 The dUMP suppression test

Rapidly dividing cells can either use preformed TMP for DNA synthesis, or can synthesize it *de novo* from dUMP (section 11.11.3.1). Isolated bone marrow cells or stimulated lymphocytes incubated with [^{3}H]TMP will incorporate label into DNA. In the presence of adequate amounts of methylene-tetrahydrofolate, the addition of dUMP as a substrate for thymidylate synthetase reduces the incorporation of [^{3}H]TMP as a result of dilution of the pool of labelled material by newly synthesized TMP and inhibition of thymidylate kinase by thymidine triphosphate

The ability of deoxyuridine to suppress the incorporation of [^{3}H]thymidine into DNA in rapidly dividing cells can be used to give an index of folate status. Bone marrow biopsy samples provide the best source, so this has been generally a research tool rather than a screening test; however, transformed lymphocytes can also be used.

In normal cells the incorporation of [^{3}H]thymidine into DNA after preincubation with dUMP is 1.4–1.8% of that without preincubation. By contrast, cells that are deficient in folate form little or no thymidine from dUMP, and hence incorporate nearly as much of the [^{3}H]thymidine after incubation with dUMP as they do without preincubation.

Either a primary deficiency of folic acid or functional deficiency secondary to vitamin B$_{12}$ deficiency will have the same effect. In folate deficiency, addition of any biologically active form of folate, but not vitamin B$_{12}$, will normalize the dUMP suppression of [^{3}H]thymidine incorporation. In vitamin B$_{12}$ deficiency, addition of vitamin B$_{12}$ or methylene-tetrahydrofolate, but not methyl-tetrahydrofolate, will normalize dUMP suppression.

11.12 *Biotin*

Biotin was originally discovered as part of the complex called *bios*, which promoted the growth of yeast and, separately, as vitamin H, the protective or curative factor in 'egg white injury' – the disease caused in man and experimental animals by feeding diets containing large amounts of uncooked egg white. The structures of biotin, biocytin and carboxybiocytin (the active metabolic intermediate) are shown in Figure 11.25.

Biotin is widely distributed in many foods. It is synthesized by intestinal flora, and in balance studies the total output of biotin in urine plus faeces is three- to sixfold greater than the intake, reflecting bacterial synthesis. It is not known to what extent this is available to the host (see also Problem 10.4).

11.12.1 ABSORPTION AND METABOLISM OF BIOTIN

Most biotin in foods is present as biocytin (ε-aminobiotinyllysine), which is released on proteolysis, then hydrolysed by biotinidase in the pancreatic juice and intestinal mucosal secretions, to yield free biotin. The extent to which bound biotin in foods is biologically available is not known.

Free biotin is absorbed from the small intestine by active transport. Biotin circulates in the bloodstream both free and bound to a serum glycoprotein which has biotinidase activity, catalysing the hydrolysis of biocytin.

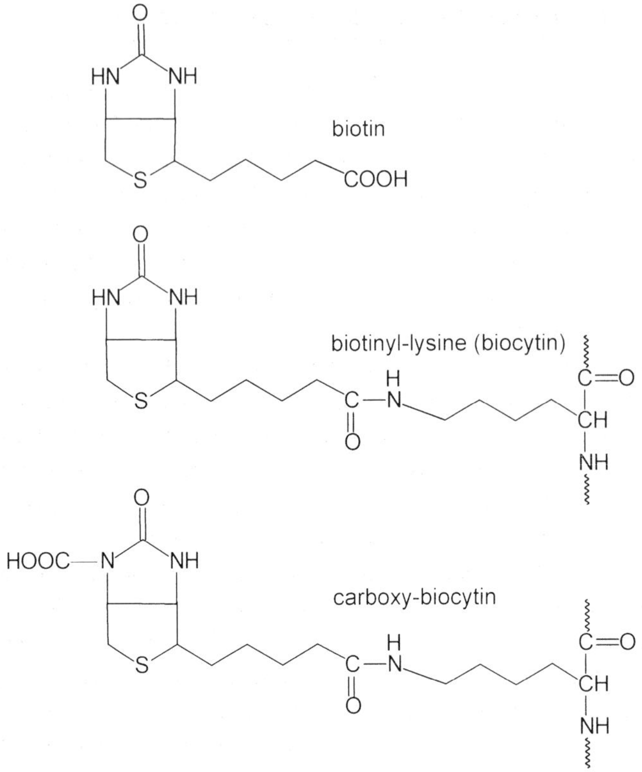

FIGURE 11.25 *Biotin, biocytin (ε-aminobiotinyllysine) and carboxybiocytin.*

Biotin enters tissues by a saturable transport system, and is then incorporated into biotin-dependent enzymes as the ε-aminolysine peptide, biocytin. Unlike other B vitamins, whose concentrative uptake into tissues can be achieved by facilitated diffusion followed by metabolic trapping, the incorporation of biotin into enzymes is relatively slow and cannot be considered part of the uptake process. On catabolism of the enzymes, biocytin is hydrolysed by biotinidase, permitting reutilization.

11.12.2 METABOLIC FUNCTIONS OF BIOTIN

Biotin functions to transfer carbon dioxide in a small number of carboxylation reactions. The reactive intermediate is 1-*N*-carboxybiocytin (Figure 11.25), formed from bicarbonate in an ATP-dependent reaction. A single holocarboxylase synthetase acts on the apoenzymes of acetyl CoA carboxylase (a key enzyme in fatty acid synthesis; section 5.6.1), pyruvate carboxylase (a key enzyme in gluconeogenesis; section 5.7), propionyl CoA carboxylase and methylcrotonyl CoA carboxylase to form the active holoenzymes from (inactive) apoenzymes and free biotin.

11.12.3 BIOTIN DEFICIENCY AND REQUIREMENTS

Biotin is widely distributed in foods, and deficiency is unknown, except among people maintained for many months on total parenteral nutrition and a very small number of people who eat abnormally large amounts of uncooked egg. There is a protein in egg white, avidin, that binds biotin extremely tightly and renders it unavailable for absorption. Avidin is denatured by cooking and then loses its ability to bind biotin. The amount of avidin in uncooked egg white is relatively small, and problems of biotin deficiency have occurred only in people eating abnormally large amounts – a dozen or more raw eggs a day – for some years.

The few early reports of human biotin deficiency all occurred in people who consumed large amounts of uncooked eggs. They developed a fine scaly dermatitis and hair loss (alopecia). Histology of the skin showed an absence of sebaceous glands and atrophy of the hair follicles. Provision of biotin supplements of between 200 and 1000 μg/day resulted in cure of the skin lesions and regrowth of hair, despite continuing the abnormal diet providing large amounts of avidin. There have been no studies of provision of modest doses of biotin to such patients, and none in which their high intake of uncooked eggs was not either replaced by an equivalent intake of cooked eggs (in which avidin has been denatured by heat, and the yolks of which are a good source of biotin) or continued unchanged, so there is no information from these case reports of the amounts of biotin required for normal health. More recently, similar signs of biotin deficiency have been observed in patients receiving total parenteral nutrition for prolonged periods after major resection of the gut. The signs resolve following the provision of biotin, but again there have been no studies of the amounts of biotin required; intakes have ranged between 60 and 200 μg/day

There is no evidence on which to estimate requirements for biotin. Average intakes are between 10 and 200 μg/day. As dietary deficiency does not occur, such intakes are obviously more than adequate to meet requirements.

11.13 *Pantothenic acid*

Pantothenic acid (sometimes known as vitamin B_5, and at one time called vitamin B_3) has a central role in energy-yielding metabolism as the functional moiety of coenzyme A and in the biosynthesis of fatty acids as the prosthetic group of acyl carrier protein (section 5.6.1). The structures of pantothenic acid and coenzyme A are shown in Figure 11.26.

Pantothenic acid is widely distributed in all foodstuffs; the name derives from the Greek for 'from everywhere', as opposed to other vitamins, which were originally isolated from individual especially rich sources. As a result, deficiency has not been unequivocally reported in human beings except in specific depletion studies, which have generally used the antagonist ω-methyl-pantothenic acid.

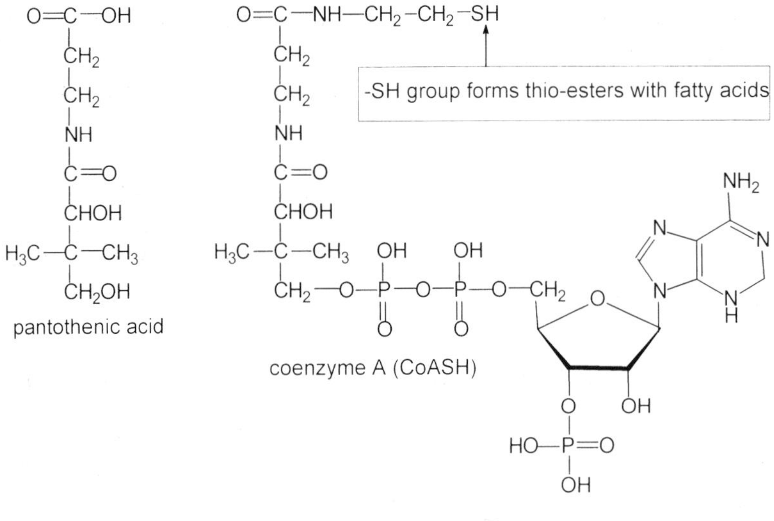

FIGURE 11.26 *Pantothenic acid and coenzyme A.*

11.13.1 ABSORPTION, METABOLISM AND METABOLIC FUNCTIONS OF PANTOTHENIC ACID

About 85% of dietary pantothenic acid occurs as CoA or phosphopantetheine. In the intestinal lumen these are hydrolysed to pantetheine; intestinal mucosal cells have a high pantetheinase activity and rapidly hydrolyse pantetheine to pantothenic acid. The intestinal absorption of pantothenic acid is by diffusion and occurs at a constant rate throughout the length of the small intestine; intestinal bacterial synthesis may contribute to pantothenic acid nutrition.

The first step in pantothenic acid utilization is phosphorylation. Pantothenate kinase is rate limiting, so that, unlike many vitamins, which are accumulated by metabolic trapping, there can be significant accumulation of free pantothenic acid in tissues.

11.13.1.1 Coenzyme A and acyl carrier protein

All tissues are capable of forming coenzyme A from pantothenic acid. CoA functions as the carrier of fatty acids, as thioesters, in mitochondrial β-oxidation (section 5.5.2). The resultant two-carbon fragments, as acetyl CoA, then undergo oxidation in the citric acid cycle (section 5.4.4). CoA also functions as a carrier in the transfer of acetyl (and other fatty acyl) moieties in a variety of biosynthetic and catabolic reactions, including:

* cholesterol and steroid hormone synthesis;

- long-chain fatty acid synthesis from palmitate and elongation of polyunsaturated fatty acids in mitochondria;
- acylation of serine, threonine and cysteine residues on proteolipids and acetylation of neuraminic acid.

Fatty acid synthesis (section 5.6.1) is catalysed by a cytosolic multienzyme complex in which the growing fatty acyl chain is bound by thioester linkage to an enzyme-bound 4′-phosphopantetheine residue, rather than to free CoA, as in β-oxidation. This component of the fatty acid synthetase complex is the acyl carrier protein.

11.13.2 Pantothenic acid deficiency: safe and adequate levels of intake

Prisoners of war in the Far East in the 1940s, who were severely malnourished, showed, among other signs and symptoms of vitamin deficiency diseases, a new condition of paraesthesia and severe pain in the feet and toes, which was called the 'burning foot syndrome' or nutritional melalgia. Although it was tentatively attributed to pantothenic acid deficiency, no specific trials of pantothenic acid were carried out; rather the subjects were given yeast extract and other rich sources of all vitamins as part of an urgent programme of nutritional rehabilitation.

Experimental pantothenic acid depletion, commonly together with the administration of ω-methyl-pantothenic acid, results in the following signs and symptoms after 2–3 weeks:

- Neuromotor disorders, including paraesthesia of the hands and feet, hyperactive deep tendon reflexes and muscle weakness. These can be explained by the role of acetyl CoA in the synthesis of the neurotransmitter acetylcholine and impaired formation of threonine acyl esters in myelin. Dysmyelination may explain the persistence and recurrence of neurological problems many years after nutritional rehabilitation in people who had suffered from burning foot syndrome.
- Mental depression, which again may be related to either acetylcholine deficit or impaired myelin synthesis.
- Gastrointestinal complaints, including severe vomiting and pain, with depressed gastric acid secretion in response to gastrin.
- Decreased serum cholesterol and decreased urinary excretion of 17-ketosteroids, reflecting the impairment of steroidogenesis.
- Decreased acetylation of *p*-aminobenzoic acid, sulphonamides and other drugs, reflecting reduced availability of acetyl CoA for these reactions.

There is no evidence on which to estimate pantothenic acid requirements. Average intakes are between 3 and 7 mg/day and, as deficiency does not occur, such intakes are obviously more than adequate to meet requirements.

11.14 *Vitamin C (ascorbic acid)*

Vitamin C is a vitamin for only a limited number of vertebrate species: man and the other primates, the guinea pig, bats, the passeriform birds and most fishes. Ascorbate is synthesized as an intermediate in the gulonolactone pathway of glucose metabolism; in those vertebrate species for which it is a vitamin, one enzyme of the pathway, gulonolactone oxidase, is absent.

The vitamin C deficiency disease, scurvy, has been known for many centuries, and was described in the Ebers papyrus of 1500 BC and by Hippocrates. The Crusaders are said to have lost more men through scurvy than were killed in battle, while in some of the long voyages of exploration of the fourteenth and fifteenth centuries up to 90% of the crew died from scurvy. Cartier's expedition to Quebec in 1535 was struck by scurvy; the local Indians taught him to use an infusion of swamp spruce leaves to prevent or cure the condition.

Recognition that scurvy was due to a dietary deficiency came relatively early. James Lind demonstrated in 1757 that orange and lemon juice were protective, and Cook maintained his crew in good health during his circumnavigation of the globe (1772–75) by stopping frequently to take on fresh fruit and vegetables. In 1804, the British Navy decreed a daily ration of lemon or lime juice for all ratings, a requirement that was extended to the merchant navy in 1865.

The structure of vitamin C is shown in Figure 11.27; both ascorbic acid and dehydroascorbic acid have vitamin activity.

Vitamin C is found in fruits and vegetables. Very significant losses of vitamin C occur as vegetables wilt, or when they are cut, as a result of release of ascorbate oxidase from the plant tissue. Significant losses of the vitamin also occur in cooking, through both leaching into the cooking water and atmospheric oxidation, which continues when foods are left to stand before serving.

11.14.1 ABSORPTION AND METABOLISM OF VITAMIN C

There is active transport of the vitamin at the intestinal mucosal brush border membrane. Some 80–95% of dietary ascorbate is absorbed at usual intakes (up to about 100 mg/day). The absorption of larger amounts of the vitamin is lower, falling from 50% of a 1.5 g dose to 25% of a 6 g and 16% of a 12 g dose.

About 70% of blood ascorbate is in plasma and erythrocytes (which do not concentrate the vitamin from plasma). The remainder is in white cells, which have a marked ability to concentrate it (section 11.14.5).

There is no specific storage organ for ascorbate; apart from leucocytes (which account for only 10% of total blood ascorbate), the only tissues showing a significant concentration of the vitamin are the adrenal and pituitary glands.

Ascorbic acid is excreted in the urine, either unchanged or as dehydroascorbate

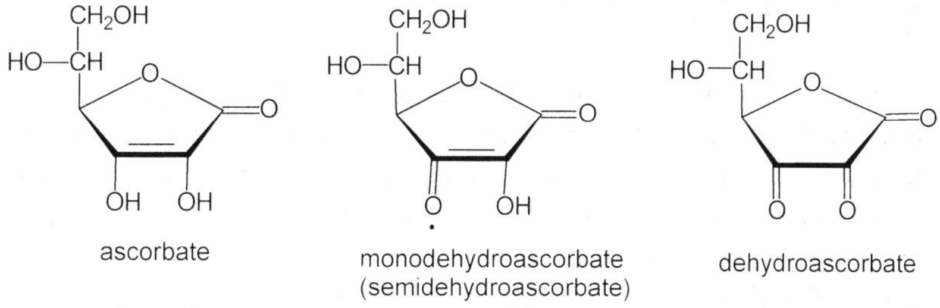

CH$_2$OH

HO—CH

OH OH

ascorbate

CH$_2$OH

HO—CH

O OH

monodehydroascorbate
(semidehydroascorbate)

CH$_2$OH

HO—CH

O O

dehydroascorbate

FIGURE 11.27 *Vitamin C.*

and diketogulonate. Both ascorbate and dehydroascorbate are filtered at the glomerulus, then reabsorbed. When glomerular filtration of ascorbate and dehydroascorbate exceeds the capacity of the transport systems, at a plasma concentration of ascorbate between 70 and 85 μmol/L, the vitamin is excreted in the urine in amounts proportional to intake.

11.14.2 Metabolic functions of vitamin C

Ascorbic acid has specific roles in two groups of enzymes: the copper-containing hydroxylases and the α-ketoglutarate-linked iron-containing hydroxylases. It also increases the activity of a number of other enzymes *in vitro*, although this is a non-specific reducing action rather than reflecting any metabolic function of the vitamin. In addition, it has a number of non-enzymic effects due to its action as a reducing agent and oxygen radical quencher (section 7.4.3.5).

11.14.2.1 Copper-containing hydroxylases

Dopamine β-hydroxylase is a copper-containing enzyme involved in the synthesis of the catecholamines noradrenaline and adrenaline from tyrosine in the adrenal medulla and central nervous system. The enzyme contains Cu$^+$, which is oxidized to Cu^{2+} during the hydroxylation of the substrate; reduction back to Cu$^+$ specifically requires ascorbate, which is oxidized to monodehydroascorbate.

A number of peptide hormones have a carboxy-terminal amide that is essential for biological activity. The amide group is derived from a glycine residue on the carboxyl side of the amino acid that will become the amidated terminal of the mature peptide. This glycine is hydroxylated on the α-carbon by a copper-containing enzyme, peptidylglycine hydroxylase. The α-hydroxyglycine residue then decomposes non-enzymically to yield the amidated peptide and glyoxylate. The copper prosthetic group is oxidized in the reaction and, as in dopamine β-hydroxylase, ascorbate is specifically required for reduction back to Cu$^+$.

11.14.2.2 α-Ketoglutarate-linked iron-containing hydroxylases

A number of iron-containing hydroxylases share a common reaction mechanism, in which hydroxylation of the substrate is linked to decarboxylation of α-ketoglutarate. Many of these enzymes are involved in the modification of precursor proteins to yield the final, mature, protein. This is a process of post-synthetic modification – modification of an amino acid residue after it has been incorporated into the protein during synthesis on the ribosome (see Problem 9.3 and section 9.2.3.4).

- Proline and lysine hydroxylases are required for the post-synthetic modification of procollagen in the formation of mature, insoluble, collagen, and proline hydroxylase is also required for the post-synthetic modification of the precursor proteins of osteocalcin and the C1q component of complement.
- Aspartate β-hydroxylase is required for the post-synthetic modification of the precursor of protein C, the vitamin K-dependent protease that hydrolyses activated factor V in the blood clotting cascade.
- Trimethyllysine and γ-butyrobetaine hydroxylases are required for the synthesis of carnitine (section 5.5.1).

Ascorbate is oxidized during the reaction of these enzymes, but not stoichiometrically with the decarboxylation of α-ketoglutarate and hydroxylation of the substrate. The purified enzyme is active in the absence of ascorbate, but after some 5–10 seconds (about 15–30 cycles of enzyme action) the rate of reaction begins to fall. At this stage the iron in the catalytic site has been oxidized to Fe^{3+}, which is catalytically inactive; activity is restored by only ascorbate, which reduces it back to Fe^{2+}. The oxidation of Fe^{2+} is the consequence of a side-reaction rather than the main reaction of the enzyme, which explains how 15–30 cycles of enzyme activity can occur before there is significant loss of activity in the absence of ascorbate, and why the consumption of ascorbate is not stoichiometric.

11.14.3 VITAMIN C DEFICIENCY: SCURVY

The vitamin C deficiency disease, scurvy, was formerly a common problem at the end of winter, when there had been no fresh fruits and vegetables for many months.

Although there is no specific organ for storage of vitamin C in the body, signs of deficiency do not develop in previously adequately nourished subjects until they have been deprived of the vitamin for 4–6 months, by which time plasma and tissue concentrations have fallen considerably. The earliest signs of scurvy in volunteers maintained on a vitamin C-free diet are skin changes, beginning with plugging of hair follicles by horny material, followed by enlargement of the hyperkeratotic follicles and petechial haemorrhage as a result of increased fragility of blood capillaries.

At a later stage there is also haemorrhage of the gums. This is frequently accompanied by secondary bacterial infection and considerable withdrawal of the gum from the necks of the teeth. As the condition progresses, there is loss of dental cement, and the teeth become loose in the alveolar bone and may be lost.

Wounds show only superficial healing in scurvy, with little or no formation of (collagen-rich) scar tissue, so that healing is delayed and wounds can readily be reopened (see Problem 9.3). The scorbutic scar tissue has only about half the tensile strength of that normally formed.

Advanced scurvy is accompanied by intense pain in the bones, which can be attributed to changes in bone mineralization as a result of abnormal collagen synthesis. Bone formation ceases and the existing bone becomes rarefied, so that the bones fracture with minimal trauma.

The name scurvy is derived from the Italian *scorbutico*, meaning an irritable, neurotic, discontented, whining and cranky person. The disease is associated with listlessness and general malaise, and sometimes with changes in personality and psychomotor performance and a lowering of the general level of arousal. These behavioural effects can be attributed to impaired synthesis of catecholamine neurotransmitters, as a result of low activity of dopamine β-hydroxylase.

Most of the other clinical signs of scurvy can be accounted for by the effects of ascorbate deficiency on collagen synthesis, as a result of impaired proline and lysine hydroxylase activity. Depletion of muscle carnitine (section 5.5.1), as a result of impaired activity of trimethyllysine and γ-butyrobetaine hydroxylases, may account for the lassitude and fatigue that precede clinical signs of scurvy.

11.14.3.1 Anaemia in scurvy

Anaemia is frequently associated with scurvy, and may be either macrocytic, indicative of folate deficiency (section 11.11.4), or hypochromic, indicative of iron deficiency (section 11.15.2.3).

Folate deficiency may be epiphenomenal, as the major dietary sources of folate are the same as those of ascorbate. However, some patients with clear megaloblastic anaemia respond to the administration of vitamin C alone, suggesting that there may be a role of ascorbate in the maintenance of normal pools of reduced folates, although there is no evidence that any of the reactions of folate is ascorbate dependent,

Iron deficiency in scurvy may well be secondary to reduced absorption of inorganic iron and impaired mobilization of tissue iron reserves (section 11.15.2.3). At the same time, the haemorrhages of advanced scurvy will cause a significant loss of blood.

There is also evidence that erythrocytes have a shorter half-life than normal in scurvy, possibly as a result of peroxidative damage to membrane lipids due to impairment of the reduction of tocopheroxyl radical by ascorbate (section 7.4.3.3).

11.14.4 VITAMIN C REQUIREMENTS

Vitamin C illustrates extremely well how different criteria of adequacy, and different interpretations of experimental evidence (section 11.1), can lead to different estimates of requirements, and to reference intakes ranging between 30 and 90 mg/day for adults.

The requirement for vitamin C to prevent clinical scurvy is less than 10 mg/day. However, at this level of intake wounds do not heal properly because of the requirement for vitamin C for the synthesis of collagen in connective tissue. An intake of 20 mg/day is required for optimum wound healing. Allowing for individual variation in requirements, this gives a reference intake for adults of 30 mg/day, which was the British RDA until 1991 and is the United Nations Food and Agriculture Organization/World Health Organization RDA.

The 1991 British RNI for vitamin C is based on the level of intake at which the plasma concentration rises sharply, showing that requirements have now been met, tissues are saturated and there is spare vitamin C being transported between tissues, available for excretion. This criterion of adequacy gives an RNI of 40 mg/day for adults.

The alternative approach to determining requirements is to estimate the total body content of vitamin C, then measure the rate at which it is metabolized, by giving a test dose of radioactive vitamin. This is the basis of both the 1989 US RDA of 60 mg/day for adults and the Netherlands RDA of 80 mg/day. Indeed, it also provides an alternative basis for the RNI of 40 mg/day adopted in Britain in 1991.

The problem lies in deciding what is an appropriate body content of vitamin C. The American studies were performed on subjects whose total body vitamin C was estimated to be 1500 mg at the beginning of a depletion study. However, there is no evidence that this is a necessary, or even a desirable, body content of the vitamin. It is simply the body content of the vitamin among a small group of young people eating a self-selected diet rich in fruit. There is good evidence that a total body content of 900 mg is more than adequate. It is three times larger than the body content at which the first signs of deficiency are observed and will protect against the development of any signs of deficiency for several months on a completely vitamin C-free diet.

There is a further problem in interpreting the results of this kind of study. The rate at which vitamin C is metabolized varies with the amount consumed. This means that, as the experimental subjects become depleted, so the rate at which they metabolize the vitamin decreases. Thus, calculation of the amount that is required to maintain the body content depends on the way in which results obtained during depletion studies are extrapolated to the rate in subjects consuming a normal diet – and on the amount of vitamin C in that diet.

An intake of 40 mg/day is more than adequate to maintain a total body content of 900 mg of vitamin C – the same as the British RNI. At a higher level of habitual intake, 60 mg/day is adequate to maintain a total body content of 1500 mg (the 1989 US RDA). Making allowances for changes in the rate of metabolism with different levels of intake, and allowing for incomplete absorption of the vitamin gives the Netherlands RDA of 80 mg/day.

The 2000 US RDA for vitamin C, shown in Table 11.3, is based on intakes required to achieve near-complete saturation of neutrophils with the vitamin, with minimal urinary loss, giving an RDA of 90 mg/day for men and an extrapolated RDA of 75 mg/day for women.

11.14.4.1 Possible benefits of high intakes of vitamin C

At intakes above about 100 mg/day the body's capacity to metabolize vitamin C is saturated, and any further intake is excreted in the urine unchanged. Therefore, it would not seem justifiable to recommend higher levels of intake. However, in addition to its antioxidant role (section 7.4.3.5), vitamin C is also important in the absorption of iron (section 4.5.1). This depends on the presence of the vitamin in the gut together with food, and intakes totalling more than 100 mg/day may be beneficial.

Inorganic iron is absorbed as Fe^{2+}, and not as Fe^{3+}; ascorbic acid in the intestinal lumen will both maintain iron in the reduced state and also chelate it, thus increasing the amount absorbed. A dose of 25 mg of vitamin C taken together with a meal increases the absorption of iron some 65%, whereas a 1 g dose gives a ninefold increase. This occurs only when ascorbic acid is present together with the test meal; neither intravenous administration of vitamin C nor intake several hours before the test meal has any effect on iron absorption. Optimum iron absorption may therefore require significantly more than 100 mg of vitamin C per day.

The safety of nitrates and nitrites used in curing meat, a traditional method of preservation, has been questioned because of the formation of nitrosamines by reaction between nitrite and amines naturally present in foods under the acid conditions in the stomach. In experimental animals, nitrosamines are potent carcinogens, and some authorities have limited the amounts of these salts that are permitted, although there is little evidence of any hazard to human beings from endogenous nitrosamine formation. Ascorbate can prevent the formation of nitrosamines by reacting non-enzymically with nitrite and other nitrosating reagents, forming NO, NO_2 and N_2. Again, this is an effect of ascorbate present in the stomach at the same time as the dietary nitrites and amines, rather than an effect of vitamin C nutritional status.

11.14.4.2 Pharmacological uses of vitamin C

A number of studies have reported low ascorbate status in patients with advanced cancer – perhaps an unsurprising finding in seriously ill patients. With very little experimental evidence, it has been suggested that very high intakes of vitamin C (of the order of 10 g/day or more) may be beneficial in enhancing host resistance to cancer and preventing the development of AIDS in people who are HIV positive. In controlled studies with patients matched for age, sex, site and stage of primary tumours and metastases, and for previous chemotherapy, there was no beneficial effect of high-dose ascorbic acid in the treatment of advanced cancer.

High doses of vitamin C have been recommended for the prevention and treatment of the common cold, with some evidence that the vitamin reduces the duration of symptoms. However, the evidence from controlled trials is unconvincing.

11.14.4.3 Toxicity of vitamin C

Regardless of whether or not high intakes of ascorbate have any beneficial effects, large numbers of people habitually take between 1 and 5 g/day of vitamin C supplements (compared with reference intakes of 30–90 mg/day), and some take considerably more. There is little evidence of any significant toxicity from these high intakes. Once the plasma concentration of ascorbate reaches the renal threshold, it is excreted more or less quantitatively with increasing intake, and there is no evidence that higher intakes increase the body pool above about 1500 mg per kg body weight. Unabsorbed ascorbate in the intestinal lumen is a substrate for bacterial fermentation and may cause diarrhoea and intestinal discomfort.

Up to 5% of the population are at risk from the development of renal oxalate stones. The risk is from both ingested oxalate and that formed endogenously, mainly from the metabolism of glycine. A number of reports have suggested that people consuming high intakes of vitamin C excrete more oxalate in the urine. However, no pathway for the formation of oxalate from ascorbate is known, and it seems that the oxalate is formed non-enzymically under alkaline conditions either in the bladder or after collection, and hence high vitamin C intake is not a risk factor for renal stone formation.

11.14.5 ASSESSMENT OF VITAMIN C STATUS

It is relatively easy to assess the state of body reserves of vitamin C by measuring the excretion after a test dose. A subject whose tissue reserves are saturated will excrete more or less the whole of a test dose of 500 mg of ascorbate over 6 hours. A more precise method involves repeating the loading test daily until more or less complete recovery is achieved, thus giving an indication of how depleted the body stores were.

The plasma concentration of vitamin C falls relatively rapidly during experimental depletion studies, to undetectably low levels within 4 weeks of initiating a vitamin C-free diet, although clinical signs of scurvy may not develop for a further 3–4 months, and tissue concentrations of the vitamin may be as high as 50% of saturation.

The concentration of ascorbate in leucocytes is well correlated with the concentrations in other tissues, and falls more slowly than plasma concentration in depletion studies. The reference range of leucocyte ascorbate is 1.1–2.8 mol/10^6 cells; a significant loss of leucocyte ascorbate coincides with the development of clear clinical signs of scurvy.

Without a differential white cell count, leucocyte ascorbate concentration does not give a meaningful index of vitamin C status. The different types of leucocyte have different capacities to accumulate ascorbate. This means that a change in the proportion of granulocytes, platelets and mononuclear leucocytes will result in a change in the total concentration of ascorbate per 10^6 cells, although there may well be no change in vitamin nutritional status. Stress, myocardial infarction, infection, burns and surgical trauma all result in changes in leucocyte distribution, with an increase in the proportion of granulocytes, and hence an apparent change in leucocyte ascorbate. This has been widely misinterpreted to indicate an increased requirement for vitamin C in these conditions.

11.15　*Minerals*

Those inorganic mineral elements that have a function in the body must obviously be provided in the diet, as elements cannot be interconverted. Many of the essential minerals are of little practical nutritional importance, as they are widely distributed in foods, and most people eating a normal mixed diet are likely to receive adequate intakes.

In general, mineral deficiencies are a problem when people live largely on foods grown in one small region, where the soil may be deficient in some minerals. Iodine deficiency is a major problem in many areas of the world (section 11.15.3.3). For people whose diet consists of foods grown in a variety of different regions, mineral deficiencies are unlikely. However, as discussed in section 11.15.2.3, iron deficiency is a problem in most parts of the world, because if iron losses from the body are relatively high (e.g. from heavy menstrual blood loss) it is difficult to achieve an adequate intake to replace the losses.

Mineral deficiency is unlikely among people eating an adequate mixed diet. More importantly, many of the minerals, including those which are dietary essentials, are toxic in even fairly modest excess. This is unlikely to be a problem with high mineral content of foods, although crops grown in regions where the soil content of selenium is especially high may provide dangerously high levels of intake of this mineral (section 11.15.2.5). The problem arises when people take inappropriate supplements of minerals or are exposed to contamination of food and water supplies.

11.15.1　CALCIUM

The most obvious requirement for calcium in the body is in the mineral of bones and teeth – a complex mixture of calcium carbonates and phosphates (hydroxyapatite) together with magnesium salts and fluorides. An adult has about 1.2 kg of calcium in the body, 99% of which is in the skeleton and teeth. This means that calcium requirements are especially high in times of rapid growth – during infancy and adolescence, and in pregnancy and lactation.

Although the major part of the body's calcium is in bones, the most important functions of calcium are in the maintenance of muscle contractility and responses to hormones and neurotransmitters. To maintain these essential regulatory functions, bone calcium is mobilized in deficiency, so as to ensure that the plasma and intracellular concentrations are kept within a strictly controlled range. If the plasma concentration of calcium falls, neuromuscular regulation is lost, leading to tetany.

The main sources of calcium are milk and cheese; dietary calcium is absorbed by an active process in the mucosal cells of the small intestine and is dependent on vitamin D. As discussed in section 11.3.3.1, the active metabolite of vitamin D, calcitriol, induces the synthesis of a calcium-binding protein, which permits the mucosal cells to accumulate calcium from the intestinal lumen, and in vitamin D deficiency the absorption of calcium is seriously impaired.

Although the effect of vitamin D deficiency is impairment of the absorption and utilization of calcium, rickets (section 11.3.4) does not seem to be simply the result of calcium deficiency. Calcium-deficient children with adequate vitamin D nutritional status do not develop rickets but have a much reduced rate of growth. Nevertheless, calcium deficiency may be a contributory factor in the development of rickets when vitamin D status is marginal.

11.15.1.1 Osteoporosis

Osteoporosis is a progressive loss of bone with increasing age, after the peak bone mass is achieved at the age of about 30. The cause is the normal process of bone turnover with reduced replacement of the tissue which has been broken down (section 11.3.3.1). Both mineral and the organic matrix of bone are lost in osteoporosis, unlike osteomalacia (section 11.3.4), in which there is loss of bone mineral but the organic matrix is unaffected.

Osteoporosis can occur in relatively young people as a result of prolonged bed rest (or weightlessness in space flight) – bone continues to be degraded, but without physical activity there is less stimulus for replacement of the lost tissue. More importantly, it occurs as an apparently unavoidable part of the ageing process. Here the main problem is the reduced secretion of oestrogens (in women) and androgens (in men) with increasing age; among other actions, the sex steroids are required for the differentiation of osteoblasts for new bone formation. The problem is especially serious in women, as there is a much more abrupt fall in oestrogen secretion at the menopause than the more gradual (and less severe) fall in androgen secretion in men with increasing age. As a result, very many more elderly women than men suffer from osteoporosis. Post-menopausal hormone replacement therapy with oestrogens has a protective effect against the development of osteoporosis.

Because there is a net breakdown of bone in osteoporosis, there is excretion of considerable amounts of calcium in the urine. There is negative calcium balance – excretion is greater than the dietary intake. This has led to suggestions that a high intake of calcium may slow or reverse the process of osteoporosis. However, the negative calcium balance is the result of osteoporosis, not the cause. There is little evidence that higher intakes of calcium post-menopausally have any effect on the development of osteoporosis.

People with higher peak bone mass are less at risk from osteoporosis, as they can tolerate more loss of bone before there are serious effects. Therefore, adequate calcium and vitamin D nutrition through adolescence and young adulthood is likely to provide protection against osteoporosis in old age. High intakes of calcium have no beneficial effect once peak bone mass has been achieved. However, there are no adverse effects either, because of the close regulation of calcium homeostasis; problems of hypercalcaemia and calcinosis (the calcification of soft tissues) occur as a result of vitamin D intoxication (section 11.2.2.6) or other disturbances of calcium homeostasis, not as a result of high intakes of calcium.

High intakes of vitamin D have no beneficial effect on the progression of osteoporosis, although the vitamin will prevent the development of osteomalacia, which can occur together with osteoporosis in the elderly.

11.15.2 MINERALS WHICH FUNCTION AS PROSTHETIC GROUPS IN ENZYMES

11.15.2.1 Cobalt

In addition to its role in vitamin B_{12} (section 11.10), cobalt provides the prosthetic group of a small number of enzymes. It is therefore a dietary essential, despite the fact that vitamin B_{12} cannot be synthesized in the body. However, no clinical signs of cobalt deficiency are known, except in ruminant animals, whose intestinal bacteria synthesize vitamin B_{12}.

11.15.2.2 Copper

Copper provides the essential functional part of a number of enzymes involved in oxidation and reduction reactions, including dopamine β-hydroxylase in the synthesis of noradrenaline and adrenaline, cytochrome oxidase in the electron transport chain (section 3.3.1.2) and superoxide dismutase, one of the enzymes involved in protection against oxygen radicals (section 7.4.3.1). Copper is also important in the oxidation of lysine to form the cross-links in collagen and elastin. In copper deficiency the bones are abnormally fragile, because the abnormal collagen does not permit the normal flexibility of the bone matrix. More importantly, elastin is less elastic than normal and copper deficiency can lead to death following rupture of the aorta.

11.15.2.3 Iron

The most obvious function of iron is in the haem of haemoglobin, the oxygen-carrying protein in red blood cells, and myoglobin in muscles. Haem is also important in a variety of enzymes, including the cytochromes (section 3.3.1.2), where it is the coenzyme in oxidation and reduction reactions. A number of enzymes also contain non-haem iron (i.e. iron bound to the enzyme other than in haem), which is essential to their function.

Deficiency of iron leads to reduced synthesis of haemoglobin, and hence a lower than normal amount of haemoglobin in red blood cells. Iron-deficiency anaemia is a major problem worldwide, especially among women. The problem is due to a loss of blood greater than can be replaced by absorption of dietary iron. In developing countries intestinal parasites (especially hookworm), which cause large losses of blood in the faeces, are a common cause of iron depletion, and hence anaemia, in both men and women. In developed countries it is mainly women who are at risk of iron deficiency anaemia, as a result of heavy menstrual losses of blood. Probably 10–15% of women have menstrual losses of iron greater than can be met from a normal dietary intake and are therefore at risk of developing anaemia unless they take iron supplements

Iron in foods occurs in two forms: haem in meat and meat products and inorganic iron salts in plant foods. The absorption of haem iron is considerably better than that of inorganic iron salts; as discussed in section 4.5.1, only about 10% of the inorganic iron of the diet is absorbed, although this is increased by vitamin C (section 11.14.4.1).

11.15.2.4 Molybdenum

Molybdenum functions as the prosthetic group of a small number of enzymes, including xanthine oxidase (which is involved in the metabolism of purines to uric acid for excretion) and pyridoxal oxidase (which metabolizes vitamin B_6 to the inactive excretory product pyridoxic acid; section 11.9.1). It occurs in an organic complex, molybdopterin, which is chemically similar to folic acid (section 11.11.1) but can be synthesized in the body as long as adequate amounts of molybdenum are available.

Molybdenum deficiency has been associated with increased incidence of cancer of the oesophagus, but this seems to be an indirect association. The problem occurs among people living largely on maize grown on soil that is poor in molybdenum. For reasons which are not altogether clear, the resultant molybdenum-deficient maize is more susceptible to attack by fungi that produce carcinogenic toxins. Thus, although the people living on this diet are at risk of molybdenum deficiency, the main problem is not one of molybdenum deficiency in the people, but rather of fungal spoilage of their food.

11.15.2.5 Selenium

Selenium functions in at least two enzymes: glutathione peroxidase (section 7.4.3.2) and thyroxine deiodinase, which forms the active thyroid hormone, tri-iodothyronine, from thyroxine secreted by the thyroid gland (see Figure 11.28). In both cases it is present as the selenium analogue of the amino acid cysteine, selenocysteine.

Selenium deficiency is widespread in parts of China, and in some parts of the United States and Finland the soil is so poor in selenium that it is added to fertilizers, in order to increase the selenium intake of the population and so prevent deficiency. In New Zealand, despite the low selenium content of the soil, it was decided not to use selenium-rich fertilizers because of the hazards of selenium toxicity.

Selenium is extremely toxic even in modest excess. The RNI for selenium for adults is 75 μg/day; signs of poisoning can be seen at intakes above 450 μg/day, and the World Health Organization recommends that selenium intakes should not exceed 200 μg/day. In some parts of the world the soil is so rich in selenium that locally grown crops would provide more than this recommended upper limit of selenium intake if they were the main source of food, and it is not possible to graze cattle safely on the pastures in these regions.

11.15.2.6 Zinc

Zinc is the prosthetic group of more than a hundred enzymes with a wide variety of functions. It is also involved in the receptor proteins for steroid and thyroid hormones, calcitriol and vitamin A. In these proteins, zinc forms an integral part of the region of the protein that interacts with the promoter site on DNA to initiate gene transcription in response to hormone action (section 10.4).

Zinc deficiency occurs only among people living in tropical or subtropical areas whose diet is very largely based on unleavened wholemeal bread. The problem is seen mainly as delayed puberty, so that young men of 18–20 are still prepubertal. This is a result of reduced sensitivity of target tissues to androgens, because of the role of zinc in steroid hormone receptors. Two separate factors contribute to the deficiency:

- Wheat flour provides very little zinc, and in unleavened wholemeal bread much of the zinc that is present is not available for absorption because it is bound to phytate and dietary fibre.
- Sweat contains a relatively high concentration of zinc, and in tropical conditions there can be a considerable loss of zinc in sweat.

Marginal zinc deficiency in developed countries may be associated with poor wound healing, increased susceptibility to infection and impairment of the senses of taste and smell.

11.15.3 MINERALS THAT HAVE A REGULATORY ROLE (IN NEUROTRANSMISSION, AS ENZYME ACTIVATORS OR IN HORMONES)

11.15.3.1 Calcium

In addition to its role in bone mineral, calcium has a major function in metabolic regulation, nerve conduction and muscle contraction. Calcium nutrition is discussed in section 11.15.1.

11.15.3.2 Chromium

Chromium is involved, as an organic complex, the glucose tolerance factor, in the interaction between insulin and cell-surface insulin receptors. The precise chemical nature of the glucose tolerance factor has not been elucidated. Chromium deficiency is associated with impaired glucose tolerance, similar to that seen in diabetes mellitus (section 10.7). However, there is no evidence that increased intakes of chromium have any beneficial effect in diabetes and, although there is no evidence of harm from organic chromium complexes, inorganic chromium salts are highly toxic.

11.15.3.3 Iodine

Iodine is required for the synthesis of the thyroid hormones, thyroxine and tri-iodothyronine. Deficiency, leading to goitre (a visible enlargement of the thyroid gland), is widespread in inland upland areas over limestone soil. This is because the soil over limestone is thin, and minerals, including iodine, readily leach out, so that locally grown plants are deficient in iodine. Near the coast, sea spray contains enough iodine to replace these losses. World-wide, many millions of people are at risk of deficiency, and in parts of central Brazil, the Himalayas and central Africa goitre may affect more than 90% of the population.

Thyroid hormone regulates metabolic activity, and people with thyroid deficiency have a low metabolic rate (section 5.1.3.1), and hence gain weight readily (section 6.3.3.7). They tend to be lethargic and have a dull mental apathy. Children born to iodine-deficient mothers are especially at risk, and more so if they are then weaned onto an iodine-deficient diet. They may suffer from very severe mental retardation (goitrous cretinism) and congenital deafness.

By contrast, overactivity of the thyroid gland, and hence overproduction of thyroid hormones, leads to a greatly increased metabolic rate, possibly leading to very considerable weight loss despite an apparently adequate intake of food. Hyperthyroid people are lean and have a tense nervous energy.

Iodide is accumulated in the thyroid gland, where specific tyrosine residues in the protein thyroglobulin are iodinated to yield di-iodotyrosine. As shown in Figure 11.28, the next stage is the transfer of the di-iodophenol residue of one di-iodotyrosine onto another, yielding protein-bound thyroxine, which is stored in the colloid of the thyroid gland. In response to stimulation by thyrotropin, thyroglobulin is hydrolysed, releasing thyroxine into the circulation. The active hormone is tri-iodothyronine, which is formed from thyroxine by a selenium-dependent deiodinase, both in the thyroid gland and, more importantly, in target tissues. Because of the role of selenium in the metabolism of the thyroid hormones, the effects of iodine deficiency will be exacerbated by selenium deficiency.

In developed countries where there is a risk of iodine deficiency, supplementation of foods is common. Iodized salt may be available, or bread may be baked using iodized salt. In developing countries, such enrichment of foods is not generally possible, and the treatment and prevention of iodine deficiency depends on periodic visits to areas at risk by medical teams who give relatively large doses of iodized oil by intramuscular injection.

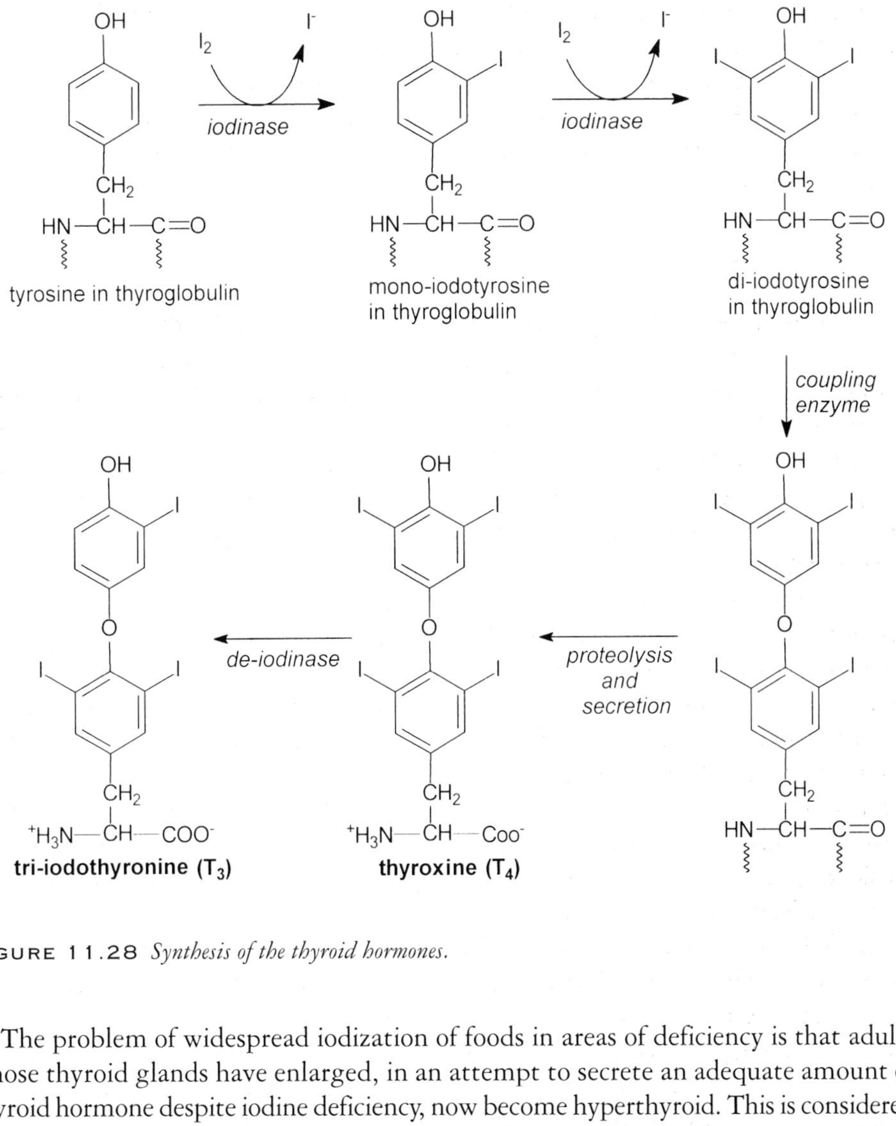

FIGURE 11.28 *Synthesis of the thyroid hormones.*

The problem of widespread iodization of foods in areas of deficiency is that adults whose thyroid glands have enlarged, in an attempt to secrete an adequate amount of thyroid hormone despite iodine deficiency, now become hyperthyroid. This is considered an acceptable risk to prevent the much more serious problems of goitrous cretinism among the young.

11.15.3.4 Magnesium

Magnesium is a cofactor for enzymes which utilize ATP and also several of the enzymes involved in DNA replication and transcription (section 9.2.2.1). It is not clear whether magnesium deficiency is an important nutritional problem, as there are no clear signs of deficiency. However, it has been clearly established that intravenous administration of magnesium salts is beneficial immediately after a heart attack.

11.15.3.5 Manganese

Manganese functions as the prosthetic group of a variety of enzymes, including superoxide dismutase, a part of the body's antioxidant defence system (section 7.4.3.1), pyruvate carboxylase in gluconeogenesis (section 5.7) and arginase in urea synthesis (section 9.3.1.4). Deficiency has been observed only in deliberate depletion studies.

11.15.3.6 Sodium and potassium

The maintenance of the normal composition of intracellular and extracellular fluids and osmotic homeostasis depend largely on the maintenance of relatively high concentrations of potassium inside cells and sodium outside. The gradient of sodium and potassium across cell membranes, is maintained by active (ATP-dependent) pumping (section 3.2.2.3). Nerve conduction depends on the rapid reversal of this transmembrane gradient to create and propagate the electrical impulse, followed by a more gradual restoration of the normal ion gradient.

There is little or no problem in meeting sodium requirements; indeed, as discussed in section 7.3.4, the main problem with sodium nutrition is an excessive intake, rather than deficiency.

11.15.4 MINERALS KNOWN TO BE ESSENTIAL BUT WHOSE FUNCTION IS NOT KNOWN

11.15.4.1 Silicon

Silicon is known to be essential for the development of connective tissue and the bones, although its function in these processes is not known. The silicon content of blood vessel walls decreases with age and with the development of atherosclerosis. It has been suggested, although the evidence is not convincing, that silicon deficiency may be a factor in the development of atherosclerosis.

11.15.4.2 Vanadium

Experimental animals maintained under very strictly controlled conditions show a requirement for vanadium for normal growth. There is some evidence that vanadium has a role in regulation of the activity of sodium/potassium pumps (section 3.2.2.3), although this has not been proven.

11.15.4.3 Nickel and tin

There is some evidence, from experimental animals maintained under strictly controlled conditions, that a dietary intake of nickel and tin is required for optimum growth and development although this remains to be conclusively demonstrated. No metabolic function has been established for either mineral.

11.15.5 MINERALS WHICH HAVE EFFECTS IN THE BODY BUT WHOSE ESSENTIALITY IS NOT ESTABLISHED

11.15.5.1 Fluoride

Fluoride has clear beneficial effects in modifying the structure of bone mineral and dental enamel, strengthening the bones and protecting teeth against decay. The use of fluoride toothpaste, and the addition of fluoride to drinking water in many regions, has resulted in a very dramatic decrease in the incidence of dental decay despite high consumption of sucrose and other extrinsic sugars (section 7.3.3.1). These benefits are seen at levels of fluoride of the order of 1 ppm in drinking water. Such concentrations occur naturally in many parts of the world, and this is the concentration at which fluoride is added to water in many areas.

Excessive intake of fluoride leads to brown discoloration of the teeth (dental fluorosis). A concentration above about 12 ppm in drinking water, as occurs naturally in some parts of the world, is associated with excessive deposition of fluoride in the bones, leading to increased fragility (skeletal fluorosis).

Although fluoride has beneficial effects, there is no evidence that it is a dietary essential. Fluoride prevents dental decay, but it is probably not correct to call dental decay a fluoride deficiency disease.

11.15.5.2 Lithium

Lithium salts are used in the treatment of manic–depressive disease; they act by altering the responsiveness of some nerves to stimulation. However, this seems to be a purely pharmacological effect, and there is no evidence that lithium has any essential function in the body, or that it provides any benefits for healthy people.

11.15.5.3 Other minerals

In addition to minerals which are known to be dietary essentials, there a number which may be consumed in relatively large amounts but which have, as far as is known, no function in the body. Indeed, excessive accumulation of these minerals may be dangerous, and a number of them are well known as poisons. Such elements include aluminium, arsenic, antimony, boron, cadmium, caesium, germanium, lead, mercury, silver and strontium.

Additional resources

PowerPoint presentation 11 on the CD.
Self-assessment quiz 11 on the CD.

Appendix: Units of physical quantities, multiples and submultiples of units

Units of physical quantities

Physical quantity	Unit	Symbol	Definition
Amount of substance	mole	mol	SI base unit
Electric current	ampere	A	SI base unit
Electric potential difference	volt	V	J/A/s
Energy	joule	J	$m^2/kg/s$
	calorie	cal	4.186 J
Force	newton	N	J/m
Frequency	hertz	Hz	s^{-1}
Length	metre	m	SI base unit
Length	ångstrom	Å	10^{-10} m
Mass	kilogram	kg	SI base unit
Power	watt	W	J/s
Pressure	pascal	Pa	N/m^2
	bar	bar	10^5 Pa
Radiation dose absorbed	gray	Gy	J/kg
Radioactivity	becquerel	Bq	s^{-1}
Temperature	degree Celsius	°C	−273.15 K
	kelvin	K	SI base unit
Time	second	s	SI base unit
Volume	litre	L (dm³)	10^{-3} m³

Multiples and submultiples of units

	Name	Symbol
$\times 10^{21}$	zetta	Z
$\times 10^{18}$	exa	E
$\times 10^{15}$	peta	P
$\times 10^{12}$	tera	T
$\times 10^{9}$	giga	G
$\times 10^{6}$	mega	M
$\times 10^{3}$	kilo	k
$\times 10^{2}$	centa	ca
$\times 10$	deca	da
$\times 10^{-1}$	deci	d
$\times 10^{-2}$	centi	c
$\times 10^{-3}$	milli	m
$\times 10^{-6}$	micro	μ
$\times 10^{-9}$	nano	n
$\times 10^{-12}$	pico	p
$\times 10^{-15}$	femto	f
$\times 10^{-18}$	atto	a
$\times 10^{-21}$	zepto	z

Glossary

In addition to the brief glossary here, the following small and reasonably priced reference books will be useful:

Concise Dictionary of Biology. Oxford University Press, Oxford, 1990.
Concise Dictionary of Chemistry. Oxford University Press, Oxford, 1990.
Concise Medical Dictionary, Oxford University Press, Oxford, 1994.
Penguin Dictionary of Biology. Penguin Books, London, 1990.
Penguin Dictionary of Chemistry. Penguin Books, London, 1990.
Bender AE and Bender DA. *Dictionary of Food and Nutrition*. Oxford University Press, Oxford, 1995.

Acid   A compound which, when dissolved in water, dissociates to yield hydrogen ions (H^+).
Acidosis   A condition in which the pH of blood plasma falls below the normal value of 7.4. A fall to pH 7.2 is life-threatening.
Acyl group   In an ester or other compound, the part derived from a fatty acid.
ADP   Adenosine diphosphate.
Alcohol   A compound with an –OH group attached to an aliphatic carbon chain. Also used generally to mean ethanol (ethyl alcohol), the commonly consumed alcohol in beverages.
Aldehyde   A compound with an HC=O group attached to a carbon atom.
Aliphatic   Containing chains of carbon atoms (straight or branched), rather than rings. Aliphatic compounds may be saturated or unsaturated.
Alkali   A compound which, when dissolved in water, gives an alkaline solution – one with a pH above 7.
Alkalosis   A condition in which the pH of blood plasma rises above the normal value of 7.4.
Amide   The product of a condensation reaction between a carboxylic acid and ammonia, a –$CONH_2$ group.
Amine   A compound with an amino (–NH_2) group attached to a carbon atom.
Amino acid   A compound with both an amino (–NH_2) and a carboxylic acid (–COOH) group attached to the α-carbon.
AMP   Adenosine monophosphate.
Amylopectin   The branched-chain structure of starch.
Amylose   The straight-chain structure of starch.

Anabolism Metabolic reactions resulting in the synthesis of more complex compounds from simple precursors. Commonly linked to the hydrolysis of ATP to ADP and phosphate.

Anaerobic Occurring in the absence of oxygen.

Anion An ion that has a negative electric charge and therefore migrates to the anode (positive pole) in an electric field. The ions of non-metallic elements are anions.

Antibiotic A substance produced by one organism to prevent the growth of another. Many are clinically useful to treat bacterial infections, whereas others are too toxic.

Anticodon The three-base region of transfer RNA which recognizes and binds to the codon on messenger RNA.

Apoptosis Programmed cell death.

Aromatic compound A cyclic compound in which the ring consists of alternating single and double bonds.

Atom The smallest particle of an element which can exist as an entity. The atom consists of a nucleus containing protons, neutrons and other uncharged particles, surrounded by a cloud of electrons.

Atomic mass The mass of the atom of any element, relative to that of carbon 12; 1 unit of atomic mass $= 1.660 \times 10^{-27}$ kg.

Atomic number The number of protons in the nucleus of an atom (and hence the number of electrons surrounding the nucleus) determines the atomic number of that element.

ATP Adenosine triphosphate.

Autocrine Produced and secreted by a cell and acting on the cell that secreted it.

Basal metabolic rate The energy expenditure by the body at complete rest, but not asleep, in the post-prandial state.

Base Chemically, an alkali. Also used as a general term for the purines and pyrimidines in DNA and RNA.

Body mass index (BMI) The ratio of body weight (in kg)/height^2 (in m). A person with a BMI over 25 is considered to be overweight and a person with a BMI over 30 is obese.

Buffer A solution of a weak acid and its salt which can prevent changes in pH as the concentration of H^+ ions changes, by shifting the equilibrium between the dissociated and undissociated acid. Any buffer system only acts around the pH at which the acid is half dissociated.

Calorie (cal) An (obsolete) unit of heat or energy. The amount of heat required to raise 1 g of water through 1 °C. Nutritionally the kcal is used; 1 kcal $= 1000$ cal; 1 cal $= 4.186$ J; 1 J $= 0.239$ cal.

Calorimetry The measurement of energy expenditure by heat output; indirect calorimetry estimates heat output from oxygen consumption.

Carbohydrate Compounds of carbon, hydrogen and oxygen in the ratio $C_nH_{2n}O_n$. The dietary carbohydrates are sugars, starches and non-starch polysaccharides.

Carboxylic acid A compound with a –COOH group attached to a carbon atom.

Catabolism Metabolic reactions resulting in the breakdown of complex molecules to simpler products, commonly oxidation to carbon dioxide and water, linked to the phosphorylation of ADP to ATP.

Catalyst Something that increases the rate at which a chemical reaction achieves equilibrium, without itself being consumed in, or altered by, the reaction.

Cation A positively charged ion which migrates to the cathode (negative pole) in an electric field. The ions of metallic elements are cations.

Cellulose   A polymer of glucose, linked by $\beta1\rightarrow4$ glycoside links, which are not digested by human enzymes.

Codon   A sequence of three nucleic acid bases in DNA or mRNA that specify an individual amino acid.

Coenzyme   A non-protein organic compound that is required for an enzyme reaction. Coenzymes may be loosely or tightly associated with the enzyme protein, and may be covalently bound to the enzyme, in which case they are known as prosthetic groups.

Condensation   A chemical reaction in which water is eliminated from two compounds to result in the formation of a new compound. The formation of esters, peptides and amides occurs by condensation reactions.

Covalent bond   A bond between two atoms in which electrons are shared between the atoms.

Deoxyribose   A pentose (five-carbon) sugar in which one hydroxyl (–OH) group has been replaced by hydrogen. The sugar of DNA.

Dietary fibre   The residue of plant cell walls after extraction and treatment with digestive enzymes. Chemically a mixture of lignin and a variety of non-starch polysaccharides, including cellulose, hemicellulose, pectin, gums and mucilages.

Disaccharide   A sugar consisting of two monosaccharides linked by a glycoside bond. The common dietary disaccharides are sucrose (cane or beet sugar), lactose, maltose and isomaltose.

Dissociation   The process whereby a molecule separates into ions on solution in water.

DNA   Deoxyribonucleic acid.

Double bond   A covalent bond in which two pairs of electrons are shared between the participating atoms.

Electrolyte   A compound that undergoes partial or complete dissociation into ions when dissolved, and so is capable of transporting an electric current. In clinical chemistry, electrolyte is normally used to mean the major inorganic ions in body fluids.

Electron   The smallest unit of negative electric charge. The fundamental particles that surround the nucleus of an atom.

Electronegative atom   An atom that exerts greater attraction for the shared electrons in a covalent bond than does its partner, so developing a partial negative charge.

Electropositive atom   An atom that exerts less attraction for the shared electrons in a covalent bond than does its partner, so developing a partial positive charge.

Element   A substance that cannot be further divided or modified by chemical means. The basic substances from which compounds are formed.

Endergonic reaction   A chemical reaction that will only proceed with an input of energy, usually as heat.

Endocrine substance   A substance produced by one organ that circulates in the bloodstream and acts on distant organs and tissues.

Endonuclease   An enzyme that hydrolyses a polynucleotide at a specific sequence within the chain, as opposed to an exonuclease.

Endopeptidase   An enzyme that hydrolyses a peptide adjacent to a specific amino acid within the sequence, as opposed to an exopeptidase.

Endothermic reaction   A chemical reaction that will only proceed with an input of heat.

Enzyme   A protein that acts as a catalyst in a metabolic reaction.

Essential amino acid   Nine of the amino acids which are required for protein synthesis and cannot be synthesized at all in the body but must be provided in the diet: histidine, lysine, methionine, phenylalanine, tryptophan, threonine, valine, leucine and isoleucine.

Essential fatty acids   Those polyunsaturated fatty acids that cannot be synthesized in the body and must be provided in the diet. Linoleic and linolenic acids are the only two that are dietary essentials, as the other polyunsaturated fatty acids can be synthesized from them.

Ester   The product of a condensation reaction between an alcohol and a carboxylic acid.

Exergonic reaction   A chemical reaction that proceeds with an output of energy, usually as heat.

Exon   A region of DNA that codes for a gene (as opposed to introns).

Exonuclease   An enzyme that removes a terminal nucleotide from a polynucleotide, as opposed to an endonuclease.

Exopeptidase   An enzyme that removes a terminal amino acid from a polypeptide, as opposed to an endopeptidase.

Exothermic reaction   A chemical reaction that proceeds with an output of heat.

Fat   Triacylglycerols, esters of glycerol with three fatty acids. Fats are generally considered to be those triacylglycerols which are solid at room temperature, whereas oils are triacylglycerols which are liquid at room temperature.

Fatty acid   Aliphatic carboxylic acids (i.e. with a –COOH group) The metabolically important fatty acids have between 2 and 24 carbon atoms (usually an even number) and may be completely saturated or have one (monounsaturated) or more (polyunsaturated) carbon–carbon double bonds in the carbon chain.

Galactose   A hexose (six-carbon) monosaccharide.

Gene   A region of DNA which carries the information for a single protein or polypeptide chain.

Genetic code   The sequence of triplets of the nucleic acid bases (purines and pyrimidines) that specifies the individual amino acids.

Gluconeogenesis   The process of synthesis of glucose from non-carbohydrate precursors.

Glucose   A monosaccharide; a hexose (six-carbon) sugar of empirical formula $C_6H_{12}O_6$.

Glycerol   A trihydric alcohol to which three fatty acid molecules are esterified in the formation of triacylglycerols (fats and oils). Glycerol has a sweet taste and is hygroscopic (attracts water); it is commonly used as a humectant in food processing.

Glycogen   A branched-chain polymer of glucose, linked by $\alpha1\rightarrow4$ links, with branch points provided by $\alpha1\rightarrow6$ links. The storage carbohydrate of mammalian liver and muscle.

Glycolysis   The metabolic pathway by which glucose is oxidized to pyruvate.

Hexose   A monosaccharide with six carbon atoms, and hence the empirical formula $C_6H_{12}O_6$. The nutritionally important hexoses are glucose, galactose and fructose.

Hydrocarbon   A compound of carbon and hydrogen only. Hydrocarbons may have linear, branched or cyclic structures, and may be saturated or unsaturated.

Hydrogen bond   The attraction between a partial positive charge on a hydrogen atom attached to an electronegative atom and a partial negative charge associated with an electronegative atom in another molecule or region of the same macromolecule.

Hydrolysis   The process of splitting a chemical bond between two atoms by the introduction of water, usually adding –H to one side of the bond and –OH to the other, resulting in the formation of two separate product molecules. The digestion of proteins to amino acids, polysaccharides and disaccharides to monosaccharides and triacylglycerols to glycerol and fatty acids are all hydrolysis reactions.

Hydrophilic   A compound that is soluble in water or a region of a macromolecule which can interact with water molecules.

Hydrophobic   Insoluble in water but soluble in lipids or, in the case of a region of a macromolecule, unable to interact with water but able to interact with lipids.

Induction   The initiation of new synthesis of an enzyme or other protein by activation of the transcription of the gene for the protein. Inducers are commonly metabolic intermediates or hormones. Induction results in an increase in the amount of enzyme protein in the cell.

Inhibition   A decrease in the activity of an enzyme with no effect on the amount of enzyme protein present in the cell.

Inorganic compound   Any chemical compound other than those carbon compounds that are considered to be organic.

Insoluble fibre   Lignin and non-starch polysaccharides in plant cell walls (cellulose and hemicellulose).

International units (iu)   Arbitrary, but standardized, units of biological activity used to express the potency of vitamins and other substances before vitamins they were purified. Now obsolete, but vitamins A, D and E are still sometimes quoted in international units.

Intron   The region of DNA in between regions that code for a gene (these are exons).

Ion   An atom or group of atoms that has lost or gained one or more electrons and thus has an electric charge.

Isomers   Forms of the same chemical compound, but with a different spatial arrangement of atoms or groups in the molecule. D- and L-isomerism refers to the arrangement of four different substituents around a carbon atom relative to the arrangement in the triose sugar D-glyceraldehyde. R- and S-isomerism refers to the arrangement of four different substituents around a carbon atom according to a set of systematic chemical rules. *Cis*- and *trans*-isomerism refers to the arrangement of groups adjacent to a carbon–carbon double bond.

Isotope   Different forms of the same chemical element (i.e. having the same number of protons in the nucleus and the same number of electrons surrounding the nucleus as each other), differing in the number of neutrons in the nucleus, and hence in the relative atomic mass.

Joule   The SI unit of energy. One joule is the work done when the point of application of a force of 1 N moves 1 m in the direction of the force. 1 J = 0.239 cal; 1 cal = 4.186 J.

Ketone   A compound with a carbonyl (C=O) group attached to two aliphatic groups.

Ketone bodies   Acetoacetate and β-hydroxybutyrate (not chemically a ketone) formed in the liver from fatty acids in the fasting state and released into the circulation as metabolic fuels for use by other tissues. Acetone is also formed non-enzymatically from acetoacetate.

Ketosis   An elevation of the plasma concentrations of acetoacetate, hydroxybutyrate and acetone, as occurs in the fasting state.

Kwashiorkor   A disease of protein–energy malnutrition in which there is oedema masking the severe muscle wastage, fatty infiltration of the liver and abnormalities of hair structure and hair and skin pigmentation.

Lactose   The sugar of milk. A disaccharide composed of glucose and galactose.

Lipid   A general term including fats and oils (triacylglycerols), phospholipids and steroids.

Lipogenesis   The metabolic pathway for synthesis of fatty acids from acetyl CoA, then the synthesis of triacylglycerols by esterification of glycerol with fatty acids.

Lipolysis   The hydrolysis of triacylglycerols to yield fatty acids and glycerol.

Lower reference nutrient intake (LRNI)   An intake of a nutrient below which it is unlikely that physiological needs will be met or metabolic integrity be maintained.

Macromolecule   A term used to describe the large molecules of, for example, proteins, nucleic acids and polysaccharides.

Maltose   A disaccharide composed of two molecules of glucose linked by an $\alpha 1 \rightarrow 4$ glycoside bond.

Marasmus   A disease of protein–energy malnutrition in which there is extreme emaciation as a result of catabolism of adipose tissue and protein reserves.

Metabolic fuel   Those dietary components that are oxidized as a source of metabolic energy: fats, carbohydrates, proteins and alcohol.

Metabolism   The processes of interconversion of chemical compounds in the body.

Minerals   Inorganic salts, so called because they can be obtained by mining.

Mitochondrion   A subcellular organelle which contains the enzymes of the citric acid cycle, fatty acid oxidation and the electron transport chain for oxidative phosphorylation of ADP to ATP.

Mole (mol)   The SI unit for the amount of material. The relative molecular mass of a compound, expressed in grams. One mol of any compound contains 6.0223×10^{23} molecules.

Molar   Concentration of a compound expressed in mol/L, sometimes abbreviated to M.

Molecular mass   The mass of a molecule of a compound, relative to that of carbon 12; the sum of the relative atomic masses of the atoms that constitute the molecule.

Molecule   The smallest particle of a compound that can exist in a free state.

Monosaccharide   A simple sugar, the basic units from which disaccharides and polysaccharides are composed. The nutritionally important monosaccharides are the pentoses (five-carbon sugars) ribose and deoxyribose and the hexoses (six-carbon sugars) glucose, galactose and fructose.

Neutron   One of the fundamental particles in the nucleus of an atom. Neutrons have no electric charge and a mass approximately equal to that of a proton. Differences in the number of neutrons in atoms of the same element account for the occurrence of isotopes.

Nitrogen balance   The difference between the intake of nitrogenous compounds (mainly protein) and the output of nitrogenous products from the body. Positive nitrogen balance occurs in growth, when there is a net increase in the body content of protein; negative nitrogen balance means that there is a loss of protein from the body.

Non-essential amino acid   Those amino acids which are required for protein synthesis but can be synthesized in the body in adequate amounts to meet requirements and therefore do not have to be provided in the diet. The non-essential amino acids are: glycine, alanine, serine, proline, glutamic acid, aspartic acid, glutamine, asparagine and arginine. In addition, tyrosine can be synthesized in the body, but only from the essential amino acid phenylalanine, and cysteine can be synthesized, but only from the essential amino acid methionine.

Non-starch polysaccharides   A group of polysaccharides other than starch which occur in plant foods. They are not digested by human enzymes, although they may be fermented by intestinal bacteria. They provide the major part of dietary fibre. The main non-starch polysaccharides are cellulose, hemicellulose (insoluble non-starch polysaccharides) and pectin and the plant gums and mucilages (soluble non-starch polysaccharides).

Nucleic acid   DNA and RNA – polymers of nucleotides which carry the genetic information of the cell (DNA in the nucleus) and information from DNA for protein synthesis (RNA).

Nucleotides   Phosphate esters of purine or pyrimidine bases with ribose (ribonucleotides) or deoxyribose (deoxyribonucleotides).

Nucleus   Chemically, the central part of an atom, containing protons, neutrons and a variety of other subatomic particles. Biologically, the subcellular organelle which contains the genetic information, as DNA, arranged in chromosomes.

Obesity   Excessive body weight due to accumulation of adipose tissue. Obesity is generally considered to be a body mass index greater than 30; between 25 and 30 is overweight.

Oil   Triacylglycerols, esters of glycerol with three fatty acids; oils are those triacylglycerols which are liquid at room temperature, whereas fats are solid. Mineral oil and lubricating oil are chemically completely different and are mainly long-chain hydrocarbons.

Oligopeptide   A chain of 2–10 amino acids linked by peptide bonds. Longer chains of amino acids are known as polypeptides (up to about 50 amino acids) or proteins.

Oligosaccharide   A general term for polymers containing about 3–10 monosaccharides.

Orbital   An allowed energy level for an electron around the nucleus of an atom, or of two atoms in a molecule.

Organic   Chemically, all compounds of carbon, other than simple carbonate and bicarbonate salts, are called organic, as they were originally discovered in living matter. Also used to describe foods grown under specified conditions without the use of fertilizers, pesticides, etc.

Overweight   Body weight relative to height greater than is considered desirable (on the basis of life expectancy), but not so much as to be considered obesity.

Oxidation   A chemical reaction in which the number of electrons in a compound is decreased. In organic compounds this is generally seen as a decrease in the proportion of hydrogen, an increase in the number of carbon–carbon double bonds or an increase in the proportion of oxygen in the molecule.

Oxidative phosphorylation   The phosphorylation of ADP to ATP, linked to the oxidation of metabolic fuels in the mitochondrial membrane.

Paracrine   Substance produced by one cell and acting on nearby cells (cf. endocrine, autocrine).

Pentose   A monosaccharide sugar with five carbon atoms, and hence the empirical formula $C_5H_{10}O_5$. The most important pentose sugars are ribose and deoxyribose (in which one hydroxyl group has been replaced by hydrogen).

Peptide bond   The link between amino acids in a protein. Formed by condensation between the carboxylic acid group (–COOH) of one amino acid and the amino group (–NH$_2$) of another to give a –CO–NH– link between the amino acids.

pH   A measure of the acidity (or alkalinity) of a solution. A neutral solution has a pH of 7.0; lower values are acid, higher values are alkaline. pH stands for potential hydrogen, and is the negative logarithm of the concentration of hydrogen ions (H^+) in the solution.

Phospholipid   A lipid in which glycerol is esterified to two fatty acids but the third hydroxyl group is esterified to phosphate, and through the phosphate to one of a variety of other compounds. Phospholipids are both hydrophilic and hydrophobic and have a central role in the structure of cell membranes.

Phosphorolysis   The cleavage of a bond between two parts of a molecule by the introduction of phosphate, yielding two product molecules. The breakdown of glycogen, to yield glucose 1-phosphate, proceeds by way of sequential phosphorolysis reactions.

Phosphorylation   The addition of a phosphate group to a compound.

Physical activity ratio   Energy expenditure in a given activity, expressed as a ratio of the basal metabolic rate.

Physical activity level   Energy expenditure, averaged over 24 hours, expressed as a ratio of the basal metabolic rate. The sum of the physical activity ratio multiplied by time spent for each activity during the day.

Polypeptide   A chain of amino acids, linked by peptide bonds. Generally up to about 50 amino acids constitute a polypeptide, while a larger polypeptide would be called a protein.

Polysaccharide   A polymer of monosaccharide units linked by glycoside bonds. The nutritionally important polysaccharides can be divided into starch and glycogen, and the non-starch polysaccharides.

Polyunsaturated   Fatty acids with two or more carbon–carbon double bonds in the molecule, separated by a methylene ($-CH_2-$) group.

Population reference intake (PRI)   An intake of the nutrient two standard deviations above the observed mean requirement, and hence greater than the requirements of 97.5% of the population. A term introduced in the 1993 EU tables of nutrient requirements.

Prosthetic group   A non-protein part of an enzyme that is essential for the catalytic activity of the enzyme and which is covalently bound to the protein.

Protein   A polymer of amino acids joined by peptide bonds.

Proton   The hydrogen ion (H^+). The positively charged subatomic particle in the nucleus of atoms. The number of protons in the nucleus determines the atomic number of the element.

Purine   Two of the bases in nucleic acids (DNA and RNA): adenine and guanine.

Pyrimidine   Three of the bases in nucleic acids: cytidine and uracil in DNA; cytidine and thymidine in RNA.

Radical   A highly reactive molecule with an unpaired electron.

Recommended daily (or dietary) allowance (or amount) (RDA)   The intake of the nutrient two standard deviations above the observed mean requirement, and hence greater than the requirements of 97.5% of the population.

Recommended daily (or dietary) intake of a nutrient (RDI)   The intake of the nutrient two standard deviations above the observed mean requirement, and hence greater than the requirements of 97.5% of the population.

Reducing sugar   A sugar which has a free aldehyde ($-HC=O$) group, which can therefore act as a chemical reducing agent. Glucose, galactose, maltose and lactose are all reducing sugars.

Reduction   A chemical reaction in which the number of electrons in a compound is increased. In organic compounds this is generally seen as an increase in the proportion of hydrogen, a decrease in the number of carbon–carbon double bonds or a decrease in the proportion of oxygen in the molecule. The opposite of oxidation.

Repression   Decreased synthesis of an enzyme or other protein as a result of blocking the transcription of the gene for that enzyme. Metabolic intermediates, end-products of pathways and hormones may act as repressors.

Respiratory quotient (RQ)   The ratio of carbon dioxide produce to oxygen consumed in the metabolism of metabolic fuels. The RQ for carbohydrates = 1.0, for fats 0.71 and for proteins 0.8.

Resting metabolic rate   The energy expenditure of the body at rest but not measured under the strict conditions required for determination of basal metabolic rate.

Ribose   A pentose (five-carbon) sugar.

Ribosome   The subcellular organelle on which the message of messenger RNA is translated into protein. The organelle on which protein synthesis occurs.

Reference nutrient intake (RNI)   A term introduced in the 1991 UK Tables of Dietary Reference Values. An intake of the nutrient two standard deviations above the observed mean requirement and hence greater than the requirements of 97.5% of the population.

Salt   The product of a reaction between an acid and an alkali. Ordinary table salt is sodium chloride.

Satiety   The state of satisfaction of hunger or appetite.

Saturated   An organic compound in which all carbon atoms are joined by single bonds, as opposed to unsaturated compounds, which contain carbon–carbon double bonds. A saturated compound contains the maximum possible proportion of hydrogen.

Soluble fibre   Non-starch polysaccharides which are soluble in water; pectin and the plant gums and mucilages.

Starch   A polymer of glucose units. Amylose is a straight-chain polymer, with 1–4 glycoside links between the glucose units. In amylopectin there are also branch points, where chains are linked through a $1\rightarrow6$ glycoside bond.

Steroids   Compounds derived from cholesterol (itself also a steroid), most of which are hormones.

Substrate   The substance or substances upon which an enzyme acts.

Sugar   Chemically, a monosaccharide or small oligosaccharide. Cane or beet sugar is sucrose, a disaccharide of glucose and fructose.

Teratogen   A compound that can cause congenital defects in the developing fetus.

Transcription   The process whereby a copy of the region of DNA containing the gene for a single protein is copied to give a strand of messenger RNA.

Translation   The process of protein synthesis, whereby the message of messenger RNA is translated into the amino acid sequence.

Triacylglycerol   The main type of dietary lipid and the storage lipid of adipose tissue. Glycerol esterified with three molecules of fatty acid. Also known as triglycerides.

Triglyceride   Alternative (and chemically incorrect) name for triacylglycerol.

Unsaturated   An organic compound containing one or more carbon–carbon double bonds and therefore less than the possible maximum proportion of hydrogen.

Urea   The main excretory end-product of amino acid metabolism.

Valency   The number of bonds which an atom must form to other atoms in order to achieve a stable electron configuration.

Van der Waals forces   Individually weak forces between molecules depending on transient charges due to transient inequalities in the sharing of electrons in covalent bonds.

Vegan   A strict vegetarian who will eat no foods of animal origin.

Vegetarian   One who does not eat meat and meat products. An ovo-lacto-vegetarian will eat milk and eggs, but not meat or fish, a lacto-vegetarian milk but not eggs; a vegan will eat only foods of vegetable origin.

Vitamin   An organic compound required in small amounts for the maintenance of normal growth, health and metabolic integrity. Deficiency of a vitamin results in the development of a specific deficiency disease, which can be cured or prevented only by that vitamin.

Index

CD Licence Agreement

The accompanying *Introduction to Nutrition and Metabolism* Third Edition CD-ROM contains:

- a PowerPoint presentation to accompany each chapter;
- a self-assessment test program;
- a series of simulations of laboratory practicals:
    - Energy Balance
    - Enzyme Assay
    - Nitrogen Balance
    - Oxygen Electrode Studies
    - Peptide Sequence
    - Radio-immunoassay of Steroid Hormones
    - Urea Synthesis.

Requires Windows 95/98/2000/NT/XP. Please see the *readme* files on the CD (*readme.rtf* or *readme.htm*) for installation instructions.

Please read this Agreement carefully before loading the CD-ROM

By loading the CD-ROM, you acknowledge that you have read and understand the following terms and conditions and agree to be bound thereby. If you do not agree with these terms and conditions, return the entire package to the following address and any payment that you have made for it will be returned to you:

Editorial Dept – Life Sciences
Taylor & Francis
11 New Fetter Lane
London EC4P 4EE
UK

Licence agreement

1 Grant of Licence. This Licence Agreement ("Licence") permits you to use one copy of the INTRODUCTION TO NUTRITION AND METABOLISM CD-ROM software product acquired with this Licence ("Software") in accordance

with the terms of this Licence. You shall not sublicence, assign or transfer the Licence or the Software.

2 Copyright. Copyright © David A. Bender 1996-2002. All rights reserved. You shall not republish, copy, modify, transfer, translate, decompile, disassemble or create derivative works of the Software, or any part thereof.

Limited warranty and disclaimer

The publishers of the Software, Taylor & Francis ("Publishers"), warrant that, for a period of ninety (90) days from the date of delivery to you, as evidenced by a copy of your receipt, the CD-ROM containing the Software will be free from defects in materials and workmanship, and the Software, under normal use, will perform without significant errors that make it unusable. Publishers' entire liability and your exclusive remedy under this warranty will be, at Publishers' option, to attempt to correct or help you around errors, or to give you a functionally equivalent Software or, upon you returning the Software to the Publishers, to refund the purchase price and terminate this Agreement.

Except for the above express limited warranties, Publishers make and you receive no warranties or conditions, express, implied, statutory or in any communication with you, and specifically disclaims any implied warranty of merchantability or fitness for a particular purpose. Publishers do not warrant that the operation of the software will be uninterrupted or error free.

Limited of liability

Taylor & Francis Ltd, and the author, shall not be liable for any damages, including loss of data, lost profits, cost of cover or other special, incidental, consequential or indirect damages arising from use of the software, under any theory of liability and irrespective of however caused. This limitation will apply even if the Publishers have been advised of the possibility of such damage. You acknowledge that the licence fee reflects this allocation of risk.

Because some jurisdictions do not allow exclusions or implied warranties or limitation or exclusion of liability for incidental or consequential damages, the above limitations may not apply to you. This warranty gives you specific legal rights. You may also have other rights which vary from jurisdiction to jurisdiction.